FREUD REAPPRAISED
A Fresh Look at Psychoanalytic Theory

FREUD REAPPRAISED
A Fresh Look at Psychoanalytic Theory

ROBERT R. HOLT
New York University

THE GUILFORD PRESS
New York *London*

To Benjamin Bjorn Rubinstein, M.D.

for his wise counsel, inspiring example, incisive criticism,
and warm friendship

© 1989 The Guilford Press
A Division of Guilford Publications, Inc.
72 Spring Street, New York, NY 10012

Printed in the United States of America

This book is printed on acid-free paper.

Last digit is print number: 9 8 7 6 5 4 3 2 1

Library of Congress Cataloging-in-Publication Data

Holt, Robert R.
    Freud reappraised.

    Includes bibliographies and index.
    1. Psychoanalysis. 2. Freud, Sigmund, 1856–1939.
I. Freud, Sigmund, 1856–1939. II. Title. [DNLM:
1. Psychoanalytic Theory. WM 460 H758f]
BF173.H737 1989   150.19′52   88-35623
ISBN 0-89862-387-1

Preface

It can hardly be doubted that the pleasure principle serves
the id as a compass in its struggle against the libido—
the force that introduces disturbances into the process
of life. (Freud, 1923b, pp. 46–47)

This passage might well be this book's epigraph, for it is the very one that caused me to throw down *The Ego and the Id* in disgust early in my graduate school years. In a sense, that was the beginning of my long struggle to understand Freud. Sooner or later, I had to start again, with a more systematic reading of Freud—I could not so easily dismiss him! And this book is the outcome. Like many a parent who works and saves so that his children won't have to go through the same struggles, I may delude myself that others can pick up where I leave off and fully profit from whatever gains I have been able to make. For one thing, of course, this book inevitably contains errors, not just omissions but inaccuracies and false insights, for which I take sole responsibility. And then, the serious scholar must of course do his own reading of Freud; this book does not pretend to substitute for it, but I do hope that it may guide and facilitate the task.

An author always hopes for a wider audience than his professional peers and the captive audience of future students. (In my case, they will have to be students of my students, since these words are being written immediately after the final lecture of my teaching career at New York University.) Freud belongs to and is part of intellectual history in the broadest sense. By that very token, my attempt to draw on resources of that history not much exploited in similar works encourages me to believe that it will be of interest to many outside the mental health professions. There must be lots of intelligent people who know something of Freud, have more or less fallen under his spell without taking the plunge into complete acceptance, and want to understand him better by seeing him against a background of some depth. I have thought of them often while writing what is planned as a sort of Baedeker for a traveler into inviting but often difficult and puzzling intellectual territory.

I hope particularly for readers who have some interest in philosophical ideas. From Freud we all have learned the importance of looking for the implicit and nonobvious causes of presenting problems. While his own bent was primarily toward uncovering unconscious motives and fantasies, it is only a slight extension of his method to search for unacknowledged assumptions. Like all of us, Freud had to take some kind of implied stand on the fundamental questions that plague metaphysicians: What is real? How is knowledge possible? How are the mind and the body related? How can we find truth? What is the nature of the universe? How can we reconcile personal freedom and scientific determinism? He grappled with such large issues only rarely in any direct way, but he was exposed to a variety of conflicting teachings and influences that shaped his orientations to them. The result was an important source of subtle confusion and contradiction in his writings. I have been able to do little more than begin what seems to me a relatively neglected kind of analysis and can only hope that the pages that follow convey some of the sense of fascination I find in pursuing it.

There will be more. I am well into a follow-up volume, in which I am trying to answer the question, "How could such an authentic genius as Freud have gotten himself into such theoretical tangles?"—namely, the ones discussed here. It will be more like an intellectual biography than the present book, which focuses on aiding the understanding and on fostering of the regeneration of psychoanalytic theory.

In the introduction, I have tried to acknowledge my indebtedness to most of the people who have helped this book to come about. I should add that the work it reports was all done during my years at New York University (1953–1989), where I came at the invitation of a wise and ideally democratic department chairman, Stuart W. Cook. His vision and administrative support made possible the creation of the stimulating and nurturing atmosphere of the Research Center for Mental Health, which for my first two decades at NYU housed and helped me in countless ways. Its research program was supported by a large grant from the Ford Foundation and smaller ones from several other sources, but notably by a series of grants from the National Institute of Mental Health. I have a special debt of gratitude to NIMH for a personal grant supporting the year (1960–61) of reflection and writing at the Center for Advanced Study in the Behavioral Sciences in Palo Alto, where a number of the ideas found here were germinated, and then for a Public Health Service Research Career Award (No. MH-K6-12,455) which supported all my work from 1962 to 1988, when the great bulk of this writing was done.

It remains to give my thanks to those who have eased the transition from manuscript to book: Seymour Weingarten and Pearl Weisinger of Guilford Press, who have been patient with my fussiness and afterthoughts; James G. Blight, who, while he was at Guilford, prodded and encouraged me to make a book out of its component papers; my old friend Morris Eagle, who read and thoughtfully commented upon the entire manuscript; and Mary Dooley, who, in her quietly cheerful and unfailingly competent manner, helped out in a myriad of ways. Of course, it would not have been written without the emotional support of my dear wife, Joan, and my equally dear children, Dorothy, Cathy, Daniel, and Michael.

Robert R. Holt
New York

Acknowledgments

Appreciation is expressed for permission to reprint, in whole or in part and with revisions, the following works:

Chapter 2—The Manifest and Latent Meanings of Metapsychology. (1982). *Annual of Psychoanalysis*, *10*, 233-255. Copyright 1982 by International Universities Press.

Chapter 3—Freud's Cognitive Style. (1965). *American Imago*, *22*, 167-179. Copyright 1965 by American Imago.

On Reading Freud. (1974). In C. L. Rothgeb (Ed.), *Abstracts of the Standard Edition of the Complete Psychological Works of Sigmund Freud* (pp. 3-79). New York: Jason Aronson. Copyright 1974 by Jason Aronson, Inc.

Chapter 4—A Critical Examination of Freud's Concept of Bound versus Free Cathexis. (1962). *Journal of the American Psychoanalytic Association*, *10*, 475-525. Copyright 1962 by the American Psychoanalytic Association.

Chapter 5—A Review of Some of Freud's Biological Assumptions and Their Influence on His Theories. (1965). In N. S. Greenfield and W. C. Lewis (Eds.), *Psychoanalysis and Current Biological Thought* (pp. 93-124). Madison: University of Wisconsin Press. Copyright 1965 by the Regents of the University of Wisconsin.

Chapter 6—Beyond Vitalism and Mechanism: Freud's Concept of Psychic Energy. (1967). In J. H. Masserman (Ed.), *Science and Psychoanalysis: Vol. 11. Concepts of Ego* (pp. 1-41). New York: Grune and Stratton. Copyright 1967 by Grune and Stratton, Inc.

Chapter 7—Drive or Wish?: A Reconsideration of the Psychoanalytic Theory of Motivation. (1976). In M. M. Gill and P. S. Holzman (Eds.), Psychology versus Metapsychology: Psychoanalytic Essays in Memory of George S. Klein. *Psychological Issues*, *9* (Monograph No. 36), 158-197. Copyright 1976 by International Universities Press.

Chapter 8—The Past and Future of Ego Psychology. (1975). *Psychoanalytic Quarterly*, *44*, 550–576. Copyright 1975 by The Psychoanalytic Quarterly, Inc.

Chapter 9—Ego Autonomy Re-evaluated. (1965). *International Journal of Psycho-Analysis*, *46*, 151–167. Copyright 1965 by the Institute of Psycho-Analysis.

On Freedom, Autonomy, and the Redirection of Psychoanalytic Theory: A Rejoinder. (1967). *International Journal of Psychiatry*, *3*, 524–536. Copyright 1967 by the International Journal of Psychiatry.

Chapter 10—The Development of the Primary Process: A Structural View. (1967). In R. R. Holt (Ed.), Motives and Thought: Psychoanalytic Essays in Memory of David Rapaport. *Psychological Issues*, *5* (Monograph 18/19), 345–383. (The chapter introduction is also reprinted from this source.) Copyright 1967 by International Universities Press.

Chapter 11—Freud's Theory of the Primary Process—Present Status. (1976). *Psychoanalysis and Contemporary Science*, *5*, 61–99. Copyright 1976 by Psychoanalysis and Contemporary Science, Inc.

Chapter 13—The Current Status of Psychoanalytic Theory. (1985). *Psychoanalytic Psychology*, *2*, 289–315. Copyright 1985 by Lawrence Erlbaum Associates, Inc.

Chapter 14—Freud's Impact upon Modern Morality and Our World View. (1984). In A. L. Caplan and B. Jennings (Eds.), *Darwin, Marx, and Freud: Their Influence on Moral Theory* (pp. 147–200). New York: Plenum. Copyright 1984 by the Hastings Center.

Chapter 12 was reprinted, with revisions, from The Death and Transfiguration of Metapsychology. (1981). *International Review of Psycho-Analysis*, *8*, 129–143. Copyright 1981 by Robert R. Holt.

Contents

PART I

Background

CHAPTER 1

A Personal Introduction

Each generation, it is said, must evaluate its heritage of cultural icons anew, for itself. Here, one such cultural hero, Sigmund Freud, is reappraised, held up to sources of light unknown in his heyday for a fresh look at the most fundamental elements of his psychoanalytic theories. The effort is to understand, to appreciate as much as to criticize, and to contribute to the revitalization of a body of thought that had as great an impact as any other on the shaping of contemporary consciousness.

Erich Fromm once remarked, in a seminar I attended over 40 years ago, that Freud and Marx had this in common: Both were the indispensable starting points for students of their respective subject matters, although practically everything they said was wrong. Fresh from my own psychoanalysis and fired with enthusiasm as I was for Freud's work, I greeted this judgment with incredulity, even scorn. As the decades have taken me deeper into the repeated study of Freud's writings, however, I have begun to feel that Fromm's statement was indeed worth remembering. In its dramatic hyperbole, it was itself a very Freudian proposition, as I shall try to demonstrate below; it made a point the validity of which could be appreciated if one saw its vehicle as rhetoric rather than as scientific weighing of evidence.

Yes, much of what Freud had to say is more or less false unless read sympathetically—not, that is, with the desire to find him right at all costs, but to learn from him. He is vulnerable to almost any diligent critic who wants to find him in error, and he has never lacked for that kind of antagonist, even though many of them have been so heavy-handed and obviously biased as to defeat their own destructive purpose. Major figures in other sciences who were Freud's contemporaries are comparably vulnerable, of course; it would be no trick for a pathologist to find many statements in the writings of Rudolf Virchow that are false by contemporary standards, or for a physiologist to do a hatchet job on Claude Bernard. But in other sciences, that kind of hostile evaluation of the great historical figures is not common, because it is taken for granted that scientific truth is always partial, relative to and limited by its historical context, and inevitably subject to correction even when not wholly superseded. It would be difficult indeed to find another scientist born in the middle decade of the 19th century whose work has not been left behind just as much as Freud's.

And yet Freud is much more than a historical figure. Again, Fromm was right: He is the indispensable starting point for *any* serious student of psychoanalysis or psychotherapy, surely, and for (at the least) *many* serious students of psychology, psychiatry, and the other behavioral sciences. Not as a source of infallible wisdom, for there is none such to be found anywhere; not as an intellectual father to be swallowed whole in a fantasied act of magical identification; and not as a generator of propositions that can be carried directly to the laboratory for rigorous verification or falsification. But read sympathetically and with appropriate caution, Freud still has an enormous amount to teach us about myriad aspects of human beings—their ways of growing up and of failing to thrive; their peculiarities, kinks, and quirks; and, above all, their secret lives.

Because I feel so strongly both that Freud has much to teach the contemporary reader and that the latter's task is unnecessarily difficult, I have brought together into the present book the results of my own struggle to gain an understanding. It is much more fragmentary than I wish it were, but I offer it in the hope that it may help others to penetrate much more deeply into Freud's meaning and to contribute more creatively to a new synthesis of psychoanalysis and the other sciences of man.

For a number of reasons, I want to begin with a personal statement about the way this book came about. I hope to make clear the nature of my psychoanalytic education and my relationship to psychoanalysis in its various meanings, and the ways in which my thinking about Freud and his theories developed. For my professional preparation and career have been unusual for a writer on psychoanalytic theory and these idiosyncrasies color many aspects of this book.

My first contact with psychoanalysis came during early adolescence when I picked up a copy of Karl Menninger's *The Human Mind* (1930), which my parents had bought through a book club. I remember being fascinated by some of the vivid clinical vignettes in which it abounds, though I doubt that I read the entire book. When I got to college, I enrolled in the introductory psychology course during my freshman year. As presented by H. S. Langfeld, then chairman of the Princeton department, psychology was so much less interesting than English literature and biology that I almost turned away from it. My attention was caught, however, by the description of a course on social psychology offered by Hadley Cantril, who had recently come from Dartmouth, and I took that during my first semester of sophomore year. I still recall the exhilarating sense of intellectual excitement and discovery this boyish, informal, shyly engaging young man conveyed as he set forth his ideas about the psychology of social movements (see Cantril, 1941). For the first time, I could get the sense of standing outside institutions of which I was a part and seeing them in the grand sweep of a mountaintop view, as well as a sense of the power of a conceptual system to integrate a host of seemingly unrelated observations. That course, more than any other I had in college, filled me with zest for a career in ideas.

It seemed natural thereafter to choose psychology as a major, and to become Cantril's devoted disciple. (Having been separated from my father at an early age by my parents' divorce, I had a sense of loss for which my devoted stepfather could never completely make up. I sought out mentors and heroes for many years—a naturalist at summer camp, a high school biology teacher, Cantril, then Gordon Allport, Henry A. Murray, and finally David Rapaport.) It was a small psychology department, and I managed to take or audit everything it offered except the experimental laboratory course, but Cantril was the only member who ever assigned any reading in Freud and spoke of him with any respect. He helped and encouraged me in many ways, got me out of the lab requirement, and enabled me to substitute for it a couple of investigations of my own. As a result, I failed to get the discipline and the feel of the laboratory, of which I was to be shy for many years, but I got hooked on research as a creative extension of the self.

Cantril sent me on to Harvard to do graduate work with Gordon Allport, the focus of his own hero worship. To my surprise and dismay, that thoughtful, scholarly, kind man proved so much more distant, so much less open than Cantril that I felt emotionally rebuffed. After a year of struggling to develop a dissertation topic that had grown out of a conversation between Cantril and Allport, I became aware of a new source of ferment and intellectual excitement: Henry A. Murray. During my first two years, he had been present only as a legend, but in the fall of 1941 he returned to the Harvard Psychological Clinic with a grant; a new scheme for the kind of collaborative, clinically oriented research that had resulted in the magnificent book *Explorations in Personality* (Murray et al., 1938); and above all his fabled, charismatic self. Quickly, his personal and intellectual magnetism drew to him a dazzling group of collaborators—such people as Robert W. White, Silvan Tomkins, Elliot Jaques, Leopold Bellak, James G. Miller, Thelma Alper, Frederick Wyatt, and O. H. Mowrer. I presented myself and my research topic, with fear and trembling, to this reputedly awesome man. To my astonishment and exhilaration, he received me with characteristic enthusiasm, urged me to join his team, and took me on as a thesis candidate. For weeks, I agonized over how to break the news to Allport, who finally approached me in Emerson Hall, told me that he had heard that I had joined Murray's group, and graciously gave me my freedom.

My most important encounter with psychoanalysis—personal treatment—had already begun over a year before, and was to continue off and on for eight years across two decades. In my first two bouts of personal treatment, I sought and found therapy for two serious psychosomatic conditions of long standing. The third go at being analyzed, which ended in 1960, enabled me to make a good marriage after an initial, unsuccessful one. I had extended contact with three Freudian analysts (one of whom was a woman) with quite different styles, personalities, and degrees of orthodoxy, and briefer periods (from a month to a year) with two others who were in their ways unique also. In retrospect, I feel that I received great therapeutic benefit from my three main analysts, as well as a direct experience of the realities behind the familiar concepts. Nothing can substitute for the personal re-evocation of oedipal longings and fears; learning the unconscious meaning of dreams, defenses, even everyday modes of behavior; experiencing the terrors of childhood traumas; literally seeing my last analyst as a horrifying hag or a beautiful woman, depending on the nature of the transference; knowing the reality of repression, as a thought would be swiftly blotted out while I was in the process of communicating it; and having my senses opened to the many-layered meanings of words and acts. I will always be grateful to Felix Deutsch, William Pious, and Charlotte Feibel for all they taught me, but especially for the ability to free myself from neurotic suffering.

To return to 1941, when I was just beginning with Deutsch (to whom my first analyst, Nils Antonisen, had referred me when he decided to leave Boston): Following the dictates of the conservative local tradition, I was under a prohibition against reading Freud. That came as a kind of relief to me, for I recall how bewildered I was by the attempt to make sense of *The Ego and the Id* during my first year of graduate work. The atmosphere of the Harvard Psychological Clinic was thoroughly psychoanalytic, but not at all orthordox. Murray and his long-time collaborator, Christiana Morgan, were among the few practicing analysts in the group (though almost everyone had had or was having some experience of being an analysand), but it was generally known that she was a thorough Jungian and that he was as much influenced by Jung as by Freud, though somewhat critical of both. Nevertheless, I was never drawn to Jung and have always found him almost unreadable. That was the time when Allport, as editor of the influential *Journal of Abnormal and Social Psychology* (see Vol. 35, Nos. 1 and 2), organized a symposium on psychoanalysis by analyzed psychologists. Imagine the sensation it created among a group of graduate students to be able to read, in current issues of the journal, personal revelations by our most senior professors, Boring and Murray, of their own neurotic struggles and their gropings toward relief and self-realization through psychoanalysis! Murray's (1940) ringing indictment of traditional academic psychology and his invitation to take the plunge into a risky alternative is still a valid and exciting statement of what psychoanalysis has to offer to psychologists.

Those years at the Plympton Street Clinic were so rich in so many ways that it is tempting to share a reliving of them. For the present purposes, however, I want mainly to stress that my first learning of psychoanalytic concepts came through *using* them in the interpretation of data from what Murray called the "multiform assessment" of human lives—those of a dozen Harvard students who were our shared, intensively studied subject pool—in a mutually supportive, intimately interacting group of students and faculty who valued theoretical innovation and empirical investigation almost equally. Silvan Tomkins was the only member of the group I can recall who had any marked bent for textual studies of psychoanalysis, and his interest was far more clinical than theoretical.

Theory meant to me then a creative rather than a critical enterprise, carried out over tea and cookies at the regular afternoon staff meetings. There Murray laid forth the new extensions of his theory of needs and press, his comprehensive taxonomic framework for describing personalities, and his slightly reshaped psychoanalytic concepts for understanding and explaining them; there, in turn, each of us set out his own attempts to contribute something, if only a translation of his experimental hypotheses into Murray's terminology. But there too we heard many challenges to Murray from his peers, which generated debates on a high level of sophistication and intellectual passion.

My next contact with psychoanalysis came during the first two years after I received my Ph.D. in February 1944. Those were war years; although I had been given an exemption from the draft, I was eager to contribute to the defeat of Hitler in any way I could. Rensis Likert's Division of Program Surveys offered "war work" in public opinion surveying (using skills I had picked up extracurricularly), mostly doing research for the Treasury Department on ways to induce people to buy more war bonds. During the evenings, there was a chance to attend many of the seminars offered by the Washington School of Psychiatry and to keep up my clinical interests. So I soon found myself speaking up as a defender of Freudian orthodoxy in seminars with Clara Thompson and (much more rarely) in those of Erich Fromm and Frieda Fromm-Reichmann. In Harry Stack Sullivan's lectures, no one spoke, except to utter little sycophantic murmurs of ecstasy. I was so repelled by his pomposity and self-importance that I developed a permanent blind spot even for the creative and insightful parts of his work. In a seminar with Ernst Schachtel, I learned for the first time what psychoanalytic understanding and sensitivity could bring to the interpretation of the Rorschach test, to which I had had the most cursory introduction in a brief set of lectures offered to the Harvard clinic staff by Jurgen Ruesch.

Once the war was over, I began to tire of sample surveys, though I had learned a great deal of permanent value from two years' immersion in such work. I wrote to Murray of my wish to get back into the kind of intensive study of individual human beings he had taught me, and soon thereafter there came an unexpected telephone call from none other than Karl Menninger: Would I be interested in joining in a bold new venture in Topeka, Kansas, working with him and David Rapaport? Would I talk it over with the latter, who was shortly coming to Washington on a recruiting trip? Soon I was sitting in a hotel room with a punctiliously polite, respectful and respect-commanding, unprepossessing yet magnetic little man. He told me about the precedent-shattering new Veterans Administration (VA) Hospital Karl Menninger was running, the grand schemes for training hordes of mental health professionals of all kinds, and the prospects of learning diagnostic testing on the job, with an ultimate chance to get into research and even psychoanalytic training if I wanted to.

Again I was quickly plunged into an atmosphere charged with intellectual and professional excitement: Great things were afoot, and one had only to join the starry-eyed throng to feel that even a neophyte clinician could soon become a pioneer. Out of a dearth of true experts, the Menningers made their own, partly by training and partly by anointment. Those who were not born to chutzpah had it thrust upon them. After six months of intensive schooling and supervision in diagnostic testing from Rapaport, the hardest taskmaster I have ever known, I was teaching and supervising the first class of graduate students in the Menninger Foundation School of Clinical Psychology. Shortly, too, came my opportunity to work directly with Rapaport as his colleague, and with Lester Luborsky, on the large-scale research on the selection of physicians for residency training in the Menninger School of Psychiatry. I was also given the chance to teach a course in theories of personality to the psychiatric residents. I had hardly learned my trade in the VA when I moved over to the Menninger Foundation's Research Department, which Rapaport headed, and where I did my principal work for the final four of the seven years I spent in Topeka.

I learned much about psychoanalysis as well as sociology, not to mention the roles of husband and father, from a brilliant young woman named Louisa Pinkham (now Howe), whom I had met in a Harvard seminar on psychoanalysis and the social sciences given jointly by Harry Murray, Clyde Kluckhohn, and Hobart Mowrer. We were married in one manic week in 1944 when I completed my psychoanalysis with Deutsch and passed my doctor's oral. When I went off to my Washington job two weeks later, she had to stay in Cambridge in a valiant but unsuccessful effort to complete her analysis with Edward Bibring and her thesis (on the feminine role) under Talcott Parsons (Holt [Howe], 1948). It was through Louisa, one of Parsons's favorite students, that I had been able to become one of three graduate students (my former roommate, Robert Freed Bales, was the third) to be admitted to an informal seminar group attempting to integrate the social sciences with psychoanalysis, which met evenings at the Parsons house in Belmont. The spokesmen for psychoanalysis there were Edward Bibring and Ives Hendrick; I attended the weekly sessions for about a year. Unlike mine, Louisa's was a training analysis. She was the first incumbent of the Boston Institute's Sigmund Freud Memorial Fellowship to train promising social scientists in psychoanalysis, and she attended a full round of seminars. After our first daughter was born in Washington, Louisa began a second thesis, finished in Topeka, which was her personal, highly original effort to synthesize sociology and psychoanalysis. I learned much from reading it and discussing it with her.

Thanks to Rapaport and his commanding influence on the intellectual scene in Topeka, Louisa and I were invited to become research members of the Topeka Psychoanalytic Society shortly after our arrival. I took advantage of my member's privilege to attend seminars, and tried to catch up to my spouse; for about five years I sampled all the offerings, doing the readings and participating on equal terms with the candidates, who were my professional peers and friends. When I found the level of discussion disappointing and the training analysts impatient with the questions I raised, I simply dropped quietly out. Theoretical and clinical seminars with Karl Menninger, Robert Knight, and Hellmuth Kaiser stand out in my memory; however, the best was a course in our School of Clinical Psychology on Chapter VII of *The Interpretation of Dreams*, given by David Rapaport. His lectures and supervisory sessions on diagnostic testing had been an unrivaled introduction to his own brand of ego psychology; now came my first real taste of metapsychology.

The "general theory" of psychoanalysis, as Rapaport called it, in distinction from the "special" or "clinical theory," was neither dull nor incomprehensible, but a superbly complex conceptual edifice, whose architectonics he limned with countless references to and parallels from his seemingly endless erudition in all the arts and sciences. As long as he was expounding metapsychology, it seemed not only internally consistent and clinically relevant, but tightly logical and amazingly sound in its selective borrowings from other sciences. My disenchantment with it, the reasons for which form the substance of this volume, began some years later.

Rapaport left Topeka in 1948, however, and I did not have continuous daily contact with him again over any extended period of time until the academic year 1959–1960, which he spent at the New York University (NYU) Research Center for Mental Health as a sabbatical from the Austen Riggs Foundation. In between, however, we were in constant correspondence, reading drafts of all of each other's papers and keeping alive through many visits what had become a close personal as well as professional friendship.

When Sigmund Koch approached Rapaport about writing the presentation of psychoanalytic theory for the American Psychological Association (APA)-sponsored encyclopedic study of the theoretical resources of psychology, Rapaport asked me whether I would join him as a collaborator. Though deeply honored and tempted, I felt (quite correctly) that I was not up to it, not having at that time read and mastered enough of the basic literature of psychoanalysis to be able to make any independent contribution. Instead, I read and made detailed suggestions about all of Rapaport's drafts, and I gained an enormous amount from that effort over a few years' span.

During that year at NYU just before his death, Rapaport offered another seminar on "the VIIth Chapter" (as he always called it), with the same format as a dozen years before but a remarkably different content. As always, he handed out each time a detailed syllabus on the next week's assignment. Everyone had to come with the book in hand, prepared to read the sentences of text containing the answer to each of the questions he had asked ("What is the first definition of the primary process?" "What is the second anticipation of the signal theory of anxiety?"). But as his own knowledge and understanding had broadened and deepened, so had the wisdom and insight he found in Freud, the latter's anticipations of the principal contributions of his epigones, and his relevance to any issue of the contemporary world. Because of the happy circumstance that his seminars on ego psychology and metapsychology in the Western New England Institute for Psychoanalysis were recorded and mimeographed, I was able to participate vicariously in several years of formal psychoanalytic training with him also, both before and after his untimely and tragic death.

My 14 years of interaction with David Rapaport gave me so much that it is hard to attempt an assessment of them. I am aware of trying to learn, and make my own, certain of his attitudes and approaches to theory: a respect for Freud's text; the need to return to it again and again as one's ability to read and understand grows, if there is to be any hope for more than a superficial grasp; an awareness that Freud's thought changed markedly as it grew, hence the necessity to study it in historical sequence; a recognition that Freud was a member of a culture and a long intellectual tradition, so that he could not be meaningfully studied in isolation from his predecessors and contemporaries or from general currents of ideas and events (see Shakow & Rapaport, 1964); knowledge of the major philosophers who helped form Freud's basic assumptions; an exegetical, closely analytical method of reading, with roots in the tradition of Talmudic scholarship (of which I never learned anything directly). For a more extended appraisal of the man, see my biographical sketch (Holt, 1967d).

To go back a bit, in the early 1950s I began to experience a growing dissatisfaction with the applied nature of the selection research (Holt & Luborsky, 1958) and a wish to get into work that was directly relevant to psychoanalytic theory, which led me to accept Stuart Cook's invitation to come to NYU and direct the Research Center for Mental Health in 1953. During those Topeka years, I had made many friends among coworkers, from whom I also learned a great deal: Roy Schafer, Margaret Brenman, Sibylle Escalona, Milton Wexler, Lester Luborsky, Benjamin Rubinstein, Merton Gill, Paul Bergman, Martin Mayman, and Gardner and Lois Murphy. I should mention my students from those years who also helped my learning in many ways, notably Philip Holzman, Herbert Schlesinger, Riley Gardner, Gerald Ehrenreich, and Arthur Kobler.

But the friendship that was to prove most professionally productive was that of George S. Klein, to whom I was greatly drawn by his combination of creative brilliance, experimental expertise, personal warmth, charm and wit, artistic sensitivity, and an aura of verve and driving ambition. We started to become good friends just before he left Topeka on a year's leave to accept a call to Harvard, which grew into a permanent departure. He had left behind an active research program, which he continued to pursue with the aid of a gifted group of students and by means of periodic visits. During one of those brief stays, we decided that we wanted to work together and agreed to make a joint search. So I went to NYU only on the condition that George join me, and together we planned and built up the Research Center.

We decided that the center would be a focus of teaching as well as research, and that our inquiry into the psychoanalytic theory of thinking—which we chose as the central topic—would be both experimental and conceptual. We had high ambitions to master and clarify the theory, making it both internally consistent and externally linked to operations, so that psychoanalytic propositions might be rigorously verified. During approximately the first half of the two decades that followed, we approached psychoanalytic theory mostly as students, awed but not daunted by the size of the task ahead, and aided by the coincidence that the *Standard Edition* was being published at just about the pace of our reading abilities.

At first it was a wrench to be separated from our immersion in a psychiatric hospital and clinic setting, with its daily contact with clinical realities. But we made the best of it, undertaking to study disordered thinking of all the kinds we could induce in the laboratory. We went after nonconscious cognition by the strategy of subliminal stimulation, studying the effects of inputs (of which the subject was not aware) on his or her simultaneous and subsequent perceptual and thought processes. On the hypothesis that continuous contact with highly structured aspects of reality was necessary for the maintenance of the secondary process, we* tried to impoverish it in several ways—principally through focusing our subjects on the indefinite configurations of Rorschach's inkblots, and through more ambitious attempts to separate them from the structure of reality as completely as possible (sensory deprivation, perceptual isolation). In altered states of consciousness, a considerable tradition suggested, primary processes might show themselves more clearly; thus we used psychedelic drugs, dreams and daydreams, imagery of all kinds, hypnosis, meditation, and biofeedback. We also tried the device of experimentally inducing intense motivational states, on the hypothesis that the primary process was drive-dominated thinking.

---

*In the rest of this paragraph, the first person plural includes all our colleagues and students, who are unfortunately too numerous to mention here.

With the aid of good fortune, happy timing, the firm institutional backing of our university and department, and the generous financial support of numerous agencies (especially the Ford Foundation and the National Institute of Mental Health [NIMH]), we were able to assemble a staff of whom we could be proud, who turned out a body of work gratifying in its size and quality. For a while, with Benjamin Rubinstein's help, Klein and I led a staff seminar that concentrated on extracting and codifying what Freud had to say about the primary and secondary processes. I recall with gratitude the contributory participation in those discussions of Donald Spence, Harriet Linton Barr, Fred Pine, Leo Goldberger, I. H. Paul, David Wolitzky, Morris Eagle, and Gudmund Smith (of the University of Lund, Sweden).

Shortly before David Rapaport's death, George Klein and I were beginning to become restive with the metapsychology we had always taken as a necessary starting point. Gradually, the difficulties we had attributed to our ignorance or the limitations of our understanding began to seem more plausibly located in the theory itself, and I began to feel an increasing need for a retreat from administrative and experimental involvements, to wrestle with purely theoretical issues. Fortunately, the financial aid of a fellowship from NIMH made it possible for me to have just such a year (1960–1961) at the Center for Advanced Study in the Behavioral Sciences in Palo Alto, California, surrounded by new and highly stimulating colleagues. There was also the happy circumstance that Merton Gill was just across the bay and was working on a theoretical monograph he had begun in collaboration with Rapaport, who died in December of 1960; Gill taught me a great deal in our discussions of his drafts.

The last influence on my thinking about psychoanalysis was a decade of teaching a graduate course on Freud's theories, which I began on my return from California in 1961. Now I was on my own: I had to integrate my thoughts about the growth of psychoanalytic ideas well enough to teach students of clinical psychology most of what they were going to get of metapsychology. That meant an intensive, analytical, and repeated reading of Freud's major theoretical works. Also, I had to field the searching questions of many classes of intellectually gifted graduate students. I have had far less (but some) experience in teaching candidates in psychoanalytic institutes, and believe that they challenge and thus instruct a teacher far less than students of clinical psychology, many of whom approach psychoanalysis without any prior commitment to it and often with skepticism bordering on hostility. To my students, I owe and am happy to express deep gratitude.

Looking back on these atypical encounters with psychoanalysis, I feel that on the whole I was fortunate in not having received my training in the ordinary, orthodox way: via medical school, psychiatric residency, and a psychoanalytic institute. That route is often criticized for taking so many years and including a good deal that is irrelevant, but mine took much longer and included at least as much learning and experience that is at best tangential to psychoanalysis. Aside from my lack of medical education, perhaps the most striking divergence from the usual pattern is my failure ever to obtain any training or experience in the therapeutic practice of psychoanalysis, or in any form of psychotherapy. I lack the *furor sanandi* of which Freud spoke; moreover, I was never encouraged by any of my analysts when I did express tentative thoughts about following in their footsteps.

I have tried to bring out some of the counterbalancing assets of my peculiar education as I have described it: the continuous encouragement I received to question and think for myself; the context of empirical research, which steadily urged an operational perspective and a regard for testability; teachers who infected me with a sense of enthusiasm for critical scholarship as a creative adventure; and an opportunity to proceed at my own pace. As a result, I was never bored by psychoanalytic theory; not prematurely committed to it; not pressured to conform or adopt attitudes of piety, overawe, personal inadequacy before a great genius, or the need to defer raising conceptual issues until I had mastered a therapeutic art; not motivated to seek premature closure (to protect the exposed position of a person whose livelihood is dependent on private practice); and not even forced to make up my mind about issues in the way demanded by teaching before I was ready to do so. My academic training and research involvement gave me the tools as well as the motivation to dissect and evaluate theory. Perhaps I was even aided by the fact that I have never developed the identity of a psychoanalyst or a sense of full belonging to the psychoanalytic movement, science, or profession. An outsider probably finds it emotionally easier than an insider to raise embarrassing questions, even to challenge the fundamental assumptions of a discipline. I am sorry if my work has at times made my friends uncomfortable, but I have never had to struggle with a feeling that I might be betraying or abandoning them or a larger cause with which we were all identified.

Just a brief postscript about philosophy is in order. I share some of Freud's ambivalence about it. As a teenager, I was strongly attracted by grandiose intellectual constructions and did my share of secret scribbling about the nature and meaning of life, the universe, and so on; yet as an undergraduate I took only a single course in the philosophy of mind, in which we read only (but all of) William James's great *Principles of Psychology* (1890). I did pick up my roommate's Whitehead (1925), however; it had a considerable influence on me. As a graduate student, too, I enrolled in only one course in philosophy, a useful but not enticing survey of modern schools. S. S. Stevens, who had recently published his positivistic manifesto (1939), indoctrinated us as well as he could in operationism and the early work of the Vienna Circle. All in all, I have not had much formal education in philosophy—just enough to glimpse some of its power and possibilities, to which I could return later on, in an unguided search for the tools of philosophical analysis that I needed.

As I reached the point in my studies of Freud where I began to feel that I was reaching conclusions worthy of being reported to others, I began to conceive various large projects: a text on metapsychology; an intellectual biography of Freud; a systematic examination of all his major philosophical presuppositions, or of the source of his ideas, or of the development and interrelations of his theoretical models of the human person; a chrestomathy of the enduringly valid passages from his works; even a restatement of psychoanalytic theory (along the lines of Rapaport's 1959 monograph), purged of all fallacies and factual errors, made internally consistent and congruent with neighboring sciences, and yet kept faithful to clinical reality. All of these schemes proved too ambitious (except perhaps the intellectual biography, which I hope to get out in a few years). Instead, starting in 1962, I published a series of papers on Freud and on psychoanalytic theory, with the general intent of somehow, sometime rewriting them all into a coherent book-length statement. But the opportunity to do so in a leisurely and thorough way has not come along, and meanwhile I have committed myself to begin a new program of empirical research, which seems to me more important than doing as good a job of synthesis as I would like.

The present volume is the result. I have not rewritten all of the chapters extensively; I have tried to hold myself to correcting what seemed clearly wrong and adding only what came readily to hand, even when a bigger job was needed and I could see a way to do it. I have tried to supply some continuity by a brief preface to each chapter, which gives the place and date of the paper's original publication.

Extensive recent additions to the text are set off by square brackets [thus], as are contemporary endnotes. In passages quoted from Freud, however, square brackets have their usual meaning of indicating editorial interpolations into the author's text. I have not usually distinguished between Strachey's and my own remarks of this kind. It would have seemed overmeticulous and obtrusive to have done so, and anyone who cares that much can readily determine who is summarizing omitted words, explaning, or otherwise commenting on Freud's text by checking against the *Standard Edition*. In all instances, italics in quotations indicate Freud's emphasis unless there is an explicit statement to the contrary—something I have done only rarely. The same goes for quotations from all other authors.

One final point having to do with the fact that these are republished papers—some dating back over 25 years—should be mentioned: The use of masculine pronouns and of "man" to indicate the generic human being has been left as it was in the original publications. I began changing "he" to "he or she" and so on, but soon found that doing so consistently throughout the text would entail much more extensive rewriting than I had realized. I therefore ask readers to accept the original usage in the understanding that no sexism is intended.

CHAPTER 2

The Manifest and Latent Meanings
of Metapsychology

In order to give the reader a preliminary overview of and an orientation toward the less familiar general theory of psychoanalysis—metapsychology—I begin with a recently published paper, not the earliest written. It is an attempt to figure out what the term "metapsychology" meant to Freud by a systematic examination of all his usages. I realized the need to do that after having become painfully aware of how little it is possible to take any of Freud's definitions literally and seriously. (The next chapter expounds and attempts to explain this idiosyncrasy of his way of working and writing.) To give him his due, it should be added that in any social/behavioral science, no important concept can easily be given a comprehensive, precise, and permanently satisfactory definition, and that this kind of analysis is necessary to elucidate any such term's functional definition in use.

Most of the chapter, however, is devoted to the early years of Freud's psychoanalytic career, the period covered by the letters to his friend Fliess (Freud, 1985). The availability—at last!—of the full text of all the letters, in translation, greatly aided my task.

The rest of the book then takes up each of the three subdivisions of metapsychology, the economic, dynamic, and structural (originally called topographic) points of view. Then we come back to another look at metapsychology as a whole—one that aims to expound what the term might (indeed, should) mean in a modern psychoanalytic theory.

An early version of this chapter was presented at a meeting of the American Psychoanalytic Association in San Juan, Puerto Rico, May 1981.

There is a good deal of confusion on the question of what metapsychology is. Marie Jahoda (1977, p. 93) has summed it up admirably:

> according to Jones (1955, p. 185), it implies "a comprehensive description of any mental process," while David Rapaport (Rapaport & Gill, 1959, pp. 795–796) reads it to mean "the study of the assumptions upon which the system of psychoanalytic theory is based"; in another publication (1960), however, he identified metapsychology as the "principles in psychoanalytic theory." Hartmann (1964, p. 328), who apparently felt uneasy about the term, defines it as

theory on the highest level of abstraction. Strachey (1957a, p. 105), in the editorial introduction to the papers on metapsychology, uses the slightly odd phrase "views on psychological theory" to characterise metapsychology, obviously implying something different from the theory itself. Hilgard (1962) seems to suggest that metapsychology is a collection of Freud's models of man, and Laplanche and Pontalis (1973, p. 249) say that "metapsychology constructs an ensemble of conceptual models which are more or less far-removed from empirical reality."

To this collection let me add only Gill's (1976) assertion that "Metapsychology is not psychology" but biology, and one more definition: "Metapsychology is a generic term which subsumes any extraclinical theory including Freud's specific metapsychology" (Rubinstein, personal communication, May 31, 1981), apparently the sense in which it is used by Smith (1982).

Faced with such diversity, we may find it helpful to begin with an effort to trace Freud's usages from the first to the last and to attempt to put them in the perspective of contemporary and antecedent intellectual movements.[1] In the process, I have developed some hypotheses about unconscious connotations that the term seems to have had for Freud, and some speculations about its nonintellectual functions.

HOW DID FREUD DEFINE
AND USE METAPSYCHOLOGY?

The term first crops up in Freud's letter to Fliess of February 13, 1896. He has just been commenting on Fliess's biological ideas about the connection between sex and the functioning of the nose ("a fine piece of objective truth"), and it seems almost by contrast that he says, after a digression into his health,

> I am continually occupied with psychology—really *meta*psychology; Taine's book *L'Intelligence* gives me special satisfaction. I hope something will come of it. The oldest ideas are really the most useful ones, as I am finding out belatedly. I hope to be well supplied with scientific interests until the end of my life. (Freud, 1985 [1887–1904], p. 172)

The first thing that must strike us about this passage, the first known usage of the neologism "metapsychology," is that Freud uses it as easily and casually as if it were well known to both of them. If it had been strange to Fliess, he might very well have asked about it; and though his letters have not survived, there is nothing in Freud's subsequent letters by way of elucidation.[2] Evidently, then, Freud must have coined the word in one of their "congresses," the most recent of which had taken place just about five months before. But that was the most notable of their meetings, the one in which Freud orally expounded what he then immediately set about writing out for his friend, his psychology for neurologists (which has come to be known as "the Project"). Indeed, Freud was occupied with this, his first major theoretical enterprise and the *fons et origo* of all his later metapsychology, in the spring and summer of 1895 and throughout the months intervening between the September meeting and the February 1896 letter. A long New Year's letter a month earlier had been devoted to a brief summary of "a complete revision" of the theory, which Freud often referred to briefly as "the psychology."

It was no ordinary psychology like the fairly conventional associationism and physiological psychology of Taine (1864), but an audacious attempt at a physicalistic, biological sketch of the human organism with particular attention to the brain and its functioning. True to the reductionist ideals of his teachers and scientific heroes—Brücke and the other members of the biophysics group of 1847 (Cranefield, 1966), the most notable of whom was Helmholtz—Freud set himself the task of explaining behavior, thought, and their aberrations without postulating any psychological entities as independent (causal) variables. The subjective phenomena of consciousness, in particular, were to be introduced only as dependent variables—that is, as the output of the apparatus, which itself was conceived in strictly anatomical and physiochemical terms. As a whole, the attempt failed; Freud could see no way of conceptualizing defense without postulating a homuncular ego, despite feats of cybernetic ingenuity which today seem astoundingly far ahead of his time. And the problem of consciousness proved insurmountable.

His situation was further confused by the evident but paradoxial necessity of postulating that all these "psychical" phenomena were often unconscious and indeed were most important and mischievous when active without the awareness of the person who in some way owned them. Despite the widespread contemporary acceptance of some concept of an unconscious, a troublesome, recurrent question remained: How could there be an unconscious idea or wish, when being present in consciousness was an accepted part of the common-sense definition of such subjective concepts? His ingenious but troublemaking answer, like that of Lipps (1883), a work he admired and which may have supplied it, was to consider consciousness and incidental and nonessential characteristic of the "psychical," which implicitly retained a separate ontological status but became a world of meanings continuing to exist even when no one was aware of them. The more usual alternative, which Freud later rejected in *The Unconscious* (1915e), though he reverted to it at times, postulates that the brain process accompanying or mediating conscious meanings can continue to operate and have effects when the correlated psychic phenomenon is absent.

Please take note of this last point, because it is an important bridge between the two principal meanings of metapsychology in this first usage:

that it is (like Taine's) first a *depth* psychology, one that explains by reference to unconscious wishes and other unconscious psychic entities; and second, that in its independent (causal) variables it is a *non*psychological theory—as Gill (1976) would have it, a neurological and biological one. And note also that these two characteristics set his theory decisively apart from the (pure) psychologies that dominated the English-speaking world.

The tentativeness of the first introduction ("psychology—it is really *meta*psychology") continued to be reflected in subsequent letters of the succeeding months when Freud was working over the Project.

The second and third usages, in two letters of 1896, make a clear distinction between clinical theory and the more general theory. In the letter of April 2, 1896: "I am making good progress on the psychology of the neuroses and have every reason to be satisfied. I hope you will lend me your ear for a few *metapsychological* questions as well" (Freud, 1985 [1887–1904], p. 180). In December, after a discussion of psychopathology, he adds: "Hidden deep within this is my ideal and woebegone child—metapsychology" (p. 216). Note the contrast in the letter of August 14, 1897: "I . . . am very satisfied with the psychology, tormented by grave doubts about my theory of the neuroses" (p. 261).

The fourth usage, a similar one, comes near the end of the dramatic letter of September 21, 1897, in which Freud renounced the seduction theory. After facing up to his error and realizing that he must give up his dreams of "eternal fame . . . certain wealth, complete independence, travel," and giving the children a better life—all of which he had been hoping his first "solution" of the problem of neurosis could bring—he says:

> I have to add one more thing. In this collapse of everything valuable, the psychological alone has remained untouched. The dream [book] stands entirely secure and my beginnings of the metapsychological work have only grown in my estimation. (Freud, 1985 [1887–1904], p. 266)

The next usage came a half-year later (in a letter of March 10, 1898). Then he was at work on his second major attempt, the conceptualization of the dreaming process:

> It seems to me [he wrote] that the theory of wish-fulfillment has brought only the psychological solution and not the biological—or rather, metapsychical— one. (I am going to ask you seriously, by the way, whether I may use the name metapsychology for my psychology that leads behind consciousness.) (Freud, 1985 [1887–1904], p. 302)

Notice that here again Freud made a clear antithesis between a psychology (implicitly, the contemporaneous science of conscious mental phenomena) and a metapsychology "which leads behind[3] consciousness." The idea of looking *behind* consciousness connotes the search for hidden causes, to which Freud was later to be quite obviously devoted. The secret, true causes of human behavior—especially the baffling pathological kind—were unconscious and ultimately biological.

Here is a clue to the reductionistic aspect of metapsychology: Freud saw his task not as supplementing the conscious surface of things by bringing to light neglected and even more important unconscious determinants, but as *discarding* the surface for the hidden truth behind it. In this respect, he could feel at one with the archeologist, digging beneath the deceptively everyday appearance of a meadow, stripping away that irrelevant overburden to expose the precious hidden remnants of a past life.

The last passage quoted is more remarkable, however, for explicitly equating "metapsychological" with "biological," and for what it shows us about the meaning this last term had for Freud. He goes right on to elaborate:

> Biologically, dream-life seems to me to derive entirely from the residues of the prehistoric period of life (between the ages of one and three)—the same period which is the source of the unconscious and alone contains the aetiology of all the psychoneuroses, the period normally characterized by an amnesia analogous to hysterical amnesia. (p. 302)

To those of us (e.g., Chapter 5, this volume; Gill, 1976, p. 74) who have been accustomed to thinking of Freud's biologizing as explaining psychological phenomena by recourse to physicalistic physiology and brain anatomy, this seems an odd explication of the biological. Yet it is entirely consistent with Freud's terminology in the Project. Near its beginning, after he has introduced his conception of the nervous system as a means of getting rid of incoming stimuli (primary function), which it does by facilitating adaptive action (secondary function), and has set forth his structural and functional conception of the neurones and contact barriers (synapses), he adds "The Biological Standpoint," as if what we had seen so far was not biology. In the new section, however, it becomes plain that he uses "biological" to mean "evolutionary," for "the biological development of the nervous system" in this context makes no sense if development signifies ontogeny: *Biological* development is phylogeny, the gradual increase in the size and complexity of the brain over geological time.

Less obvious in this fourth section of the first part of the Project is the antithesis Freud draws between "a Darwinian line of thought" which he rejects, and another which he prefers. The former ("to appeal to the fact of impermeable neurones' being indispensable and to their surviving in consequence" (Freud, 1950 [1895], p. 303) may be read as natural selection: Since chance variations in the permeability of certain neurones gave an adaptive advantage, their possessors survived and bred better than those who had only one class of neurones. What Freud preferred as "more fruitful and more modest" was "learning from biological experience." It is little more than a version of Lamarck's "law" of modification through use. Just as straining for high leaves supposedly lengthened the giraffe's neck, much use lowered the synaptic resistance in certain neural pathways, and in both conceptions, this effect of experience was passed on to future generations by heredity, an important added assumption. The idea, upheld by most evolutionists including Darwin himself, was very widespread at the time, and is undeniably more attractive than Darwin's notion of random genetic variation as the source of change. Surely Freud found no appeal in the idea of stochastic processes when something more purposive and directional could be conceived.

In any event, in over a dozen places throughout the Project Freud continued to invoke biological considerations, always with reference to phylogenetic adaptiveness and frequently in a Lamarckian sense. Early on (Freud, 1950 [1895], p. 305, n.3), Strachey points out that "by 'biological' he means that it is determined genetically—by its survival value for the species," though the editor seems to have missed the implied reliance on inheritance of acquired characters. Sulloway's (1979) careful and detailed discussion of then-current evolutionary biology is a most useful supplement and corrective. Surprisingly few other writers on Freud have noticed what a large and growing role biology, in its large, evolutionary sense, played in the development of psychoanalytic theory [but see also Sjöbäck, 1988].

Returning to the 1898 letter, we see at once that while Freud uses "biological" to mean "evolutionary," as in the Project, he is now implying an evolutionary principle that plays no role in the 1895 document. He clearly does not develop his argument by showing that dreaming is "expedient" (adaptive) or that it is something "learned from biological experience." Rather, Freud here seems to be saying that dreaming is a repetition of something from infancy, which in turn is a recapitulation of a "prehistoric" phase in phylogenesis before the emergence of consciousness. Not all of that is there on the surface in this condensed passage, which becomes intelligible only after we begin (with Sulloway's help) to recognize how pervasively Freud had begun to use the notion of a biologically determined *recapitulation*.

His second crucial theorem of evolutionary biology was supplied for Freud by a man who played the role for Darwin in Germany that Huxley did in England: Ernst Haeckel, still famous for his so-called biogenetic law that ontogeny recapitulates phylogeny (Gould, 1977b). As Freud understood it, that implied some law of nature whereby the contemporary individual had to go through the same stages of development in a few years as his remotest prehuman and human ancestors did over centuries.

I deliberately emphasize the idea of a "law of nature," because by one of the ironies of history, Darwin's great champion promulgated a principle which he thought quite in keeping with the master's materialistic and mechanistic theorizing, but which as used by such enthusiasts as Freud became just the kind of historicist principle that Darwin devoted all his efforts to opposing.[4] The idea that everything changes and evolves was prominent in *Naturphilosophie* [see Chapter 6, this volume], but has ancient roots indeed. The biblical account of creation is one such: The world and all that is in it did not come into being just as we see it today, in an instant of divine fiat. Instead, Genesis tells us that God did it in stages, apparently executing a divine plan. As a young man, Darwin encountered the idea that biological species change in accordance with a plan; that idea, in fact, came to be called "evolution," a term Darwin never—well, hardly ever—used because of this supernatural connotation (Gould, 1977a; oddly enough, neither Lamarck nor Haeckel used it either). His contribution was not that species change, but that there was a nonteleological mechanism for it—a natural selection of adaptive, inherited, random variations. And despite Freud's reverence for Darwin, I have seen no evidence anywhere that he was attracted to or made any use of this explanatory idea or any transformation of it. Instead, he was attracted to "historicism," the attempt to find general laws of history and build from them a science. He probably first encountered it in a history of England by H. T. Buckle (1871), about which he was highly enthusiastic as an adolescent.[5] Buckle speaks frequently and confidently about the laws of history and of the mind.

Popper (1957) makes several subtle and highly useful distinctions in discussing the way that evolution became a historicist doctrine, adapting his argument slightly to the example of biogenesis. Let us note first that there was an observed regularity (which some call an empirical generalization): All macroscopic living forms grow in a short time from small and simple infantile beginnings (a spore, a seed, an egg cell) to large, more complex adult individuals. There is also a striking similarity between this individual developmental course and the reconstructed sequence of living species across geological time, even to the point that the human embryo and fetus morphologically resemble a number of remote hypothetical ancestors— think of the "gill slits" and tail that appear and disappear before birth.

Haeckel exaggerated this similarity and then expressed it by the empirical generalization that individual development often seems to repeat (recapitulate) phyletic development. He extended this generalization to a hypothesis, which by definition was universally applicable. Even if true, Popper (1957) points out, such a "hypothesis is not a universal law. . . . It has, rather, the character of a particular (singular or specific) historical statement" (p. 107). If we were able to observe the origin and development of life on many other planets, and found that this (or any other evolutionary hypothesis) was repeatedly verified, Popper goes on, we could promote it to the status of a scientific law. But since, so far as we know, "the evolution of life on earth, or of human society, is a unique historical process" (p. 108), Popper argues there can be no laws of evolution, biological or social. "The fact that all laws of nature are hypotheses must not distract our attention from the fact that not all hypotheses are laws," he warns, a point not grasped by either Haeckel or Freud. Yet confusion on this point made historicism possible. Like most intellectuals of his time, notably including Marx, Freud never doubted that there were laws of history, and mistook the somewhat different real achievements of evolutionary biology as the discovery of just such laws.

Notice that Haeckel's "law" differed from Darwin's explanation of the origin of species in one critical rrespect: Darwin—especially as aided by Weismann, father of modern genetics—provided an intelligible, point-by-point, materialistic explanation of the evolutionary regularities he observed; whereas Haeckel's principle is lacking precisely on the score of mechanism, or the question of *how* it worked. The reasoning of historicists has been simple and apparently logical enough: How could such regularities (e.g., the rise and fall of civilizations) occur if not in response to the workings of some general law? It is precisely the kind of thinking that seeks to explain any observed regularity of behavior by postulating an instinct. We and so many other vertebrates act parentally because of a parental instinct; if people everywhere (and many other mammals too) collect things so avidly, we and they just have an instinct of acquisition, or a "drive to amass wealth" (Fenichel, 1938); if all forms of life struggle to stay alive, there must be some life instinct or motive for survival, and if they all die, why not also a death drive? (For further discussion of the fallacies of this kind of reasoning as applied to motivation, see Chapter 7, this volume.)

Briefly, the error in all this kind of thought is the assumption that a regularity can come about only in response to some specific cause. Yet similar effects may have quite different causes; genetics gives us the terminology to express the principle that the same phenotype may have different genotypes and also provides familiar examples from Mendel's studies of dominant and recessive traits in peas of pure and mixed heredity. "Like begets like" is a roughly true empirical generalization, but it is no law and is not an explanation at all—only a digression into the strange world of chromosomes and genes, mitosis and DNA, begins to supply explanatory laws.

To hark back briefly to the Project, there Freud uses two basic types of explanation, which he calls "mechanical" and "biological." Ideally, they mesh, and a problem can be resolved by both means, as when he notes with evident satisfaction that the difference between the Φ and Ψ neurones "in respect of permeability is explained biologically and mechanically" (Freud, 1950 [1895], p. 305). Here Strachey makes this point in a footnote:

It is worth noticing that all through the present work Freud groups the explanations of the phenomena he is studying under two headings: 'mechanical' and 'biological.' . . . By 'mechanical' (for which he sometimes uses 'automatic' as a synonym) he means that the phenomenon in question is detemined directly by contemporary physical events; by 'biological' he means that it is determined genetically—by its survival value for the species. (p. 305, n.3)

My impression is that Freud felt the former to be a sounder type of explanation; he seems uncomfortable when he admits, in a later discussion of attention:

> I find it hard to give a mechanical (automatic) explanation of its origin. For that reason I believe that it is biologically determined—that is, that it has been left over in the course of psychical evolution because any other behavior by Ψ has been excluded owing to the generation of unpleasure. (Freud, 1950 [1895], pp. 360-361)

Surely this passage makes it perspicuous that he saw these as two alternative explanatory resources, not easily synthesized into one single, consistent system. Here we have the incompatibility between Freud's two sets of borrowings from the nonpsychological sciences: Considerations of forces and energies operating quantitatively in some structural network (either an explicitly neural one, in the Project, or an implicit one in later topographical and structural models) are "mechanical," coming ultimately from physics by route of physicalistic physiology; and evolutionary, phylogenetic propositions are "biological," stemming mainly from Lamarck and Haeckel. Interestingly, if Freud had studied his Darwin closely enough, he would have seen that the latter's basic explanatory conception was materialistic and mechanistic, not teleological or historicist, and as such *not* incompatible with the outlook of metapsychology. *There was no available way for Freud to integrate these two kinds of theoretical resources, even though both were drawn from branches of biology,* either in 1895 or at any later time in his career. It is true that in some works, notably *Beyond the Pleasure Principle*, he interwove propositions of both kinds, but they remain incommensurate and unarticulated.

Only 16 months after the letter in which metapsychology seems to mean an application of recapitulation theory, when he had almost finished *The Interpretation of Dreams*, Freud (1985 [1887-1904]) wrote to Fliess:

> At any rate, a part of the first third of the large task will have been accomplished, that of placing the neuroses and psychoses in [the sphere of] science by means of the theory of repression and wish-fulfillment. (1) The organic–sexual; (2) the factual–clinical; (3) the metapsychological. . . . (p. 362)

Now metapsychology does *not* include "the organic–sexual," the realm in which Freud most extensively relied on evolutionary biological ideas. (For a detailed expansion of that last proposition, see Sulloway, 1979.)[6]

In no later place that I have been able to find does Freud make such a threefold division of his "great task," but his statement deserves to be strongly highlighted. Metapsychology is clearly differentiated not only from the clinical theory of neurosis (so much closer to factual observation), but from evolutionary biological theories. The last-named, though they first came to the center of the stage in *Totem and Taboo* (1912–1913), never ceased to play a vital role in Freud's attempts to understand several basic theoretical problems (Sulloway, 1979). All three kinds of theorizing can be found combined in various proportions, throughout Freud's works, even though metapsychology came to the fore during a brief period, approximately 1915 through 1917.

There remains one more undiscussed usage, in a letter of August 26, 1898:

> I have set myself the task of building a bridge between my germinating metapsychology and that contained in the literature, and have therefore immersed myself in the study of Lipps, who I suspect has the clearest mind among present-day philosophical writers. (Freud, 1985 [1887–1904], p. 324)

The unexpected word "philosophical" should serve to remind us of a number of other passages in letters to Fliess where it crops up incongruously to a modern ear. At the height of his early excitement over the Project (letter of October 16, 1895), he refers to what he has already sent as "a few pages of philosophical stammering"! In a couple of later letters, he clears up this puzzle:

> I see how, via the detour of medical practice, you are reaching your first ideas of understanding human beings as a physiologist, just as I most secretly nourish the hope of arrive, via these same paths, at my initial goal of philosophy. For that is what I wanted originally, when it was not yet at all clear to me to what end I was in the world. (p. 159; letter of January 1, 1896)

> As a young man I knew no longing other than for philosophical knowledge, and now I am about to fulfill it as I move from medicine to psychology. (p. 180; letter of April 2, 1896)[7]

Lipps was indeed a professor of philosophy in that era when psychology was only beginning to detach itself from its mother-discipline, though he figures in the history of the "new (experimental) psychology." As Boring (1929, p. 427) notes, he was a peripheral act psychologist, "by temperament more of a logician than an experimentalist," and is best known for his theory of empathy in aesthetics. It is possible that Brentano, a much more central figure in act psychology, had first called Lipps to Freud's attention during the period of his university years when he was seriously considering becoming a philosopher (Clark, 1980, p. 34).

In any event, this tangential reference to philosophy should serve to remind us that, to the extent that metapsychology was a kind of psychology, it tended to connote philosophy. Moreover, for Freud, work on the Project had one important structural similarity to philosophy: It was as close as he ever came to building a comprehensive, deductive system, the very aspect of philosophy Freud so often condemned in later years.

A second indication of similar import is to be found in the first published use of metapsychology, in *The Psychopathology of Everyday Life* when Freud (1901b) was discussing superstition and religion. Noting that "the mythological view of the world . . . *is nothing but psychology projected into the external world*," he observes that

> the construction of a *supernatural reality* . . . is destined to be changed back once more by science into the *psychology of the unconscious*. One could venture to explain in this way the myths of paradise and the fall of man, of God, of good and evil, or immortality, and so on, and to transform *metaphysics* into *metapsychology*. (pp. 258-259)

Here his theories of the unconscious are explicitly to take the place of philosophy—indeed, to explain the profoundest problems with which philosophers and religionists have grappled throughout all the ages.[8] A grandiose conception, and doubtless an enthralling one!

Oddly enough, Freud did not mention metapsychology in *The Interpretation of Dreams*; its only appearance there is in a footnote interpolated in 1919. He was silent about it for 14 productive years (though of course he continued to use dynamic and economic concepts) until the great flowering of 1915.

The implication that metapsychology was not merely to be a "psychology of the unconscious" but a *system* became explicit in a footnote to one of the last-published metapsychological papers and indeed the only one with the adjective in its title (Freud, 1917d [1915], p. 222). After saying that he had originally intended to publish "a collection . . . in book form" as "Preliminaries to a Metapsychology," he says, "The intention of the series is to clarify and carry deeper the theoretical assumptions on which a psychoanalytic system could be founded" (p. 222 n.). N.B.: Not to discover, extend, or elaborate, the assumptions; he apparently believed that he had already set them forth completely enough. What was needed was to clarify them (unexceptionable enough), and to "carry them deeper," a more obscure phrase. It reiterates the metaphor of *depth* psychology, a spatial allusion to what is fundamental, old, covered-over, perhaps because it is dirty or evil, but perhaps also because it is wise and precious. For in his paper *The Antithetical Meaning of Primal Words*, Freud (1910e) expressed the conviction that many words connote their opposites, simultaneously suggesting both sides of an antithesis.

The collection that was to have been a book comprised 12 papers: the five that he reprinted in collections of his own works as "metapsychological papers" (written in an average of ten *days* each between March 15 and May 4, 1915!), and seven more written during the following three months.

Not until the third paper, *The Unconscious*, did Freud define metapsychology afresh. Discussing the topography and dynamics of repression, he began by saying that there must be "a *withdrawal* of cathexis" (1915e, p. 180). After pursuing this idea awhile, ending with the idea of anticathexis, the "permanent expenditure" (note the metaphor) of cathectic energy in a primal repression, he remarks:

> We see how we have gradually been led into adopting a third point of view in our account of psychical phenomena. Beside the dynamic and the topographical points of view, we have adopted the *economic* one. This endeavors to follow out the vicissitudes of amounts of excitation and to arrive at least at some *relative* estimate of their magnitude.
>
> It will not be unreasonable to give a special name to this whole way of regarding our subject-matter, for it is the consummation of psycho-analytic research. I propose that when we have succeeded in describing a psychical process in its dynamic, topographical and economic aspects, we should speak of it as a *metapsychological* presentation. (1915e, p. 181)

The consummation of psychoanalytic research! Aside from its sexual connotation, this phrase strikes the eye, for with it Freud puts metapsychology at the pinnacle of his endeavors. From the tone of this passage, one would expect that he would have given high priority to completing and refining his metapsychology, or at least that he would have been constantly preoccupied with attaining the objective of systematically treating any subject about which he theorized from these three points of view. Yet he blew hot and cold about it, occasionally making the attempt in an explicit way but often neglecting one or another of the points of view in his theoretical works. Even when he revised *The Interpretation of Dreams* in 1919, he neglected to link its seventh chapter explicitly to the metapsychological enterprise.

Contrary to Strachey's statement that after 1915 it came into "frequent use," in his remaining years of prolific writing, Freud used the word "metapsychology" (or any variant of it) less than once a year, on average, and in only nine works. In these, he makes several illuminating points, however. First, metapsychology was an attempt "to arrive at some more general points of view on the basis of psychoanalytic observations" (Freud, 1925d, p. 58); he repeats several times his claim that however speculative it might be, it always had a clinical foundation. Then, it affords "the most complete description of [mental processes] of which we can at present conceive" (1920g, p. 7), "the furthest goal that psychology could attain." He contrasts it with "mere description" (1926d, p. 109), making it repeatedly clear that metapsychology is an *explanatory* theory.

Yet the ambivalence in that early characterization ("my ideal and woebegone child") remained right to the end. In a letter to Abraham of August 1, 1915, he characterized the unpublished metapsychological papers as "wartime atrocities, like a lot of other things. Several, including that on consciousness, still require thorough revision" (Freud & Abraham, 1965, p. 228). Frequently Freud apologized for "the indefiniteness of all our discussions on . . . metapsychology" (1920g, p. 30); he disclaimed any intent "to disguise or gloss over the uncertain and tentative character of these metapsychological discussions" (1917d [1915], p. 234 n.), noting that he had engaged in them "not sufficiently often" (1927d, p. 164). In a few places (notably in *Group Psychology and the Analysis of the Ego*, 1921c, p. 138) he noted the difficulty of carrying out the metapsychological program. And in his autobiography, he seemed satisfied that the published metapsychological papers "remained no more than a torso . . . I broke off, wisely perhaps, since the time for theoretical predications of this kind had not yet come" (1925d, p. 59).

In Freud's last great original work, *Analysis Terminable and Interminable* (1937c), occur some most interesting final references to metapsychology. Near the beginning of the third section he begins considering theoretical aspects of the problem of what psychoanalytic treatment can accomplish, and brings up the concept of the "taming" of an instinct:

> That is to say, the instinct is brought completely into the harmony of the ego, becomes accessible to all the influences of the other trends in the ego and no longer seeks to go its independent way to satisfaction. If we are asked by what methods and means this result is achieved, it is not easy to find an answer. We can only say: "So muss denn doch die Hexe dran!" ["We must call the witch to our help after all!"—Goethe, *Faust*]—the Witch Metapsychology. Without metapsychological speculation and theorizing—I had almost said "phantasying"—we shall not get another step forward. Unfortunately, here as elsewhere, what our Witch reveals is neither very clear nor very detailed. (p. 225)

The Witch Metapsychology—what an unexpected, astonishing image! Where could it have come from? Freud taught us that unconscious wishes and fantasies often determine figurative turns of thought, particularly unusual ones; notice in this passage his near-equating of theorizing and fantasying. Surely the witch is a potent participant in many an infantile fantasy, as the embodiment of the "split image" of the bad mother. That is, unable to comprehend how the same person can at times be warm, loving, protecting, and sensuously exciting, and at others harsh and painfully punitive, arousing guilt and the deepest anxiety, the young child finds it easier to develop images of all-good, ideal goddess and uncannily evil witches. There are a number of reasons to believe that in the last year of his infantile Freiberg era, the three-year-old child Freud formed a fantasy of having two mothers—his real mother, all good and loving, and his witchlike Nana (nurse), of whom he wrote: "Her treatment of me was not always excessive in its amiability, and her words could be harsh if I failed to reach the required standard of cleanliness" (Freud, 1900a, pp. 247-248). As I plan to argue in detail at a later time, Nature, as described in Goethe's *Fragment*, played an important part as an idealized mother-image at the very beginning of Freud's career; now, at its end, it seems appropriate that the other, more usually repressed part of the split image should appear, again ushered in by Goethe. The context is the *taming* of an instinct, itself a metaphor in which desires are treated as wild animals and their control as a process of domestication.⁹ But such desires are those—especially the secret and shameful ones—of a young child, who "seeks to go its independent way" to satisfaction but is "brought completely into the harmony of" the household by a series of confrontations with the mother.¹⁰ Since struggles over toilet training are the first such crises of taming, when the loving mother becomes a demanding and threatening witch, it is understandable that the witch is mythologically associated with anal and urethral imagery.

At any rate, that is what Freud tells Fliess in a series of three remarkable letters written in the space of two weeks during January 1897. In the first of these, he says with evident excitement that he is enclosing two "red-hot" ideas, "based, of course, on the results of analyses" (Freud, 1985 [1887-1904], p. 221). One is the hypothesis that a "psychosis of being overwhelmed" is precipitated instead of a neurosis if the incestuous "sexual abuse" occurs in the first 18 months; he backed the generalization by a story of a patient's seducing, perverse father-figure. The second is the idea that perversions "have an animal character." The sense of smell is dominant in animals, so "urine, feces, and the whole surface of the body, also blood, have a sexually exciting effect. The heightened sense of smell in hysteria presumably is connected with this" (p. 223). As Strachey footnotes, he was beginning "his understanding of the psychological importance of anal material" (Freud, 1950 [1892-1899], p. 242 n.) and developed it further in the other letters of this series.

In the second, he raises the question,

why did the Devil who took possession of the poor things invariably abuse them sexually and in a loathsome manner [apparently a reference to anal intercourse]? Why are their confessions under torture so like the communications made by patients in psychic treatment? (Freud, 1985 [1887-1904] p. 224)

A few days later:

[Wtiches'] "flying" is explained; the broomstick they ride probably is the great Lord Penis. . . . I read one day that the gold the Devil gives his victims regularly turns into excrement. . . . I dream, therefore, of a primeval devil religion, with rites that are carried on secretly, and understand the harsh therapy of the witches' judges. (p. 227)

(Notice the implicit equating of therapy with severely punitive control.)

Judging by these letters, the witch seems to have had several unconscious meanings to Freud: She is the evil mother, both because she forbids infantile gratification with phallic punitiveness, thus taming the animal-like child, and because she is the (projective) embodiment of forbidden anal and sexual desires which she acts out secretly with that other wicked parental figure, the Devil. Moreover, witches are the victims of (sexual) possession by the bad father and therefore suggest Freud's bothersome hysterical female patients. But as adepts in magic, they partake of the "omnipotence of thought" and the power to accomplish such wonders as the transformation of human beings by means of words—thus they foreshadow the therapeutic work and role of the psychoanalyst.

In suggesting that Freud's ambivalence may have been in part a reaction to unconscious, infantile, sexual, and other bodily connotations of metapsychological concepts, I am adopting a hypothesis put forward by Gill (1978, pp. 362–363) and Schafer (1976, p. 6). Let me now advance one further speculative implication.

Recall the occupational hazard of psychoanalysis: that the analyst must listen all day to just the fantasies and wishes and fears that no one else would tolerate in conversation—because, on the simplest level, such stuff is upsetting. In the course of our own "taming," we have learned not to "talk dirty," not to introduce shocking images of a raw, instinctual nature into everyday social interactions. We censor them out as a way of keeping our own impulses under control, in part by not letting incestuous, sadistic, or other unacceptable wishes consciously form in our minds. No matter how well analyzed a psychoanalyst may be, no matter how much desensitized by the daily repetition of talk about this infantile underworld, it can readily jar his or her equilibrium, stirring up unruly fantasies, occasionally even to the point where the analyst acts them out with the patient.

Because he was the first to be subjected to this combination of sexual temptation, provocation of anxiety and anger, and reawakening of personal infantile conflicts, Freud had no less need for defenses than a contemporary psychoanalyst—probably more. He needed all the help he could get in dealing with these unwelcome, intrusive, mischievous emotions and impulses. And let us not delude ourselves with the heroic myth of his Olympian serenity and preternatural maturity: A strong strain of prudery in his nature is plain from his many comments about his patients and the disgusting things they told him.

Near the beginning of the Dora case (1905e [1901], pp. 48–49), Freud writes:

This short piece of the analysis may perhaps have excited in the medical reader . . . feelings of astonishment and horror . . . The astonishment is probably caused by my daring to talk about such delicate and unpleasant subjects to a young girl . . . It is possible for a man to talk to girls and women upon sexual matters of every kind without doing them harm and without bringing suspicion upon himself. . . . The best way . . . is to be dry and direct. . . . I have certainly heard of some people—doctors and laymen—who are scandalized by a thera-peutic method in which conversations of this sort occur, and who appear to envy either me or my patients the titillation which, according to their notions, such a method must afford. . . . As regards the second kind of emotional reaction . . . which regards the perverse nature of her phantasies as horrible, I should like to say emphatically that a medical man has no business to indulge in such passionate condemnation.

He goes on to deplore the practice among writers on sexual "aberrations" to "seize every opportunity of inserting into the text expressions of [their] per-sonal repugnance at such revolting things. . . . We must learn to speak without indignation of what we call the sexual perversions" (p. 50), because we all have some degree of such impulses, and so on. Yet two pages later he remarks: "So we see that this excessively repulsive and perverted phantasy of sucking at a penis has the most innocent origin" (p. 52). Similarly, in his great work of that period on sexuality (1905d), he spoke about the "horrifying result" of the mental work in certain of "the most repulsive perversions" (p. 161).

In a letter to Reik, Freud (1928b) remarked that he did not really like Dostoevsky as a person: "That is because my patience with pathological natures is exhausted in analysis. In art and in life I am intolerant of them" (p. 196).

He was quite capable of describing a patient being discussed by a fellow analyst as "an absolute swine, a case of infantile and homologously inflated sexuality; we have so many repressions within ourselves that, when faced with that, we feel aversion" (quoted in Nunberg & Federn, 1967, p. 379). Notice particularly the final, self-revealing comment. Thus at the least, the surprisingly moralistic tone with which he characterized "per-verse" material suggests that he found it personally repugnant.

Metapsychology, therefore, seems to have been one important way that Freud used to come to terms with this dangerous and potentially ruinous aspect of his work. Its very property of replacing the data-close terms of the clinical theory with the more abstract, impersonal, and austere language of natural science and mathematics is the intellectualizing form of isolation put to work in the service of "taming." It enabled him to live with a rather extraordinarily stressful kind of everyday work.

Just as a symptom expresses both a forbidden wish and a defense against it, a creative intellectual product may usefully be examined from the same dual standpoint. In addition to the infantile wishes and fears that seem to be connoted by the various points of view, the metapsychological enterprise as a whole seems to have been the partial gratification of Freud's wish for a godlike comprehensiveness of knowledge and for the power that such near-omniscience would entail. That recurrent Freudian phrase, "the omnipotence of thought," sums up the dream of possessing magic, the source of the witch's uncanny power. Perhaps Freud had to abjure philosophy so vigorously and repeatedly after his adolescent flirtation with it because it came too close to these forbidden infantile fantasies. He may have sensed that to enter seriously on an attempt to solve the great problems of existence—man's place in the cosmos, and the nature of good and evil (committing Adam's sin)—and to do so merely by the exercise of the intellect without the patient collection of data, would threaten to lift his repressive defenses against very early, overweening wishes. Those are transparently Promethean derivatives of the oedipal wishes to kill and replace the father, seizing not only his sexual prerogatives but his seemingly endless power. The figure of the Witch Metapsychology condenses, then, symbols both of forbidden wishes and of threatening controlling parental authority.

It may be reasonable to suppose that metapsychology serves some of the same wishful and defensive functions for many a Freudian psychoanalyst of today who loyally clings to it. Still hoping that it will unlock some great storehouse of knowledge, he or she may harbor unconscious wishes to become a potent magus or witch, and may refuse to give it up despite many demonstrations that Freud's metapsychology fails to serve effectively any specific scientific purpose—only the general one of being a technical language. Unlike the scientifically less pretentious terms of the clinical theory of the neuroses, it helps the psychoanalyst to keep his or her intellectual cool; it is a badge of loyalty to Freud and his movement, a shibboleth of the in-group member; and it implicitly confirms the analyst's self-image as a scientist. Unfortunately, it accomplishes this last objective at the cost of implying a scientific world view limited to that of 19th-century reductionism, mechanism, and physicalism, supplemented by equally anachronistic remnants of vitalistic, romantic humanism and evolutionary historicism. I shall briefly indicate some of the sources from which Freud imbibed those notions in the following section, [developing some of the ideas at greater length in subsequent chapters.]

SOME INTELLECTUAL ANTECEDENTS OF METAPSYCHOLOGY

In this review of Freud's usages, I hope to have made it clear that he always thought of metapsychology as something distinct from his clinical theorizing about psychopathology and its treatment: It was more general, more explanatory, and closer to an ideal of psychology as a natural science. At times he hoped to combine ideas from evolutionary biology with the mostly physicalistic conceptions, but he seems to have realized that it was difficult if not impossible to do so and left metapsychology as a predominantly mechanistic amalgam of concepts from physics, economics, and philosophy.

And where did he get the idea of building such a theory? One can approach that question by demonstrating in a more or less scholarly manner the similarity of each principal metapsychological concept to ideas of predecessors. Dorer (1932) led the way by showing the many striking parallels between Freud's concepts and those of J. F. Herbart, which we know he studied in a textbook by Lindner during his last Gymnasium year; and Ellenberger (1956) has shown the equally impressive antecedents of metapsychology in the works of G. H. Fechner, whose influence Freud explicitly acknowledged. I can add two names: (Büchner (1855) and Buckle (1871), whom he read before going to the university [see Holt, 1988].

But I think that it is much more important to point out the fact that similar ideas were all around, and that from the beginning of Freud's contact with scientific ideas, he learned one consistent mode of theorizing about psychological topics: Brücke, Meynert, Exner, Breuer, and Fliess were all influenced by Herbart and Fechner, and were all under the influence of the anti-vitalistic biophysics movement of 1847 (mislabeled "the school of Helmholtz"), with its avowed program of *reducing* physiology to physics and chemistry. That theoretical mode was physicalistic, borrowing specific concepts from physics as well as imitating its style of theoretical thinking; analytic and atomistic, looking for simple units to work with and seeking to understand a whole subject by dissecting it concretely or abstractively; reductionistic, assuming that the older, subbiological natural sciences were somehow closer to Truth and more explanatory; and mechanistic, using the analogy of the organism as a machine that functions automatically without the need to assume that it has any special constituents or aspects other than those of a very complicated clockwork mechanism (see also Yankelovich & Barrett, 1970).

The foregoing properties describe an ideal type of *nomological science*, which was generally dominant in the 19th century and had high prestige, especially in German-speaking countries. Freud was no stranger to it when he began work in the exciting atmosphere of the Physiological Institute, which was devoted to precisely this kind of science, and he gave up his dream of being a university scientist like his contemporary ideal, Ernst Brücke, only reluctantly. When he felt that he had a good enough grasp of the new field of neurotic psychopathology into which his practice led him so that he might begin to make contributions to scientific theory, it was natural for him to draw on *this* ideal type, as his guiding image for what his own new science was to be.

Metapsychology, therefore, allured him as a way of attaining his early ambition of becoming a great contributor to a rigorous natural science. At the same time, it frustrated him by leading him away from the firmer observational ground of clinical data into vague abstractions, and by its intrinsic difficulty: the difficulty of integrating into it the alien ideas of Lamarck and Haeckel, which—unknown to Freud—were regressive revivals of nature-philosophy masquerading as modern evolutionary biology.

CHAPTER 3

Freud's Cognitive Style

Freud had a number of idiosyncrasies as a writer and theory builder, with which we do well to familiarize ourselves before undertaking a detailed critique of metapsychology.

As I got seriously into the self-assigned task of understanding psychoanalytic theory, I began to collect notes on the topic of this chapter. In the atmosphere of the NYU Research Center for Mental Health, where I was working, the concept of cognitive style was everywhere—part of the air one breathed. It was natural for me, therefore, to apply it to Freud, and to try to figure out what kind of unique individual he was in this respect.

Since this essay was first published, there have been several books and papers on Freud's style, most notably that of Mahony (1982). No one I know of has tried an analysis of the type presented here, however, and after the lapse of over 20 years I have found relatively little to change about it.

For the modern reader, a major source of difficulty in understanding Freud is his cognitive style. Anyone who has read Freud at all may react to that proposition with astonishment, for Freud's literary style is much admired for its limpid elegance and clarity. Even in translation, Freud is vivid, personal, and charmingly direct in a way that makes him highly readable; he uses imaginative and original figures of speech, and often leads the reader along by a kind of stepwise development that enables him to penetrate into difficult or touchy areas with a minimum of effort. Anyone who has read much of his writing can easily understand why he received the Goethe Prize for literature.

Nevertheless, there are stylistic difficulties in understanding him; but these are matters of *cognitive*, not literary style. George Klein [1970] coined the term "cognitive style" to mean the patterning of a person's ways of taking in, processing, and communicating information about his world. Freud has an idiosyncratic way not just of writing but of thinking, which makes it surprisingly easy for the modern reader to misinterpret his meaning, to miss or distort many subtleties of his thought. To some degree, I may myself be subtly distorting Klein's concept, for he operationalized it in the laboratory, not the library, presenting subjects with hidden figures to be extracted from camouflage, series of squares to be judged for size, and other unusual tasks (some of his own, some of others' devising). By contrast, the methods I have used are more like those of the literary critic. I have collected notes on what struck me as characteristic ways in which Freud observed, processed data, obtained ideas by means other than direct observation, thought about them, argued their merits, and put his personal stamp on them. In doing so, however, I have been guided by my long association with Klein and his way of approaching cognitive processes and products; so I trust that I have been true to the spirit of this contribution of his, which is now so widely used as to be virtually a part of psychology's common property.

CHARACTER STYLE

Perhaps as good a place to start as any is with Ernest Jones's well-known biography. Much of the little that he has to say on this topic can be organized in the form of antitheses or paradoxes. First of all, there was a great deal about Freud that was compulsively orderly and hard-working. He led a stable, regular life, in which his work was a basic necessity. As he wrote to Pfister (Freud & Pfister, 1963, p. 35): "I cannot face with comfort the idea of life without work; work and the free play of the imagination are for me the same thing, I take no pleasure in anything else." Yet he went on, "That would be a recipe for happiness but for the appalling thought that productivity is entirely dependent on a sensitive disposition." As his biographers have attested, he did indeed work by fits and starts, not quite so steadily and regularly as, say, Virgil or the psychologist Wilhelm Wundt, but when the mood was on him.

Again, Jones remarks on "Freud's close attention to verbal detail, the striking patience with which he would unravel the meaning of phrases and utterances" (1955, p. 398). On the other hand,

> His translators will bear me out when I remark that minor obscurities and ambiguities, of a kind that more scrupulous circumspection could have readily avoided, are not the least of their trials. He was of course aware of this. I remember once asking him why he used a certain phrase, the meaning of which was not clear, and with a grimace he answered: *"Pure Schlamperei"* (sloppiness). (Jones, 1953, p. 33–34)

He was himself not a meticulous translator, though a highly gifted one.

> Instead of laboriously transcribing from the foreign language, idioms and all, he would read a passage, close the book, and consider how a German writer would have clothed the same thoughts . . . His translating work was both brilliant and rapid. (Jones, 1953, p. 55)

Similarly, Jones remarks on Freud's "quickness of thought and observation" generally, and the fact that "His type of mind was such as to penetrate through the material to something really essential beyond rather than to dally or play with it" (1955, p. 399). In short, he was intuitive rather than ploddingly systematic.

This particular paradox can be resolved, I believe, by the recognition that Freud was basically an obsessive–compulsive personality, in which this type of ambivalence is familiar. He had a good measure of certain traits of a kind he himself called "anal"—orderliness and compulsive attention to detail. Yet when it came to his mode of working with such details as the turn of a phrase in the telling of a dream (which only a compulsive would have noticed in the first place), an intuitive gift showed itself. For he was undoubtedly a genius, a man of extraordinary intelligence.

NATURE OF FREUD'S INTELLECT

What *kind* of intelligence was it, then? If we adopt the frame of reference of the Wechsler (1939) intelligence tests, it was first of all predominantly a verbal rather than a performance sort of ability. I have seen no evidence that Freud was specially gifted with his hands; he failed as a chemical experimenter (Jones, 1953, p. 54), and though he was a good microscopist and invented a new tissue stain during his years of scientific apprenticeship in Brücke's physiological laboratory, there is no evidence that he was skilled at the mechanical end of it. He was never what we call "an apparatus man," an ingenious tinkerer.[1] The only sports he engaged in—if they may be called such—were walking and gathering mushrooms.

Incidentally, the usual implication of a markedly higher verbal IQ than performance IQ would be borne out in Freud's case: He was surely never given to acting out, but was always an intellectualizer and internalizer. Moreover, "That there was a pronounced passive side to Freud's nature is a conclusion for which there is ample evidence," Jones (1953, p. 53) notes; "He once remarked that there were three things to which he felt unequal: governing, curing, and educating." He gave up hypnosis as "a coarsely interfering method" and soon abjured the laying on of hands, despite the fact that he treated several of the ladies in *Studies on Hysteria* by physical massage. Sitting quietly and listening to free associations, responding only verbally (largely by interpretations), is the method *par excellence* of a man with verbal gifts and a disinclination to manipulate.

Within the realm of verbal intelligence, we can make some more specific statements as well. "He had an enormously rich vocabulary," Jones (1955, p. 402) attests, "but he was the reverse of a pedant in words." He knew eight languages, having enough mastery of English and French to write scientific papers in those tongues. There is a fair amount of evidence between the lines of Freud's writings that the modality of his thought was largely verbal, as opposed to imageless, visual, auditory, or kinesthetic. His theory that thought becomes conscious by means of verbal residues (1915e, p. 210) implies a striking overvaluation of the prevalence and importance of thinking in terms of words, as does his statement that

> Thinking in pictures is, therefore, only a very incomplete form of becoming conscious. In some way, too, it stands nearer to unconscious processes than does thinking in words, and it is unquestionably older than the latter both ontogenetically and phylogenetically. (1923b, p. 21)

Freud did, in fact, place great value on words, especially as a means of treatment:

> Words were originally magic and to this day words have retained much of their ancient magical power. By words one person can make another blissfully happy or drive him to despair, by words the teacher conveys his knowledge to his pupils, by words the orator carries his audience with him and determines their judgements and decisions. Words provoke affects and are in general the means of mutual influence among men. Thus we shall not depreciate the use of words in psychotherapy and we shall be pleased if we can listen to the words that pass between the analyst and his patient. (1916–1917, p. 17)

He gives testimony that he had once had visual imagery of a vividness that sounds eidetic:

> . . . for a short period of my youth some unusual feats of memory were not beyond me. When I was a schoolboy I took it as a matter of course that I could repeat by heart the page I had been reading; and shortly before I entered the University I could write down almost verbatim popular lectures on scientific subjects directly after hearing them. (1901b, p. 135)

His auditory imagery could be extraordinarily vivid, too, at least up until a few years later, when he was studying with Charcot in Paris. During these days, he reports, "I quite often heard my name suddenly called by an unmistakable and beloved voice," which he goes on to refer to unblinkingly as a "hallucination" (1901b, p. 261).[2] Yet he writes about these experiences in such a way as to indicate that, like most other eidetic imagers, he gradually lost the ability as he grew older. True, his dreams remained vividly visual, his writing is full of visual imagery (in the rhetorical sense of that last term), and he occasionally was able to get a sharp visual image in waking life, but he emphasized that such occasions were exceptional:

> For example, in the *Signorelli* case, so long as the painter's name remained inaccessible, the visual memory that I had of the series of frescoes and of the self-portrait which is introduced into the corner of one of the pictures was *ultra-*

clear—at any rate much more intense than visual memory-traces normally appear to me. In another case, also described in my 1898 paper, which concerned a visit which I was very reluctant to pay to an address in a strange town, I had forgotten the name of the street beyond all hope of recovery, but my memory of the house number, as if in derision, was ultra-clear, whereas normally I have the greatest difficulty in remembering numbers. (1901b, p. 13 n.)

By contrast, I have never found any indication that Freud was even aware that such a phenomenon as imageless thought exists, though investigators from Galton to Anne Roe have found that it characterizes many leading figures in such disciplines as mathematics and theoretical physics—disciplines that Jones specifically says (1953, p. 33) Freud could never have excelled in.

Perhaps there is a hint here that Freud's mind was not at the very forefront as far as highly abstract thinking is concerned. Surely he was not much of a mathematician; he once characterized himself as following:

I have very restricted capacities or talents. None at all for the natural sciences; nothing for mathematics; nothing for anything quantitative. But what I have, of a very restricted nature, was probably very intensive. (Letter to Marie Bonaparte, 1926; quoted in Jones, 1955, p. 397)

As we shall see a little later, this relative weakness in quantitative ability had a number of noticeable effects on Freud's manner of thinking.

To shift for a moment to the frame of reference of Guilford (1967) and his structure-of-intellect model, Freud's strength lay in *semantic* (verbal) and *behavioral* (psychological, interpersonal) abilities, not *figural* (spatial) or *symbolic* (mathematical) ones. In terms of operations, he was most outstanding in *divergent production* (creative activity), and least so in *convergent production* (conventional problem solving) and *evaluation* (judgment), in that he can occasionally be faulted on matters that involve those mental processes even though his overall level might well have been highly superior. Jones (1955) and Roazen (1975) have pointed to a number of motivated lapses in his memory, also. Finally, in terms of the third dimension of Guilford's model, products, Freud clearly excelled in some aspects of *transformations* and *implications* of semantic or verbal data, while his relative weakness of synthetic ability might have shown up in relation to *systems*.

To summarize so far, in terms of abilities: Freud had a predominantly verbal intelligence and mode of thinking. He was extraordinarily gifted at memory; concentration; passive (or as he put it, "evenly-suspended") attention; creative concept formation; and deciphering the transformed implications of words, gestures, and expressions. His gift was more analytic than synthetic, just as his preference was for the former over the latter aspect of thinking. He had no notable gifts along sensorimotor, manipulative, or quantitative lines, nor in the most abstract types of thought. Above all, he was divergently productive and original.

STYLE OF THINKING AND WRITING

Self-Critical Doubts versus Self-Confident Determination

In moving on to some more stylistic aspects of his thought, I shall continue to pursue antitheses. One such is the cognitive side of a prominent theme in Freud's personality: a self-critical, even retiring and self-doubting modesty versus a largely covert and negated thirst for fame coupled with great self-confidence. A number of the quotations both from Freud and from Jones have touched on his self-critical side, and the evidence for his deep-seated longing to see his name carved on a rock for the ages is omnipresent in Jones's three volumes, though the disciple outdid the master in protesting that it wasn't so. Both of these facets of Freud's mind come out in relation to the ideas he set forth in *Beyond the Pleasure Principle*. There he wrote:

> It may be asked whether and how far I am myself convinced of the truth of the hypotheses that have been set out in these pages. My answer would be that I am not convinced myself and that I do not seek to persuade other people to believe in them. Or, more precisely, that I do not know how far I believe in them. . . . Since we have such good grounds for being distrustful, our attitude towards the results of our own deliberations cannot well be other than one of cool benevolence. (1920g, p. 59)

He was speaking, of course, about his most controversial speculations, concerning the death instinct. Yet only a few years later, he wrote:

> To begin with it was only tentatively that I put forward the views I have developed here, but in the course of time they have gained such a hold upon me that I can no longer think in any other way. To my mind, they are far more serviceable from a theoretical standpoint than any other possible ones; they provide that simplification, without either ignoring or doing violence to the facts, for which we strive in scientific work. (1930a, p. 119)

In short, he had a tendency to become so accustomed to his own ideas as to consider them indispensable and finally as established, even though they were originally presented with great modesty. Indeed, he looked back on the shaky speculations of *Beyond the Pleasure Principle* as a basis for supporting his fundamental assumption that there had to be two classes of instinctual drives:

> Over and over again we find, when we are able to trace instinctual impulses back, that they reveal themselves as derivatives of Eros. If it were not for the

considerations put forward in *Beyond the Pleasure Principle*, and ultimately for the sadistic constituents which have attached themselves to Eros, we should have difficulty in holding to our fundamental dualistic point of view [in instinct theory]. (1923b, p. 46)

Here we have the first hint of one of the basic problems with which Freud struggled, and which helped shape the nature of his thought: Working as he did in a new field, with no conventional criteria for establishing valid knowledge, he had to be sustained against the inevitable self-doubts— even the despair that what he was doing could lead anywhere—by an irrational confidence in himself, a faith that his intuitions and hypotheses would be vindicated, and even a certain degree of self-deception that he had established points more firmly than he in fact had been able to do.

His determination to persist in the face of his recognition that progress was difficult is well expressed in the following quotation:

It is almost humiliating that, after working so long, we should still be having difficulty in understanding the most fundamental facts. But we have made up our minds to simplify nothing and to hide nothing. If we cannot see things clearly we will at least see clearly what the obscurities are. (1926d, p. 124)

One of the positive aspects of Freud's ability to be self-critical was his willingness to change his ideas: "We must be patient and await fresh methods and occasions of research. We must be ready, too, to abandon a path that we have followed for a time, if it seems to be leading to no good end." (1920g, p. 64).

If he was not always able to live up to this brave program, if he failed to recognize that many of his unquestioned assumptions were not as axiomatically true as he thought, these are the necessary consequences of being human. Freud was surely sustained in his long quest by a passionate interest in penetrating the mysteries of nature and a capacity to care deeply about his ideas; all the more natural, therefore, that he should have tended at times to lose scientific detachment and confuse his concepts with realities. Thus, he would refer to "the 'super-ego,' one of the later *findings* of psychoanalysis" (1900a, p. 558, n. 1), or to "the *discovery* that the ego itself is cathected with libido" (1930a, p. 118; emphasis added in both quotations).

When I spoke above about his unquestioned assumptions, I had principally in mind the passive reflex model of the organism, which is today demonstrably false [see Chapter 5, this volume]. Yet to Freud—along with most of his contemporaries—it seemed so self-evidently true that he referred to it as a fact on which he could found one of his most questionable constructs:

The dominating tendency of mental life, and perhaps of nervous life in general, is the effort to reduce, to keep constant or to remove internal tension due to stimuli . . .—a tendency which finds expression in the pleasure principle; and our recognition of that *fact* is one of our strongest reasons for believing in the existence of death instincts. (1920g, pp. 55–56; emphasis added)

Another aspect of this same antithesis was Freud's conviction that the essence of what he was setting forth was *truth*, which would be fully appreciated only by future generations, versus his expectation that much of what he taught would be quickly overthrown, as in the following 1909 letter to Jung in response to the latter's expressed fear that Freud's writings would be treated as gospel: "Your notion that after my retirement from the ranks my errors may come to be worshiped as relics amused me a good deal, but I don't believe it. I believe on the contrary that the younger men will demolish everything in my heritage that is not absolutely solid as fast as they can" (Freud & Jung, 1974, p. 277). Freud shows here the strength of his faith that there would be kernels of eternal truth as well as chaff in the harvest of his labors. And, so far as we can see today, his faith was justified.

Analysis versus Synthesis

Another familiar antithesis in the realm of thinking is analysis versus synthesis. In this realm, the preference of the inventor and namer of psychoanalysis was clear and marked. In 1915 he wrote to Lou Andreas-Salomé:

> I so rarely feel the need for synthesis. The unity of this world seems to me something self-understood, something unworthy of emphasis. What interests me is the separation and breaking up into its component parts what would otherwise flow together into a primeval pulp. . . . In short, I am evidently an analyst and believe that synthesis offers no obstacles once analysis has been achieved. (Freud, 1960, p. 310)

Yet in spite of the fact that the concept of the synthetic function of the ego is associated less with Freud than with Nunberg, the latter's paper by this name (Nunberg, 1931) is in large part simply a drawing together of points Freud made in passing in many contexts. Freud could perform remarkable feats of synthesizing many disconnected facts—see, for example, his masterly review of the scientific literature on dreams (1900a, Chapter I) —and he taught us a great deal about synthetic functioning; nevertheless, his ability and his predilection ran predominantly along the lines of analysis.

In this respect [as I shall show in Chapter 5], Freud thought in a manner typical of 19th-century scientists. He is not greatly different from the vast majority of his contemporaries in having an analytic orientation and in particular the kind I shall describe as "dissectional"—a preference to analyze into constituent parts instead of into abstract properties. I chose this term partly because of Freud's fondness for this surgical metaphor; for example:

Analogies of this kind are only intended to assist us in our attempt to make the complications of mental functioning intelligible by dissecting the function and assigning its different constituents to different component parts of the apparatus. So far as I know, the experiment has not hitherto been made of using this method of dissection in order to investigate the way in which the mental instrument is put together, and I can see no harm in it. (1900a, p. 536)[3]

Dialectic Dualism

One reason I have adopted the antithetical method in this exposition is that a preference for opposed binary concepts was itself highly characteristic of Freud's thinking.[4] In his theories, it is surely an impressive and well-known fact that his major concepts come in matched opposing pairs. Perhaps the most striking is his motivational theory in its various guises. Fairly early, he pitted unconscious wish against preconscious cathexis, then the libidinal versus the ego instincts, going on to narcissistic versus object libido, to Eros versus the death instincts (or love against hate); in any case, it was always a dual-drive theory. Or recall *"the three great polarities that dominate mental life"*: activity–passivity, ego–external world, and pleasure–unpleasure (1915c, p. 140). Many other such oppositions come to mind: masculine versus feminine, quantity versus quality, autoplastic versus alloplastic, ego-syntonic versus ego-alien, pleasure principle versus reality principle, free versus bound cathexis, and the primary process versus the secondary process. Even when he proposed triads of concepts (*Cs.*, *Pcs.*, and *Ucs.*; ego, superego, and id), Freud had a strong tendency to reduce them to binary form—for example, usually speaking of *Cs.-Pcs.* or *Pcs.(Cs.)* as against *Ucs.* The 1923 work is, after all, entitled merely *The Ego and the Id*; and the distinction between conscious and unconscious always impressed Freud as "our one beacon-light in the darkness of depth-psychology" (1923b, p. 18). Terms like "ambivalence" and "conflict" conceptualize this dualism as fundamental facts of psychology. Indeed, one might argue that many of the antithetical dynamic concepts are a direct consequence of Freud's recognizing how important conflict was in both normal and pathological development.

Freud's thinking was saved from the crudity usually entailed by such reliance on dichotomous concepts by the aid of what he knew as the "complemental series." That is, a contrasting pair (e.g., primary and secondary process) were treated as the defining endpoints of a continuum, along which all manner of intermediate forms could be ranged.

As regards their causation, instances of neurotic illness fall into a series within which the two factors—sexual constitution and experience . . .—are represented in such a manner that if there is more of the one there is less of the other.

At one end of the series are the extreme cases of which you could say with conviction: these people, in consequence of the singular development of their libido, would have fallen ill in any case, whatever they had experienced and however carefully their lives had been sheltered. At the other end there are the cases, as to which, on the contrary, you would have had to judge that they would certainly have escaped falling ill if their lives had not brought them into this or that situation. In the cases lying within the series a greater or lesser amount of predisposition in the sexual constitution is combined with a lesser or greater amount of detrimental experience in their lives. . . .

I propose, Gentlemen, that we should name a series of this kind a "complemental series." (1916–1917, p. 347)

This conception gave him an intellectual tool which he applied with cogency to several issues—for example, heredity–environment (1895f, pp. 135–138), normal–abnormal (1905d, p. 171)—and even to the distinction between such antithetical concepts as the ego and the id: "The ego is not sharply separated from the id; its lower portion merges into it" (1923b, p. 24). It is not easy to specify just where this way of softening the starkness of dichotomies is useful and where it creates fresh problems.

For the moment, let us simply note it as a stylistic peculiarity that Freud did have a marked preference for opposed pairs of sharply contrasted concepts, but was able to handle the failure of the resulting map to fit reality by invoking the complemental series. Thereby, he was able to summon the whole range of grays to supplement the dramatic blacks and whites with which he liked to paint.

Reason versus Intuition; Realism versus Occultism

Another striking antithesis in Freud's makeup has been noted by many observers (but particularly well summarized by Roazen, 1975, pp. 232–241): his alternation between a rigorously rational and realistic, antimystical orientation, and an attraction to parapsychological phenomena and the occult. Much could be said about Freud's ambivalent relationship to philosophy in general and *Naturphilosophie* in particular [see Chapter 6, this volume]. Here I want to emphasize a few stylistic aspects of the present antithesis. Freud was for the most part an heir of the Enlightenment—a devotee of reason, clear thinking, precise speech, and a no-nonsense pragmatism and practicality. He was always put off by mystics and obscurantists; he warned against "an exaggerated respect for the 'mysterious unconscious.' It is only too easy to forget that a dream is as a rule merely a thought like any other" (1923b, p. 112). When in this vein, he could downgrade intuition:

. . . there are no sources of knowledge of the universe other than the intellectual working-over of carefully scrutinized observations—in other words, what we call research—and alongside of it no knowledge derived from revelation, intuition or divination. . . . Intuition and divination would be . . . [methods of research] if they existed; but they may safely be reckoned as illusions, the fulfillments of wishful impulses. (1933a, p. 159)

Speaking about constructing theories, he remarked: "I do not think a large part is played by what is called 'intuition' in work of this kind" (1920g, p. 59). And near the end of his life, in opposing the kind of direct mystical communion with extrascientific sources of truth that Jung had advocated, he stated:

The riddles of the universe reveal themselves only slowly to our investigation; there are many questions to which science today can give no answer. But scientific work is the only road which can lead us to a knowledge of reality outside ourselves. It is . . . an illusion to expect anything from intuition and introspection; they can give us nothing but particulars about our own mental life, which are hard to interpret, never any information about the questions which religious doctrine finds it so easy to answer. (1927c, pp. 31–32)

This last passage helps resolve some of the paradox, for here Freud clearly did not reject intuition and introspection in their proper role, as sources of self-knowledge. It remains ambiguous how he felt about intuitive understanding of others; he was at times envious of Stekel's "good flair for the meaning of the hidden and unconscious" (Jones, 1955, p. 62) while downgrading his theoretical thinking and charging him with relying "exclusively on his inspirations, instead of submitting them to the control of conscious thinking" (Nunberg & Federn, 1967, p. 10). As Strachey notes [in a footnote to *Introductory Lectures on Psycho-Analysis*,] "it was relatively late before . . . he realized the full importance of dream symbolism, largely under the influence of Wilhelm Stekel. It was not until the fourth (1914) edition of *The Interpretation of Dreams* that a special section was devoted to the subject" (1916–1917, p. 149 n.), by which time the break with Stekel was complete.

It would be a mistake, however, to view Freud as a purely rational thinker who was closed off from intuitive or empathic kinds of nonverbal, direct knowledge of others. His gift for making deep interpretive constructions of episodes in the early childhood of patients, which were later independently confirmed, was frequently demonstrated and documented (though of course we have no record of his misses and no way to compute a hit–miss ratio). The romantic movement of the 19th century had left an unmistakable mark on him. He was undeniably possessed of a natural psychological insightfulness which was greatly sharpened by long and intense practice. And much as he might cultivate a self-image as a cool, impartial scientist, he was a man of intense passions, attracted to the demonic aspect of human nature.

In speaking of Freud's similar attraction for paranormal or occult ("psychical") phenomena, Jones groups it together with some other evidences of credulousness as a gullibility that was a necessary consequence of Freud's being open-minded enough to make his epochal discoveries. Be that as it may, in several papers on telepathy written in the last 20 years of his life, Freud (1941d [1921], 1922a, 1925i) at last revealed his ambivalent belief in "thought-transference" (as he liked to call it), especially in dreams. Speaking about such things in 1933 (1933a, p. 54), he said that "they first came into my range of vision more than ten years ago"; 32 years earlier, in 1901, he had told an anecdote from his stay in Paris during 1885–1886:

> During the days when I was living alone in a foreign city . . . I quite often heard my name suddenly called by an unmistakable and beloved voice; I then noted down the exact moment of the hallucination and made anxious enquiries of those at home about what had happened at that time. Nothing had happened. (1901b, p. 261)

The "anxious enquiries" are a testament to his having shared the common belief that such hallucinatory experiences were not wish-fulfillments but what were then called "phantasms of the living," extranormal communications from loved persons (here, his fiancée) at a time of crisis.

Jones has documented Freud's superstitious fears of his own impending death, which lasted at least throughout his adult life. Despite his opposition to superstition and his derogation of it on many occasions, he confessed that in "unconscious thought-operations with numbers I find I have a tendency to superstition. . . . I generally come upon speculations about the duration of my own life and the lives of those dear to me" (1901b, p. 250, n. 2). This tendency must have made him as uncritically accepting as he was for years to Fliess's numerological system. After the final rupture of their friendship, Freud turned sharply against speculation, superstition, the occult, and similar matters for about two decades, during which time anything he said in public was negative. Looking back on this time later, he wrote: "I too felt a dread of threat against our scientific *Weltanschauung*, which, I feared, was bound to give place to spiritualism or mysticism if portions of occultism were proved true. Today I think otherwise" (1933a, p. 54).

To a degree, then, Freud managed to prevent a collision between his Apollonian devotion to reason and the more Dionysian pull of his will to believe in the occult, by suppressing the latter for a good part of his life. By and large, however, he did so in just the way he described as characteristic of obsessive–compulsives: by keeping the ideas segregated in logic-tight compartments, a form of the defense of isolation.

Tolerated Contradiction
(Synthesis Deferred)

In general, Freud's thinking is characterized by an unusual *tolerance for inconsistency*. If you went through the works of any author as prolific as he was, you would doubtless find many mutually contradictory statements, and many propositions that are actually incompatible with his basic assumptions. But it is not difficult to find other reasons for the presence of inconsistencies in Freud's work besides its sheer size, which is enormous.

A first such reason was Freud's orientation toward the accumulating bulk of his own writings, with the accompanying changes in his views. He preferred to think of it, I believe, as a steadily growing corpus of findings, rather than as in part a set of reformulations of essentially similar observations. If his implicit model was the work of a scientific institute like Brücke's, such an output might be somewhat disorderly, but it did not demand to be synthesized in order to be valuable. One worker's findings might seem unrelated or even contradictory to the results obtained by another pursuing a different problem by different techniques, but one could be confident that eventually the pieces would fall into place within a larger scheme. Freud was of course aware that he had changed his mind on many issues, and justifiably defended his right to do so: "only believers, who demand that science shall be a substitute for the catechism they have given up, will blame an investigator for developing or even transforming his views" (1920g, p. 64). But scrutiny of his way of working and writing indicates that he did not conceive of himself as making anything like "paradigm shifts" (Kuhn, 1970) or fundamental changes of a kind that would require reconsideration and reworking of what he had said up to such a point of change. He seems instead to have viewed most of what he wrote as the setting forth of *data*, factual findings of permanent value.

One way in which this outlook shows itself is in his way of writing and revising.

> He wrote easily, fluently, and spontaneously, and would have found much rewriting irksome. . . . one of his main characteristics [was] his dislike of being hampered or fettered. He loved to give himself up to his thoughts freely, to see where they would take him, leaving aside for the moment any question of precise delineation; that could be left for further consideration. (Jones, 1953, pp. 33–34)

True, he did rewrite and revise several of his books many times. Fortunately, the *Standard Edition* provides a variorum text and scrupulously informs us of every change, edition by edition. It is not difficult, therefore, to characterize Freud's style of revision by studying *The Interpretation of*

Dreams, The Psychopathology of Everyday Life, and *Three Essays on the Theory of Sexuality.* These books, first published from 1900 to 1905, went through eight, ten, and six editions, respectively, all of them containing additions from at least as late as 1925. Thus, each spans two or more major periods in the development of Freud's thought, including a far-reaching change in his metapsychology. Yet one statement covers the vast majority of the revisions: He added things. There was never any fundamental reconsideration of these works, precious little synthesis of earlier and later theories.

Hanns Sachs, who had had many years of opportunity to observe his "master and friend," described him as disinclined to make minor revisions in rewriting: "In his writing Freud never blotted out a [i.e., only one] line . . . he cancelled the whole thing and started to re-write it. . . . He always hated to patch up things, whether in the intellectual or emotional sphere" (Sachs, 1945, pp. 95–96).

Perhaps if Freud had not had such a superb command of written communication, so that he rarely had even to polish his first drafts, he would have reworked his books more thoroughly as they went through new editions. At most, he added an occasional footnote pointing out the incompatibility of a statement with later doctrines. Even Chapter VII of *The Interpretation of Dreams,* Freud's most ambitious and important work, was left virtually untouched except for interpolations—after the innovations of 1915 and 1917 that undid the possibility of topographical regression, and even after the jettisoning of the whole topographic theory in 1923 and its replacement by the structural theory, which makes no provision for the conceptualization of *any* complete cognitive process. Indeed, to the end, Chapter VII contained anachronistic carryovers from the neurological scheme of the unpublished "Project," which had preceded it by four years; throughout all the revisions, Freud never eliminated the lapses into reference to "neurones," "pathways," and "quantity."

A second source of cumulative inconsistency was Freud's attitude of modesty, as a hard-working plodder who humbly contented himself with the dogged pursuit of one thing at a time, in a kind of *piecemeal empiricism.* For example: "You are aware of my preference for the fragmentary treatment of a subject, with emphasis on the points which seem to me best established" (1912f, p. 246). A dozen years later, he wrote: ". . . it is plain that a science based upon observation has no alternative but to work out its findings piecemeal and to solve its problems step by step" (1925d, p. 58). Or witness his self-characterization in the following letter to Andreas-Salomé in 1917; he had been contrasting himself with "the system-builders" Jung and Adler: ". . . you have observed how I work, step by step, without the inner need for completion, continually under the pressure of the problems immediately on hand and taking infinite pains not to be diverted from the path" (1960, p. 319). Seven years earlier, he had written to Jung:

I see that you go about working in the same way as I do; rather than take the obvious path that leads straight ahead, you keep your eye peeled for one that strikes your fancy. This is the best way, I think; afterwards one is amazed at the logical sequence in all these digressions. (Freud & Jung, 1974, p. 358)

To follow one's nose empirically, adding to the theory whatever bits and pieces might accrue along the way—this was the procedure with which Freud felt at home, with his faith that ultimately the truth would prevail.

CONCEPTION OF SCIENTIFIC METHOD AND CONCEPTS

This attitude was of a piece with Freud's basic conception of scientific work. Science was first and foremost a matter of empirical observation, which he usually contrasted with speculation to the latter's discredit.[5] As Freud conceived it, a speculative, or philosophical, system started with "clear and sharply defined basic concepts" (1915c, p. 117), and built on this "smooth, logically unassailable foundation" (1914c, p. 77) a "complete and ready-made theoretical structure" (1923b, p. 36) which could "easily spring into existence complete, and thereafter remain unchangeable" (1906a, p. 271). But "no science, not even the most exact," operates this way:

> The true beginning of scientific activity consists rather in describing phenomena and then in proceeding to group, classify and correlate them. Even at the stage of description it is not possible to avoid applying certain abstract ideas to the material in hand, ideas derived from somewhere or other but certainly not from the new observations alone. . . . They must at first necessarily possess some degree of indefiniteness; . . . we come to an understanding about their meaning by making repeated references to the material of observation from which they appear to have been derived, but upon which, in fact, they have been imposed. . . . It is only after more thorough investigation of the field of observation that we are able to formulate its basic scientific concepts with increased precision, and progressively so to modify them that they become serviceable and consistent over a wide area. Then, indeed, the time may have come to confine them in definitions. The advance of knowledge, however, does not tolerate any rigidity even in definitions. (1915c, p. 117)

When tackling a new topic, therefore,

> Instead of starting from a definition, it seems more useful to begin with some indication of the range of the phenomena under review, and to select from among them a few specially striking and characteristic facts to which our enquiry can be attached. (1921c, p. 72)

Thereafter, any psychoanalytic inquiry must "find its way step by step along the path towards understanding the intricacies of the mind by making an analytic dissection of both normal and abnormal phenomena." (1923b, p. 36). But because of the complexity of its subject matter, psychoanalysis cannot hope for quick successes:

> The extraordinary intricacy of all the factors to be taken into consideration leaves only one way of presenting them open to us. We must select first one and then another point of view, and follow it up through the material as long as the application of it seems to yield results. Each separate treatment of the subject will be incomplete in itself, and there cannot fail to be obscurities where it touches upon material that has not yet been treated; but we may hope that a final synthesis will lead to a proper understanding. (1915d, pp. 157–158)

The truth, when attained, will be simple:

> . . . we have no other aim but that of translating into theory the results of observation, and we deny that there is any obligation on us to achieve at our first attempt a well-rounded theory which will commend itself by its simplicity. We shall defend the complications of our theory so long as we find that they meet the results of observation, and we shall not abandon our expectations of being led in the end by those very complications to the discovery of a state of affairs which, while simple in itself, can account for all the complications of reality. (1915e, p. 190)

Freud thus demonstrated a capacity to tolerate, in addition to inconsistency and delay, considerable conceptual indefiniteness or, in the terminology of today, ambiguity. "It is true," he was ready to admit, "that notions such as that of an ego-libido, an energy of the ego-instincts, and so on, are neither particularly easy to grasp, nor sufficiently rich in content." Nevertheless, psychoanalysis would "gladly content itself with nebulous, scarcely imaginable basic concepts, which it hopes to apprehend more clearly in the course of its development, or which it is even prepared to replace by others" (1914c, p. 77).

Note the obligation stated here, which follows clearly enough from his position regarding definition, for a periodic conceptual stocktaking; if consistent and useful definitions never precipitate out, the concept should be abandoned. As we have seen, however, such a process of regular review was quite incompatible with Freud's style of working and thinking, and he rarely discarded concepts when he added new ones. It is a little sad, but not surprising, to find that instinct, which in 1915 (1915c, pp. 117–118) were "at the moment . . . still somewhat obscure," were characterized 18 years later as "mythical entities, magnificent in their indefiniteness" (1933a, p. 95). Yet there was also something heroic in such tenacity despite the refusal of simple solutions to emerge [see quotation from 1926d, p. 40 above].

Some years ago, I decided to try my hand at this winnowing process, taking one of Freud's central but tantalizing ill-defined concepts (the binding of cathexis; see Chapter 4) and following it through his writings to see what kind of definition emerged. The labor of finding and collating the contexts in which it occurred, and educing the 14 different meanings that I was able to discern, was great enough to make me realize that if Freud had undertaken to work his own theories over continuously in this way, after a few years he would not have had time to analyze any more patients, much less write anything new! For psychoanalysis, however, the long-run consequence has been unfortunate. As Hartmann, Kris, and Loewenstein (1946) put it, the fact that a

> concern with clarification of terms is unpopular among psychoanalysts and rare in psychoanalytic writing is partly due to Freud's example. Semantics could hardly be the concern of the great explorer, and some inconsistency in the usage of words may well be considered the prerogative of genius. [Serious difficulties arise, however] . . . when a generation or two of scientists assume a similar prerogative. (p. 11)

So far, I have emphasized the knowingly provisional, tentative nature of Freud's theorizing—his deliberate abjuring of any attempt to build a complete and internally coherent system, in favor of piecemeal empiricism instead. Quite some contrast to the view of Freud as the dogmatic systematist who would brook no deviation from a rigid "party line" of theory! Yet this popular conception has its roots in fact also. For one thing, Freud seems to have had a fluctuating, never-explicit set of standards about what parts of psychoanalysis had been proved, which only he might change with impunity, and what parts were modifiable by others. True to his agglutinative principle of revision, he welcomed additions so long as they did not explicitly call for reconsideration of concepts and propositions that had come to seem basic and necessary. Thus, Adler's ideas about organ inferiority and the will to power were acceptable until the disciple started insisting that they clashed with the libido theory and demanded the latter's drastic revision.

STYLE OF THEORIZING

Quite aside from Freud's relation to the contributions of others (a matter that is obviously a great deal more complicated than the brief discussion above might seem to imply), there are bases for the conception of Freud as a doctrinaire dogmatist in certain stylistic peculiarities of his own theorizing. Let me summarize first and then expand, with examples. Freud was fond of stating things "as it were, dogmatically—in the most concise form and in the most unequivocal terms" (1940a, p. 144); indeed, hyperbole was one of his favorite rhetorical devices. As his early colleague Breuer put it, in a letter of 1907, "Freud is a man given to absolute and exclusive formulations: this is a psychical need which, in my opinion, leads to excessive generalization" (quoted in Cranefield, 1958, p. 320). When he thought that he glimpsed a law of nature, he stated it with sweeping universalism and generality. He was likewise fond of extending concepts to the limit of their possible applicability, as if stretching the realm of phenomena spanned by a concept was a way to make it more abstract and useful. His device for escaping the dangers of oversimplification to which this pattern exposed him was to follow one flat statement with another that qualified it by partial contradiction. Therefore, the inconsistency in many of Freud's propositions is only apparent: He was perfectly well aware that one statement undid another, and used such sequences as a way of letting a richly complicated conception grow in the reader's mind as considerations were introduced one at a time.

Here, then, is one reason why Freud is at once so delightfully easy to read and so easy to misunderstand, particularly when statements are taken out of context. His view of human behavior was unusually subtle, complex, and many-layered; if he had tried to set it forth in sentences of parallel complexity and hierarchical structure, he would have made Dr. Johnson look like Hemingway. Instead, he writes simply, directly, forcefully; he dramatizes by grand overstatement, setting out in hard black outlines what he considers the basic truth about a matter as the reader's initial orientation. Then he fills in shadows; or, by another boldly simple stroke, suddenly shows that forms are disposed on different planes. Gradually, a three-dimensional reality takes shape before the eyes of the one who knows how to read Freud.

Here is an example of an initial flat statement, followed by qualifications:

> The way in which dreams treat the category of contraries and contradictories is highly remarkable. It is simply disregarded. 'No' seems not to exist so far as dreams are concerned. (1900a, p. 318)

> I have asserted above that dreams have no means of expressing the relation of a contradiction, a contrary or a 'no.' I shall now proceed to give a first denial of this assertion. [The idea of "just the reverse" is plastically represented as something turned around from its usual orientation.] (p. 326)

> . . . the 'not being able to do something' in this dream was a way of expressing a contradiction—a 'no'—; so that my earlier statement that dreams cannot express a 'no' requires correction. (p. 337)

(A third "denial" appears on p. 434.)

Perhaps an even more familiar sweeping generalization is the following: "Psycho-analysis is justly suspicious. One of its rules is that *whatever interrupts the progress of analytic work is a resistance*" (1900a, p. 517). Less often quoted is Freud's footnote, in which he makes that statement—so infuriating to many an analysand!—more palatable:

The proposition . . . is easily open to misunderstanding. It is of course only to be taken as a technical rule, as a warning to analysts. It cannot be disputed that in the course of an analysis various events may occur the responsibility for which cannot be laid upon the patient's intentions. His father may die without his having murdered him; or a war may break out which brings the analysis to an end. But behind *its obvious exaggeration* the proposition is asserting something both true and new. Even if the interrupting event is a real one and independent of the patient, it often depends on him how great an interruption it causes; and resistance shows itself unmistakably in the readiness with which he accepts an occurrence of this kind or the exaggerated use which he makes of it. (1900a, p. 517 n.; emphasis added)

All too often (and unfortunately difficult to illustrate by quotation), the softening statement following the initial overgeneralization is not explicitly[6] pointed out, may not follow very soon, or is not obviously related. For Freud, this was a conscious strategy of scientific advance, however:

The transformations of scientific opinion are developments, advances, not revolutions. A law which was held at first to be universally valid proves to be a special case of a more comprehensive uniformity, or is limited by another law, not discovered till later; a rough approximation to the truth is replaced by a more carefully adapted one, which in turn awaits further perfectioning. (1927c, p. 55)

Many examples of statements formulated with arresting exaggeration can easily be cited.

The analysis of cases of neurotic abasia and agoraphobia removes all doubt as to the sexual nature of pleasure in movement. (1905d, p. 203 n.)

The doctrine of reward in the afterlife . . . is nothing other than a mythical projection of this revolution in the mind. (1911b, p. 223)

. . . hysteria . . . is concerned only with the patient's repressed sexuality. (1906a, p. 278)

. . . no one can doubt that the hypnotist has stepped into the place of the ego ideal. (1921c, p. 114)

It is certain that much of the ego is itself unconscious, and notably what we may describe as its nucleus; only a small part of it is covered by the term 'preconscious'. (1920g, p. 19)

Strachey appends the following rather amusing footnote to the last passage quoted above:

In its present form this sentence dates from 1921. In the first edition (1920) it ran: 'It may be that much of the ego is itself unconscious; only a part of it, probably, is covered by the term "preconscious".' (1920g, p. 19 n.)

In this case, it took only a year for a cautious probability to become a certainty.

In other instances, hyperbole takes the form of the assertion of an underlying unity where only a correlation is observed:

> All these three kinds of regression [topographical, temporal, and formal] are, however, one at bottom and occur together as a rule; for what is older in time is more primitive in form and in psychical topography lies nearer to the perceptual end. (1900a, p. 548)

All too often, the sweeping formulation takes the form of a declaration that something like the Oedipus complex is *universal*. I believe that Freud was less interested in making an empirical generalization from his limited data than in groping in this way for a basic law of nature. He put it thus in a letter to Fliess of October 15, 1897:

> A single idea of general value dawned on me. I have found, in my own case too, [the phenomenon of] being in love with my mother and jealous of my father, and I now consider it a universal event in early childhood. . . . If this is so, we can understand the gripping power of *Oedipus Rex*. (Freud, 1985 [1887–1904], p. 272)

Again, four years later, he generalized universally from his own case:

> There thus runs through my thoughts a continuous current of 'personal reference' of which I generally have no inkling, but which betrays itself by such instances of my forgetting names. It is as if I were obliged to compare everything I hear about other people with myself; as if my personal complexes were put on the alert whenever another person is brought to my notice. This cannot possibly be an individual peculiarity of my own: it must rather contain an indication of the way in which we understand 'something other than ourself' in general. I have reasons for supposing that other people are in this respect very similar to me. (1901b, pp. 24–25)

To the contemporary psychologist, trained to be cautious in generalizing from small samples, it seems audacious to the point of foolhardiness to jump from self-observation to a general law. But Freud was emboldened by the very fact that he was dealing with vital issues:

> I thoroughly dislike the notion that my opinions are correct, but only in regard to a part of the cases. . . . That is not possible. It must be one thing or the other. These characteristics are fundamental, they can't vary from one set of cases to another. . . . Either a case is our kind or nothing is known about it. I am sure that basically you agree with me. There. Now I have avowed the full extent of my fanaticism. (Letter to Jung, April 19, 1908; Freud & Jung, 1974, p. 141)

Remember, also, the fact that Freud's initial scientific efforts considerably antedated the invention of statistics, sampling theory, or experimental design. In his early days, when he was most secure in his role as scientist, Freud was studying neuroanatomy at the microscope, and like his respected teachers and colleagues, generalizing freely and automatically from samples of one![7]

Then, too, recall Freud's principle of exceptionless determinism in psychology: All aspects of behavior are lawful, he believed, which made it easy for him to confuse (1) the universal applicability of abstract laws and concepts with (2) the universal occurrence of empirically observable behavioral sequences. Thus, the concept of sex-role differentiation is general enough to be applied to every known culture, but that is quite different from assuming that the particular sharing of labor between the sexes characteristic of our culture is universal—which it clearly is not.

Finally, we are so used to considering Freud a "personality theorist" that we forget how little interested he was in individual differences as against general principles. He once wrote to Abraham: "'Personality' . . . is a rather indefinite expression taken from surface psychology, and it doesn't contribute much to our understanding of the real processes, i.e., metapsychologically" (quoted in Jones, 1955, p. 438). Despite the fact that he wrote great case histories, he used them to illustrate his abstract formulations, and had no conviction about the scientific value or interest of the single case except as a possible source of new ideas.

The inclination to generalize sweepingly may be seen also in Freud's tendency to stretch the bounds of his concepts. The best-known, not to say most notorious, example is that of sexuality. In his earliest papers, the "sexual etiology of neurosis" meant literal child abuse ("seduction"), always involving the stimulation of the genitals. Rather quickly, in the *Three Essays on the Theory of Sexuality*, the concept was expanded first to include all of the "partial drives," based on the oral, anal, and phallic–urethral erogenous zones, plus the eye (for voyeurism and exhibitionism). In the decade following the first publication of the *Three Essays*, he found cases in which other parts of the body seemed to serve the function of sexual organs. Accordingly, he added a footnote to the 1915 edition, saying: "After further reflection and after taking other observations into account, I have been led to ascribe the quality of erotogenicity to all parts of the body and to all the internal organs" (1905d, p. 184 n.). In addition, he thought, "all comparatively intense affective processes, including even terrifying ones, trench upon sexuality" (p. 203). And finally, "It may well be that nothing of considerable importance can occur in the organism without contributing some component to the excitation of the sexual instinct" (p. 205).

A similar process seems to have gone on in Freud's blurring the distinctions among the various ego instincts, and that between ego instincts and narcissistic libido, resolved by his finally putting everything together in the notion of Eros, the life instinct.

USE OF FIGURES OF SPEECH

One of the notable features of Freud's literary style is his frequent and effective use of figurative language. Since metaphors, analogies, and other such tropes may serve a number of functions, it is worth our while to examine the ways he used them. The editors of the *Standard Edition* have made the task relatively easy by index entries, for each volume, under the heading "Analogies." Picking two volumes more or less at random (12 and 14), I looked up the 31 analogies so indexed and attempted to see in what way Freud employed them.

As one professor of rhetoric (Genung, 1900) has said

> The value both of example and of analogy is after all rather illustrative than argumentative; they are in reality instruments of exposition, employed to make the subject so clear . . . that men can see the truth or error of it for themselves. (p. 615)

For the most part, in these two volumes Freud used analogies as "instruments of exposition," added *after* an argument had been completely stated in its own terms, to supply lively, visualizable concreteness; some of them are little jokes, adding a touch of comic relief to lighten the reader's burden. At times, however, the analogy moves into the mainstream of the argument and serves a more direct rhetorical purpose; this is true, surprisingly enough, a good deal more often in Volume 14, which contains the austere metapsychological papers, than in Volume 12, largely devoted to the case of Schreber and the papers on technique. It turns out, however, that the argumentative use of analogy occurs largely in the polemical passages where Freud is attempting to refute the principal arguments with which Jung and Adler severed their ties to classical psychoanalysis; mostly, it takes the form of ridicule, a form of discrediting an opponent by making his argument appear ludicrous rather than meeting it on its own grounds. It is not difficult to understand how angry Freud must have felt at the apostasies of two of his most gifted and promising adherents in rapid succession, so that strong affect had its usual effect of degrading the level of argument.

Freud used analogies in two other kinds of ways in the metapsychological papers, however. In a few instances, the analogy seems to have played the role of a model. That is, when he wrote that "The complex of melancholia behaves like an open wound, drawing to itself . . . 'anticathexes' . . . from all directions, and emptying the ego until it is totally impoverished" (1917e [1915], p. 253), he revived an image that he had used in an unpublished draft, written and sent to Fliess 20 years earlier (Freud, 1985 [1887-1904], pp. 103-104); moreover, he was to use it again five years later in the theory of traumatic neurosis (1920g, p. 30). Interestingly enough, in none of these versions did Freud say explicitly what there is about a wound that makes it a

useful analogue. Obviously, however, he had in mind the way that leucocytes gather around the margins of a physical lesion, one of those medical
mechanisms of defense that may well carry ancestral responsibility for the
concept of psychic defense mechanisms.[8]

The other use of an extended figure of speech does not employ an
analogy in the strict sense and so is not indexed. (Indeed, the vast majority
of Freud's analogies were not indexed; only the protracted ones that resemble epic similes were. But the text is so dense with tropes of one kind or
another that a complete index would be impractically enormous.) I am
referring to an example of a characteristic Freudian device—the "scientific
myth," as he called the best-known example, the legend of the primal horde.
Near the beginning of *Instincts and Their Vicissitudes* (1915c), after considering the drive concept quite abstractly from the standpoint of physiology,
and in relation to the concept of "stimulus," he suddenly says: "Let us
imagine ourselves in the situation of an almost entirely helpless living organism, as yet unorientated in the world, which is receiving stimuli in its
nervous substance" (p. 119).

What an arresting image! And note that this is no mere conventional
figure of speech, in which man is compared point by point to a hypothetical
primitive organism. Instead, here we are given an invitation to
identification: Freud encourages us to anthropomorphize, to picture how it
would be if we, as adult and thinking people, were in the helpless and
exposed position he goes on to sketch so graphically. It seems easy to follow
him, therefore, when he attributes to the little animalcule not only consciousness but self-awareness—an attribute we realize, on sober reflection,
to be (most likely) uniquely human and a rather sophisticated achievement.
His introductory phrase, however, invites us at once to suspend disbelief
and waive the usual rules of scientific thinking. It is like a child's "let's
pretend"; it leads us to expect that this is not so much a way of pushing his
argument forward as a temporary illustrative digression—like his usual
analogies, a pictorial holiday from hard theoretical thinking. We soon discover that he uses this suspension of the rules as a way of allowing himself a
freedom and fluidity of reasoning that would not otherwise be acceptable.
And yet he proceeds thereafter as if the point had been proved in a rigorous
way.

The conception of a completely vulnerable organism swimming in a
sea of dangerous energies was another recurrent image that seems to have
made a profound impression on Freud. It plays an even more critical role in
the development of his argument in *Beyond the Pleasure Principle*, though it
is introduced in a somewhat soberer fashion ("Let us picture a living
organism in its most simplified possible form as an undifferentiated vesicle
of a substance that is susceptible to stimulation"; 1920g, p. 26). Yet he does
not explicitly present it as a hypothesis about the nature of the first living
organism; in fact, it never becomes quite clear just what kind of existential

status this "vesicle" has. Freud proceeds with some digressions to suppose that the organism would be killed by the "most powerful energies" that surround it if it remained unprotected, and that the cooking of its outer layer formed a crust that protected what lay underneath. Suddenly, Freud takes a mighty leap from this original, partly damaged living cell:

> In highly developed organisms the receptive cortical layer of the former vesicle has long been withdrawn into the depths of the interior of the body, though portions of it have been left behind on the surface immediately beneath the general shield against stimuli. (pp. 27–28)

Implicitly, he has assumed that his unicellular Adam has been fruitful and has populated the earth, always passing along its original scabs by the inheritance of acquired characters.

Just when you think that Freud is presenting a highly fanciful, Lamarckian theory about the origin of the skin and senses, he switches the metaphor. First, however, he hypothesizes that

> The specific unpleasure of physical pain is probably the result of the protective shield having been broken through. . . . Cathectic energy is summoned from all sides to provide sufficiently high cathexes of energy in the environs of the breach. An 'anticathexis' on a grand scale is set up, for whose benefit all the other psychical systems are impoverished. (p. 30)

Along about here, the sharp-eyed reader will do a double take: It sounded as if Freud was talking about a physical wound in the skin, but what get summoned to its margins are not the white blood cells but quanta of psychic energy! Then on the next page, we learn that "preparedness for anxiety and the hypercathexis of the receptive systems constitute the last line of defence of the shield against stimuli" (p. 31). This shield, which seemed so concrete and physical, turns out to be a metaphor wrapped in a myth.

It is true that this whole fourth chapter is introduced by the following disarmingly candid paragraph:

> What follows is speculation, often far-fetched speculation, which the reader will consider or dismiss according to his individual predilection. It is further an attempt to follow out an idea consistently, out of curiosity to see where it will lead. (1920g, p. 24)

In light of the later development of Freud's theories, in which (as we have seen) he came to lean on this tissue of speculations as if it were a stoutly supportive fabric, it seems that this modest disclaimer is another way of persuading the reader to relax usual critical standards in order to let creativity run free.

As usual, however, it is possible to find contrary examples—instances in which Freud used a figure of speech explicitly as a model and in a controlled and responsible way. A celebrated instance is his likening the psychic apparatus to a telescope. Among the sensible comments he makes in that context, the following remarks appear:

> I see no necessity to apologize for the imperfections of this or of any similar imagery. . . . We are justified, in my view, in giving free rein to our speculations so long as we retain the coolness of our judgement and do not mistake the scaffolding for the building. (1900a, p. 536)

If only he could have taken his own good advice!

FREUD'S RHETORIC

The upshot of my survey of the means Freud used in his search after truth is that he relied heavily on all the classical devices of rhetoric. The effect is not to prove, in any rigorous sense, but to persuade, using to some extent the devices of an essayist but even more those of an orator or advocate, who writes his brief and then argues the case with all the eloquence at his disposal. Notice that I have based this conclusion primarily on a survey of Freud's most technical, theoretical papers and books. In such masterly works for the general reader as his two series of introductory lectures (1916–1917, 1933a) or *The Question of Lay Analysis* (1926e), the rhetorical form is even more explicit; the last-named work is actually cast in the form of an extended dialogue, harking directly back to the classic Greek texts of which Freud was so fond.

There is a tendency today to take "rhetoric" as a pejorative term. Except in the minds of the Platonists, it had no such connotation in classical times. As Kennedy (1963) points out,

> One of the principal interests of the Greeks was rhetoric. . . . In its origin and intention rhetoric was natural and good: it produced clarity, vigor and beauty, and it rose logically from the conditions and qualities of the classical mind. Greek society relied on oral expression. . . . Political agitation was usually accomplished or defeated by word of mouth. The judicial system was similarly oral. . . . All literature was written to be heard, and even when reading to himself a Greek read aloud. (p. 3–4)

Rhetoric, as the theory of persuasive communication, was necessarily a good deal more than that; it was the only form of criticism in Greek thought. In one of Aristotle's definitions, rhetoric is "a process of criticism wherein lies the path to the principles of all inquiries" (*Topics I*; quoted in McBurney, 1936, p. 54).

Since science was not as sharply differentiated from other methods of seeking truth then as it later became, rhetoric was the closest thing to scientific methodology that the Greeks had. In Aristotle's presentation, there were two kinds of truth, exact or certain, and probable; the former was the concern of science, which operated by means of syllogistic logic or complete enumeration. All other kinds of merely probabilistic knowledge were the realms of argumentative inquiry, which operated by means of dialectic and rhetoric. But the only discipline to which Aristotle's criterion of "unqualified scientific knowledge" applies is mathematics (today construed to include symbolic logic); only in such a purely formal science can strict deductive procedure be used and certainty attained.

I go into this much detail about Greek rhetoric because it suggests to me a possibly illuminating hypothesis. About all I can do to make it plausible is to point out that Freud did know Greek well and read the classics in the original; and among the five courses or seminars he took with Brentano were one on logic and at least one on "the philosophy of Aristotle" (Bernfeld, 1951). If Freud received any formal training in methodology, the critical philosophy of science, it was with the Aristotelian philosopher-psychologist Brentano. I have not found anywhere in Freud's works any references to Aristotle's *Rhetoric* or any direct evidence that he knew it; the best I can do is to offer these bits of circumstantial evidence (or, as Aristotle would have put it, to make an argument from signs). It is, then, possible that Freud was in this way introduced to the devices of rhetoric and enthymemetic or probabilistic reasoning as the legitimate instruments of inquiry into empirical matters. His rejection of speculative, deductively exact system building may indicate that he was accepting the Aristotelian dichotomy between exact (or mathematical) and probable truth and choosing to work in the real and approximate world, where rhetoric was the appropriate means of approaching an only relative truth.

The way I have put this point of view deliberately blurs a fine but important distinction between two kinds of probabilism: that of rhetoric, in which the technical means of plausible reasoning are used to enhance the subjective probability in the mind of the listener that the speaker's thesis is true; and that of modern skeptical science, which uses the most exact and rigorous methods possible to measure the probability of a thesis—that is, the amount of confidence we can have that it is a good approximation to a reality that can be approached only asymptotically. For the former, proof is the establishment of belief; for the latter, verification is the rejection of a surely false null hypothesis and the temporary acceptance of an alternative as the best one available at the moment. I do not believe that Freud saw this distinction clearly; at any rate, he did not write as if he thought in these terms.

Surely he was a superb rhetorician, whether he was a conscious one or not. He was a master of all its five parts, invention, arrangement, style, memory, and delivery. We have discussed so far primarily aspects of the first, invention, which includes the modes of proof: direct evidence, argumentation from the evidence, and indirect means of persuasion by the force of personal impression or presence (*ethos*) or by "the emotion he is able to awaken by his verbal appeals, his gestures," and so on (*pathos*) (Kennedy, 1963, p. 10). Freud's excellence at ethos and pathos, and at the last two of the parts, memory and delivery, is described by Jones:

> He was a fascinating lecturer. The lectures were always enlightened by his peculiar ironic humor. . . . He always used a low voice, perhaps because it could become rather harsh if strained, but spoke with the utmost distinctness. He never used any notes, and seldom made much preparation for a lecture. (1953, p. 341)

The biographer goes on to state that "He never used oratory," but he seems to be using the term in the modern sense as synonymous with "bombast," which was surely not what the ancient Greeks meant. What Jones's description conveys is a very effective kind of personal presence. Freud

> talked intimately and conversationally. . . . One felt he was addressing himself to us personally. . . . There was no flicker of condescension in it, not even a hint of a teacher. The audience was assumed to consist of highly intelligent people to whom he wished to communicate some of his recent experiences. (Jones, 1953, p. 342)

With respect to the remaining two parts in the Aristotelian five-part division of rhetoric, arrangement and style, much could be written, but it would trench on literary criticism. The Greeks analyzed style evaluatively in terms of the four virtues of correctness, clarity, ornamentation, and propriety; I will merely record my impression that Freud would earn top grades on all of these counts.

Freud prided himself on having held aloof from the brawling controversy of polemics. Only once, he says with some pride in his *An Autobiographical Study* (1925d), did he directly answer a critic, in 1894. Yet it is obvious that he wrote in a polemical mood much of the rest of his life, always with a consciousness that the reader might be hostile. He was explicit about it in many letters to his followers. For example, he wrote to Jung in 1909:

> We cannot avoid the resistances, why not face up to them from the start? In my opinion attack is the best form of defense. Perhaps you are underestimating the intensity of these resistances if you hope to disarm them with small concessions. (Freud & Jung, 1974, p. 28)

And to Pfister two years later:

> Public debate of psycho-analysis is hardly possible; one does not share common ground, and against the lurking affects nothing can be done. Psycho-analysis is

a deep-going movement, and public debates are bound to be as useless as the theological disputations of the time of the Reformation. (Freud & Pfister, 1963, p. 80)

Feeling this strongly, Freud could not have done other than to approach the task of exposition as one of argument. The amazing thing is that the skilled verbal swordsman let the scientist in Freud have the floor as much as he did.[9]

To set matters in some perspective, I should call the reader's attention to the fact that an analysis like the foregoing is bound to give a false impression because of the lack of any control data. It seems not only possible but likely that an equally close and critical reading of any great figure in psychology would uncover many of the same errors in reasoning, similar idiosyncrasies of thought and writing, and analogous reliance on rhetorical devices in scientific argument. In such a series, Freud's personal style could be studied with an emphasis on what was quantitatively outstanding as well as on what was qualitatively idiosyncratic. Without it, all too many lapses, which he probably shares with many another, are bound to seem unique to him.

In this connection, I am reminded of an experience in the course of research comparing the cognitive effects of sensory deprivation and of LSD (Goldberger & Holt, 1961; see also Barr, Langs, Holt, Goldberger, & Klein, 1972). Looking for cognitive tests that might be sensitive to the pronounced but evanescent impact of several hours of perceptual isolation on thought processes, Leo Goldberger and I tried out a task requiring logical argumentation. We posed some common social issues (e.g., monogamy, racial discrimination), asking normal adult subjects to talk about each for five minutes, giving arguments pro and con. To our dismay, when we analyzed the quality of reasoning used under control conditions—before any experimental intervention, under no stress—we found it so poor that there was literally no room for regression, no way for an impairment to be manifested in our scoring system. (See also Shneidman's [1961] study of the reasoning used by Kennedy and Nixon in their televised debate of 1960.)

All such allowances being made, I still have the impression that as compared with William James, a contemporary on his same level, Freud's scientific reasoning is less impressive than his rhetorical skill. An additional explanatory hypothesis springs to mind: It would have been amazing indeed if Freud's style of thinking and writing had not been affected by the special situation of psychoanalysis as compared to every other science I can think of. Typically, in recent centuries, the sciences have grown up in universities and other publicly endowed institutions of learning and research. In that protected setting, scientists have developed a set of shared values concerning their work, which have been admirably codified by Bronowski (1965). He writes (in part):

... they do not make wild claims, they do not cheat, they do not try to
persuade at any cost, they appeal neither to prejudice nor to authority, they are
often frank about their ignorance, their disputes are fairly decorous, they do not
confuse what is being argued with race, politics, sex or age . . . (p. 59)

Scientists are "trained to avoid and organized to resist every form of persuasion but the fact" (p. 59).

Perhaps the last remark is an overstatement. Science is not without its bitter controversies, and psychology in particular has known a number of polemicists who have made the air crackle at scientific meetings. Scientists are people, often passionate people with the capacity to get deeply involved in their work—a reality that should not be deplored. For the kind of entailment of self-esteem in the fortunes of a theory that motivates a scientist to argue with all the resources of rhetoric also produces the commitment that sustains him through the frustrations and failures that are a necessary part of his work.

Yet there is a difference between psychoanalysis and academic psychology in the quality of debate. Part of it doubtless stems from the fact that the latter discipline has well-delineated methods of putting theories to empirical test, whether experimental or psychometric, and thus has developed a tradition of persuasion by the fact. I suggest that the difference in the economic base of the two professions is also a powerful determinant. Academic psychology, like any other university-based science, gets its money through governmental and other essentially public channels. To the tenured professor, it matters little whether his salary is paid directly by the state or from private gifts and educational fees. Only under exceptional circumstances does his livelihood depend in any way on the outcome of his scientific controversies. Hence, the latter tend to have the degree of decorum Bronowski described.

Whatever the prestige of the kind of *a.o.* (adjunct) professorship Freud dreamed of so often and finally attained in 1902, it paid him nothing. Up to his dying days, he was dependent on money he received from patients in direct payment for therapeutic services, supplemented in only a minor way by royalties. When he fought for psychoanalysis, therefore, he was almost literally fighting for his life. His students and followers, too, at first joined him at considerable financial risk if not sacrifice.

But was the same not true of neurology and the other branches of medicine? Were they not also simultaneously sciences and professions, whose practitioners earned their bread in private practice? To a much smaller degree. For generations the scientific arm of medicine has been separated from the arm that ministers directly to the public, and medical scientists have been based in hospitals, research institutes, and medical schools, where most of their income and all the costs of their scientific work come from impersonal sources. The promulgator of a new medical theory with therapeutic implications does not have the incentive to found his own professional schools, much less a "movement" with ideological and political aspects as well as scientific and professional ones.

The argument of economic determinism should not be pushed too far. Fromm (1959) makes a convincing showing that Freud's "mission" had deep personal roots, being closely connected with his largely warded-off thirst for fame and power. In an almost religious sense he had a vocation, to reform nothing less than civilization at large, to take as his patient "the whole human race" (1925e, p. 221). The aim was grandiose, but not in the clinical sense. When Freud saw himself as, like Copernicus and Darwin, one who had troubled the sleep of mankind by undermining its narcissism, who can deny that his self-estimation was realistic?

Fueled from such various sources, the fire within Freud made him a formidable antagonist indeed. An attack on his ideas hit directly at his pride, his identity, and his pocketbook, but it was also an act of counterrevolution. As is so often the case with more or less persecuted religious sects and political splinter parties, the bitterest hatred got directed against followers who strayed from the Way. It is impossible to understand the nature of Freud's split with Adler, Jung, and Rank (as well as some others of less fame) unless one appreciates the intensity of Freud's devotion to "the cause," as he called it—the psychoanalytic movement—and the depth and complexity of passionate wishes and fears that were interwoven with it. Unfortunately, it has become traditional in Freudian circles to take the master's side in these disputes almost entirely, at the cost of a realistic understanding of the movement's history [see, however, Gay, 1988]. But now that those who had direct contact with his charismatic presence are dying, this tradition is weakening. It cannot hurt psychoanalysis to face the truth about some of the less admirable sides of the extraordinarily complex and truly great man who founded it.

SUMMARY

And now let me return to cognitive style in its contemporary technical sense. As Klein used the term, a cognitive style characterizes a person and his unique way of processing information. There are, of course, similarities among people in these respects, and the dimensions into which cognitive styles may be analyzed are called "cognitive control principles." (The most nearly definitive statement of the principles discovered by Klein and his collaborators is contained in the monograph by Gardner, Holzman, Klein, Linton, & Spence, 1959.)

We have seen that Freud had, to an unusual degree, a tolerance for ambiguity and inconsistency. He needed it. As I argued in earlier sections above, his thinking always took place in the context of pervasive conflicts [(see also Chapter 12, this volume). A penchant for tender-minded, speculative, wide-ranging, and fantasy-like thinking, deriving from Freud's humanistic heritage, was pitted against the disciplined, empirical, physicalistic (reductionist), analytical methods of contemporary mechanistic science. These patterns seem to have been part of two opposing world views, entailing a humanistic and a scientistic image of man—one artistic, literary, and philosophical; the other grounded in a reductionistic ideal of science and its promise of progress through objectivity and rigor (Holt, 1972a). Moreover, as we shall see in later chapters,] Freud's metapsychology clashes at many crucial points with reality; so a further conflict took place between one set of Freud's basic orienting assumptions and his growing knowledge of the facts about behavior.

Because of these and other conflicts, I believe that he had to operate in his characteristically loose-jointed way. If he had had a compulsive need for clarity and consistency, he would probably have had to make choices and resolve his intellectual conflicts. If he had followed the way of hard-headed science, he would have been the prisoner of the methods and assumptions he learned in his medical school and its laboratories—another, more gifted Exner, who might have written a series of excellent neurological books like the one on aphasia, but who would probably have emulated his cautious contemporaries in steering clear of hysterical patients. And if he had turned his back on the effort at scientific discipline and had opened the floodgates of his speculative inventiveness, we might have had a spate of nature-philosophical essays but nothing like psychoanalysis; or if the humanist in him had decisively won over the mechanist, he might have written brilliant novels and never have made his great discoveries.

But because Freud was able to keep one foot in literature and one in science, because he could comfortably retain the security of a set of ideas and principles inherited from respected authorities without letting it wholly blind him to the aspects of reality that it had no place for, he was able to be extraordinarily creative. Productive originality in science involves a dialectic of freedom and control, flexibility and rigor, speculation and self-critical checking. Without some loosening of the chains of conventional, safe, secondary-process thinking, there can be little originality; Pegasus must have a chance to take wing. But liberation alone is not enough. If flexibility is not accompanied by discipline, it becomes fluidity, and then we have a visionary, a *Phantast* (as Freud once called himself and Fliess) instead of a scientist. It was just this possibility that Freud feared in himself. The daring but fruitful ideas must be sorted from the merely daring or positively harebrained ones; insights must be painstakingly checked; new concepts must be worked into a structure of laws so that they fit smoothly into, buttress, and extend the edifice. All of this takes an attitude that is antithetical to the earlier, more strictly creative one. It is asking a great deal of a person, therefore, to be adept in both types of thinking and able to shift appropriately from the role of dreamer to that of critic. Perhaps that is one reason why we have so few truly great scientists.

This first major characteristic of Freud's cognitive style is strikingly reminiscent of the principle of cognitive control called by Klein and his associates "tolerance for instability" or for unrealistic experiences. "'Tolerant' subjects [as compared to intolerant ones] seemed in equally adequate contact with external reality, but were much more relaxed in their acceptance of both ideas and perceptual organizations that required deviation from the conventional" (Gardner et al., 1959, p. 93). It is a relaxed and imaginative kind of mind, opposed to the kind that rigidly clings to a literally interpreted reality. And Freud (1933a) was unusually willing to entertain parapsychological hypotheses that go well beyond scientifically conventional concepts of reality. Telepathy, "the fact of thought-transference" (letter to Weiss; quoted in Roazen, 1975, p. 240), is quite literally an "unrealistic experience."

If Freud was tolerant of ambiguity, inconsistency, instability, and unrealistic experiences, there was one similiar-sounding state that he could *not* tolerate: meaninglessness, the assumption that a mental process was stochastic or that a behavioral phenomenon occurred because of random error. In discussing slips of the tongue and other errors (1901b, p. 257), he wrote: "I believe in external (real) chance, it is true, but not in internal (psychical) accidental events." Not doubt this attitude led him at times into overinterpreting data and reading meaning—especially dynamic or motivational meaning—into behavior unwarrantedly. But it also spurred his basic discoveries, such as the interpretability of dreams and of neurotic and psychotic symptoms.

Let us see how well the remaining five dimensions described by Gardner et al. (1959) serve as a framework for summarizing Freud's manner of thinking. It surely seems probable that Freud was strongly *field-independent*. Inner-directed he surely was, and Graham (1955) has shown an empirical connection between Riesman's (1950) and Witkin's (1949) concepts. Here is the Gardner et al. (1959) description of the kind of person who is field-independent—*not* markedly dependent on the visual field for orientation to the upright: He is characterized by "(a) activity in dealing with the environment; (b) . . . 'inner life' and effective control of impulses, with low anxiety; and (c) high self-esteem, including confidence in the body and a relatively adult body-image" (p. 67). It sounds a good deal like Freud, except possibly for his ambivalent and rather hypochondriacal attitudes towards his body—"poor Konrad," as he wryly called it. Linton (1955) has further shown that field-independent people are little susceptible to group influence, surely true of Freud.[10]

In his preference for a small number of extremely broadly defined motivational concepts, Freud seems to have had a broad *equivalence range*. And on Klein's dimension of *flexible versus constricted control*, Freud would assuredly have scored well over at the flexible end. Was he not "relatively comfortable in situations that involved contradictory or intrusive cues . . . not overimpressed with a dominant stimulus organization if . . . another part of the field [was] more appropriate"? And surely he "did not tend to suppress feeling and other internal cues." This is the description of the flexibly controlled subject (Gardner et al., 1959, pp. 53–54).

The other two dimensions of cognitive control seem less relevant. *Scanning* (as against *focusing*) as a way of using attention might seem to suggest the way Freud attended to his patients, but it is qualitatively different. Scanning is accompanied by the ability to concentrate on what is important, but at the cost of isolation of affect and overintellectualization; it is not so much passively relaxed attending as a restlessly roaming search for everything that might be useful. And so far as I can determine, Freud was not either a *leveler* or a *sharpener*, he neither habitually blurred distinctions and oversimplified, nor was he specially alert to fine differences and always on the lookout for slight changes in situations, though he tended in the latter direction.

It is fair to conclude, I think that some of these principles of cognitive control seem quite apt and useful, though a good deal of the flavor of Freud's uniqueness as a thinker is lost when we apply them to him.

In addition, several other aspects of cognitive style have been suggested by other authors as characterizing Freud. Kaplan (1964) begins a general discussion of the cognitive style of behavioral scientists thus: " . . . thought and its expression are surely not wholly unrelated to one another, and how scientific findings are formulated for incorporation into the body of knowledge often reflects stylistic traits of the thinking behind them" (p. 259). He goes on to describe six principal styles, and mentions Freud in connection with the first two of them: the literary and the academic styles. The literary style is often concerned with individuals, interpreted "largely in terms of the specific purposes and perspectives of the actors, rather than in terms of the abstract and general categories of the scientist's own explanatory scheme. . . . Freud's studies of Moses and Leonardo . . . exhibit something of this style" (p. 259). The academic style, by contrast, is

much more abstract and general. . . . There is some attempt to be precise, but it is verbal rather than operational. Ordinary words are used in special senses, to constitute a technical vocabulary. . . . [Treatment of the data] tends to be highly theoretical, if not, indeed, purely speculative. System is introduced by way of great "principles," applied over and over to specific cases, which illustrate the generalization rather than serve as proofs for it. (pp. 259–260)

Ellenberger (1970, p. 466) undertakes the related task of listing Freud's attributes as a great writer: "First he had linguistic and verbal gifts, the love of his native language, a richness of vocabulary, the *Sprachgefühl* (feeling for the language) that infallibly led him to choose the appropriate word." Second, he had "that gift of intellectual curiosity that impels a writer to observe his fellow men to try to penetrate their lives, their loves, their intimate attitudes." Third, he loved writing and did a great deal of it. In this connection, Ellenberger makes the apposite remark that "For a man of letters to write down one's thoughts and impressions is more important than to check their exactness." Fourth, he had credibility, the ability to "make the most implausible story seem true." Despite differences in our frames of reference, I trust it will be apparent how well these descriptions summarize much of what I have tried to bring out about Freud.

A DECALOGUE FOR THE READER OF FREUD

To conclude, let me come back to my original statement that a better understanding of Freud's cognitive style would help the contemporary reader to read him with insight rather than confusion, and try to give it substance in the form of ten admonitions. Like another decalogue, they can be reduced to one golden rule: Be empathic rather than projective—learn what the man's terms are and take him on his own terms.

1. Beware of lifting statements out of context. This practice is particularly tempting to textbook writers, polemical critics, and research-minded clinical psychologists who are more eager to get right to the testing of propositions than to undertake the slow study of a large corpus of theory. There is no substitute for reading enough of Freud to get his full meaning, which is almost never fully expressed in a single paragraph, no matter how specific a point is.

2. Don't take Freud's extreme formulations literally. Treat them as his way of calling your attention to a point. When he says "never," "invariably," "conclusively," and the like—read on, for the qualifying and softening statements. Remember the change that has taken place in the general atmosphere since Freud wrote his major works; social acceptance and respectability have replaced shock and hostility, which made Freud feel that his was a small and lonely voice in a cold wilderness, so that he had to shout in order to be heard at all.

3. Look out for inconsistencies; don't either trip over them or seize on them with malicious glee, but take them as incomplete dialectic formulations awaiting the synthesis that Freud's cognitive style made him consistently draw back from.

4. Be on the watch for figurative language, personification in particular (reified formulations of concepts as homunculi). Remember that it is there primarily for color even though it did at times lead Freud astray himself, and that it is fairest to him to rely primarily on those of his statements of issues that are least poetic and dramatic.

5. Don't expect rigorous definitions; look rather for the meanings of his terms in the ways they are used over a period of time. And don't be dismayed if you find a word being used at one place in its ordinary, literary meaning, at another in a special technical sense which changes with the developmental status of the theory. An enterprise like the *Dictionary of Psychoanalysis*, put together by a couple of industrious but misguided analysts (Fodor & Gaynor, 1950) who lifted definition-like sentences from many of Freud's works, is completely mistaken in conception and betrays a total misunderstanding of Freud's style of thinking and working.

6. Be benignly skeptical about Freud's assertions of proof that something has been established beyond doubt. Remember that he had different standards of proof than we do today; that he rejected experiment partly from a too-narrow conception of it and partly because he had found it stylistically incompatible long before even the first works of R. A. Fisher (1945); and that he tended to confuse a replicated observation with a verified theory of the phenomenon in question.

7. In general, don't assume that the theory is invalidated by its being stated much of the time in methodologically indefensible form. Freud was overfond of dichotomies, even when his data were better conceptualized as continuous variables.

8. Be wary of Freud's persuasiveness. Keep in mind that he was a powerful rhetorician in areas where his scientific footing was uncertain. Though he was often right, it was not always for the reasons he gave, which are almost never truly sufficient to prove his case, and not always to the extent that he hoped.

Finally, be particularly cautious not to gravitate towards either of two extreme and equally untenable positions: that is,

9. Don't take Freud's every sentence as a profound truth, which may present difficulties but only because of our own inadequacies—our pedestrian difficulty in keeping up with the soaring mind of a genius who did not always bother to explicate steps that were obvious to him, but which we must supply by laborious exegetical scholarship. This is the temptation of the scholars working from within the psychoanalytic institutes, those earnest Freudians who, to Freud's annoyance, had already begun to emerge during his lifetime. For most of us in the universities, the corresponding temptation is the more dangerous one:

10. Don't let yourself get so offended by Freud's lapses from methodological purity that you dismiss him altogether. Almost any psychologist can learn an enormous lot from Freud, if he will listen carefully and sympathetically, and not take his pronouncements too seriously.

PART II

Psychic Energy: The Economic Point of View

CHAPTER 4

A Critical Examination
of Freud's Concept
# of Bound versus Free Cathexis

When I first began seriously working on trying to understand psychoanalytic theory, George Klein and I had started the Research Center for Mental Health at NYU with the explicit aim of making it a center of psychoanalytic research. Our plan was simple, with the audacity of youth. Being trained as empirical research psychologists, we intended to do quantitative, controlled investigations, as rigorously as might be consistent with fidelity to the spirit of the issues, their clinical foundations, and the theory we had found so useful in our clinical work. Both of us had started work elsewhere on different types of investigation (his experimental, mine psychometric—representing the "two disciplines of scientific psychology" of which Cronbach [1957] was shortly to speak), which we pursued interactively and collaboratively, following leads in our data. Yet we wanted to do more than simply invoke psychoanalytic concepts after the fact to rationalize whatever findings we chanced upon. Our goal was to implement the ideal we had been taught in graduate school, of a hypothetical–deductive approach to research. That implied extensive theoretical work, clarifying and systematically elaborating theoretical propositions to the point where in a deductive way they could be made to yield predictions about the outcome of studies before they were done.

So we began a continuing theoretical enterprise at the same time as we pushed ahead empirically, Klein in the laboratory and I emphasizing tests. For a few years, we had a staff seminar on the psychoanalytic theory of thinking, which was our common focus; we read the volumes of the Standard Edition and of the Jones biography as they appeared, trying to extract and systematize the theory of primary and secondary processes. Very soon, it became apparent to me that there was an intimate relation between "the free and bound states of $Q\mathring{\eta}$ [quantity], [and] the primary and secondary processes" (Freud, 1985 [1887–1904], p. 146). For Freud, it seemed evident that "the whole thing held together" as "a machine [sic] that shortly would function on its own"; yet neither in the letter (October 20, 1895) from which these phrases are quoted nor anywhere else did he ever make it very clear just what that connection was, and how the whole system functioned. Surely it must be there somewhere; if one were only a good enough scholar, it would turn up.

After five years, I thought that I had found the place to get hold of this large and sticky problem: If I could only get straight about what binding was, that might clear up a good deal. My mentor, David Rapaport, had taught me (more by example than by precept) how to work at theoretical clarification. First of all came the word, the Freudian text; that had to be mastered, and in historical order. Close textual exegesis in the Talmudic tradition was the next step. One had to find and excerpt all the key passages in which Freud used a term, compare them carefully, and figure out what he was doing with it in each context. The elusive meaning would then become clear. The present chapter was the product of such an effort. I put the final touches on the original version of it during my first few weeks at the Center for Advanced Study in the Behavioral Sciences in the fall of 1960, and it was published two years later.

When in the early months of 1982 I decided to include this paper in the present book, and I started going over it carefully, at first I felt a strong temptation to rewrite it completely. In the intervening years, I had occasionally come across (and had noted down) passages I had missed in my original effort. Then a concordance (Guttman, Jones, & Parrish, 1980) appeared, making it quite possible to do a truly comprehensive job. Most of all, I felt embarrassed by my own theoretical errors and sins, of the very kind I had meanwhile been discovering in Freud, and it seemed only prudent to expunge them quietly.

On reflection, aided by the advice of several friends and colleagues, I have decided to reprint the text with very few changes. I have, however, added an afterword to explain my present point of view more clearly.

A final word of warning: This chapter is the most technical and difficult part of the book, yet it deals with only one aspect of the economic third of metapsychology. Therefore, any reader who is not particularly interested in the concept of bound/free cathexis may profitably skip (or skim) to the Summary and the first two sections of the Afterword, leaving the details to the specialists.

On a number of occasions when Freud invoked the concept of bound cathectic energy to explain some phenomenon, he spoke of it in such a way as to indicate that he considered it highly important to his general theory. The concept recurs a number of times in his writings on general psychological theory, and has also been rather widely used by other analysts since him. Kris (1952, p. 424, n. 2) said: "The distinction between 'bound' or 'quiescent' psychical energy on the one hand and 'free' or 'mobile' psychical energy on the other is one of Freud's most fundamental concepts," and Rapaport (1951a, p. 353) commented: "The conception of 'bound cathexes,' though it is central to the cathectic theory of psychoanalysis, refers to one of the least understood psychoanalytic observations."

One thing that must strike the student of psychoanalytic theory is the shifting meanings that the terms "bound," "free," and "mobile" accrue in various contexts. Rapaport (1951a) speaks of the "mobility of counter-cathexes"; and it would not be difficult to adduce many other examples from recent psychoanalytic writings that indicate how little unanimity there is on the exact meaning of these terms. It seems high time for re-examination of the underlying concept, its origins, and its development in Freud's thought.[1]

BREUER'S AND FREUD'S USES OF THE CONCEPT

In a number of places where Freud used the concept of bound versus free cathexis—for example, in *The Unconscious* (1915e) and in *Beyond the Pleasure Principle* (1920g)—he attributed it to his former friend and collaborator, Breuer. It is true that in the theoretical part of their joint book, *Studies on Hysteria* (1895), Breuer had used similar terms, and this published usage antedates by several years the first time Freud used the concept in print (in *The Interpretation of Dreams*). This generous attribution of an important concept to Breuer was a characteristic act on Freud's part: In doing so, he expressed a benevolent temper and at the same time probably strove to make up for negative feelings he had toward the older man (Jones, 1953). But he overlooked the fact that his was a distinctly different concept from Breuer's, and his later usage bore more resemblance to his own early ideas than it did to the passage of Breuer's to which he twice referred. A good place to begin the investigation of the concept of binding, therefore, is to examine the discrepancy between Breuer and Freud.

In his sober, common-sense attempt to theorize about hysteria and the method of psychotherapy that Freud and he had developed for it, Breuer followed a generally organic line, though not an extreme one; it is essentially neuropsychology. In the second part of his chapter (headed "Intracerebral Tonic Excitations—Affects"), Breuer set himself the task of explaining the various levels of consciousness that could be distinguished, ranging from dreamless sleep to a clear waking state. He postulated that nerve cells could not be traversed in sleep, while in the waking state they were completely traversable (i.e., a current could pass through them unimpeded).

> The existence of these two different conditions of the paths of conduction can, it seems, be made intelligible only if we suppose that in waking life these paths are in a state of tonic excitation (what Exner [1894, p. 93] calls 'intercellular tetanus'), that this intracerebral excitation is what determines their conductive capacity, and that the diminution and disappearance of that excitation is what sets up the state of sleep. (Breuer & Freud, 1895, p. 193)

In a footnote to this passage, he made the far-seeing statement: "We usually think of the sensory nerve-cells as being passive receptive organs.

This is a mistake . . . these sensory nerve-cells also send out excitation into the nerve fibres . . . a state of tension must exist" in them. He compared it to the electric tension (i.e., potential or voltage) in a physical system as contrasted to the electric current that might pass along wires of the system. He made it clear that he did not mean the potential energy of "the chemical substance of the cell" but a continuous state of slight excitation, comparable to the continuous slight contraction of healthy muscles, which is called tonus. Indeed, Breuer suggested that the state of "tonic excitation" was directly experienced as a state of phenomenal tension.[2]

Incidentally, subsequent neurophysiological discoveries have established the existence of a complexity in the electrical activity of the nerves very similar to the duality Breuer postulated:

> There is now clear evidence that the dendrite has a "slow-burning" activity which is not all-or-none, tends not to be transmitted, and lasts 15 or 30 milliseconds instead of the spike's one millisecond. It facilitates spike activity, but often occurs independently and may make up the greater part of the EEG record. (Hebb, 1955, p. 248)

There is then, a nontransmitted, "quiescent" nerve activity which does facilitate the transmission of the more important and obvious, evoked spike potential. But the kind of large-scale facilitation of psychic activity Breuer had in mind is today understood in terms of a different neurological finding: the reticular systems of Magoun and Jasper. Again, Breuer's formulation has a pretty modern sound. The differences between sleep and wakefulness are attributed by many neurophysiologists to a state of generalized excitation (activation) of the cortex, from the reticular formations of the brain stem and hypothalamus. The structure and functions of these parts of the brain have been elucidated only in recent decades; it is now demonstrated that cortical activation does depend on diffuse discharges from these lower centers, which have just the kind of facilitating effect on informational inputs from the senses that Breuer suspected. The difference is that the source of activation is not inherent to the cortical neurones.

Turning to Freud and the passage in which he most handsomely credited Breuer, we find him dealing with quite a different kind of question. In Section V of his paper "The Unconscious" (1915e), he set forth the special characteristics of the system *Ucs.*, as contrasted with the other half of the psychic apparatus, the system *Pcs.* (including *Cs.*). One of the principal points of difference is as follows:

> The cathectic intensities [in the *Ucs.*] are much more mobile [*Beweglichkeit*]. By the process of *displacement* one idea may surrender to another its whole quota of cathexis; by the process of *condensation* it may appropriate the whole cathexis of several other ideas. I have proposed to regard these two processes as

distinguishing marks of the so-called *primary psychical process.* In the system *Pcs.* the *secondary process* is dominant. (p. 186)

[Elaborating the last point a few paragraphs later, he went on:]

The processes of the system *Pcs.* display—no matter whether they are already conscious or only capable of becoming conscious—an inhibition of the tendency of cathected ideas towards discharge. When a process passes from one idea to another, the first idea retains a part of its cathexis and only a small portion undergoes displacement. Displacements and condensations such as happen in the primary process are excluded or very much restricted. This circumstance caused Breuer to assume the existence of two different states of cathectic energy in mental life: one in which the energy is tonically 'bound'[3] and the other in which it is freely mobile [*frei beweglichen*] and presses towards discharge. In my opinion this distinction represents the deepest insight we have gained up to the present into the nature of nervous energy, and I do not see how we can avoid making it. A metapsychological presentation would most urgently call for further discussion at this point, though perhaps that would be too daring an undertaking as yet. (p. 188)

What are the differences and similarities here? Note first the subtle change in terminology that Freud introduced: Breuer had spoken of "tonic excitation," while Freud changed it to "tonic binding" (and gradually dropped the word "tonic")—Breuer never used the word "binding" at all.[4] For him, tonic excitation was a necessary assumption to account for the facts of different states of consciousness—something that Freud did not allude to directly, though inferentially he associated free cathexis with the *Ucs.* and the dream work, and thus with a state specifically mentioned by Breuer as lacking in a free transmission of excitation.

Several other points of difference are plain enough. Breuer was talking hypothetical but rather concrete neurophysiology; Freud was constructing an ostensibly abstract psychological theory, [though in fact it too is an implicit neuropsychology, with occasional references to neurones and their excitations]. In Breuer's conception, the tonic neural activity occurred simultaneously with and made possible the free, rapid transmission of impulses in larger amounts. For Freud, the two are antithetical, and binding *hinders* the free transmission of cathexis in large amounts.

Despite these differences, there are also notable similarities. Both men were talking about two conditions of energy, differentiated in terms of negative freedom of its movement. Moreover, the two terms, "tonic excitation" and "binding," both refer to the cathectic state of affairs in waking, rational thought: the secondary process.[5] But each man was concerned with a different aspect of rational thinking: Freud with the stability of its contents, Breuer with its flexibility. Both observations are valid; in different ways, ordinary waking thought is more stable and reliable, *and* more freely manipulable, than dream thinking. Freud ultimately resolved this paradox by assuming that two types of energy were involved in the secondary process: a motivating energy derived ultimately from drive, which was bound to the contents of thought; and a mobile, freely manipulable energy of attention and consciousness, hypercathexis. Binding and hypercathexis were, as we shall see, closely associated in Freud's mind, so that it should not be surprising that he slipped slightly in identifying Breuer's "tonic excitation" with bound cathexis instead of with hypercathexis, his own concept for the energy associated with consciousness and with the flexibility of the secondary process. Furthermore, as we shall see, at the time that Freud was building a neurological theory, he actually used Breuer's conception if not his terminology.

THE CONCEPT IN THE *PROJECT FOR A SCIENTIFIC PSYCHOLOGY*

In Draft E, a manuscript sent to Fliess apparently in June 1894, Freud was trying to understand how anxiety arises. In anxiety neuroses, he suggested, when sexual excitement occurs,

> The physical tension increases, reaches the threshold level at which it can arouse a psychical affect . . . [Ordinarily, to summarize his argument, it would arouse libido which would then lead to copulation.] . . . but for some reasons the psychical linkage offered to it remains insufficient: a *sexual affect* cannot be formed, because there is something lacking in the psychical determinants. Accordingly, the physical tension, not being psychically bound, is transformed into—anxiety. (1950 [1892-1899], p. 193)

Here he was saying that in the ordinary state of affairs, when (somatic) sexual impulses become (psychic) sexual desires, this [nonempirical] transformation acts to *bind* the excitation and prevent an alternative psychic transformation into anxiety. Here binding implies a normal state of affairs ending in direct sexual gratification, which is closer to the primary process than to the secondary. Thus, at this moment when his contact with his older friend was still close, Freud's concept was like Breuer's, in that both described processes of *facilitation* of the neuronal flow.

A few months and a few drafts later, Freud was wrestling with the problem of melancholia, and its relation to sexual anesthesia. He made another reference, this time more obscure (possibly in the sense of "time binding"?), to the general theory of "the 'binding' of excitation in the memory" (1950 [1892-1899], p. 203).[6] But these ideas were elucidated later the same year, when

> the barriers suddenly lifted, the veils dropped, and everything became transparent—from the details of neurosis to the determinants of consciousness . . .

The three systems of n[eurones], the free and bound states of $Q\dot{\eta}$ [quantity], the primary and secondary processes . . . all that was correct, and still is today. Naturally, I can scarcely manage to contain my delight. (Letter of October 20, 1895; Freud, 1985, p. 146)

These exciting insights were set forth in the longest draft of all, which Kris calls the "Project for a Scientific Psychology" (Freud, 1950 [1895]).

It will be worth our while to take up the way the concept is used in the Project in some detail, for in this respect, as in so many others, it contains in germ many of the ideas Freud developed during the rest of his life. It is a work of truly astonishing originality and audacity, being no less than an attempt to produce a complete neurological model of the functioning of the mind in health and in neurosis. Working with concepts of the newly discovered neurone and synapse, Freud wove an elaborate theory that bears many family resemblances to Chapter VII of *The Interpretation of Dreams*.

The dynamic element of the system is quantity—a word Freud used to signify excitation of the neurone. Ordinarily, quantity (often abbreviated as Q or $Q\eta$), passes through the neurones from peripheral sense organs through the projection system, which he called Φ, and into the central mass of the brain (Ψ) where the contact barriers (his term for synapses) are much more effective and transmission is slower, ultimately affecting a third system (W) of perceptual neurones and completing the reflex arc on through to efferent motor nerves. After learning, passage of the neural current through Ψ is facilitated through modification of the contact barriers. As Amacher (1965) has shown, so far this theory was quite conventional and was distinguished from those of his teachers Brücke and Meynert and his older colleagues Exner and Breuer only by the number of separate neural systems Freud described. Even in distinguishing part of the Ψ system as an ego (*Ich*), Freud had a model in Meynert's *Psychiatry* (1884, Part I, p. 168; quoted by Amacher, 1965).

Quite early in the Project, Freud introduced the conception of "a cathected neurone filled with a certain $Q\dot{\eta}$ while at other times it may be empty" (1950 [1895], p. 298). He contrasted this condition of cathexis with "the hypothesis of a *current*" of quantity, only rarely (and apparently accidentally) speaking of cathexis when referring to moving charges of excitation.[7] So far as I know, this is the first introduction of the term "cathexis" (*Besetzung*), and it is important to note that at this time Freud was using it in a restricted, static sense. Although the German word derives from *sitzen*, "to sit" (Pinloche, 1922)—a static enough term!—it is easy to overlook the fact that "cathexis" was being used in this narrower sense if we approach the Project after familiarity with Freud's later works, in which "cathexis" is used for the energy of psychic apparatus, whether attaching to particular presentations or flowing in a current.

In the very conception of cathexis, then, Freud was using Breuer's idea of tonic excitation. Or was it Breuer's? Pribram (1962) tells us that at that time neurophysiologists commonly assumed that there was, in addition to the transmitted neural impulse, also a nontransmitted, quantitatively varying kind of excitation. Even Breuer's use of a term analogous to muscular tonus was not unique: Hartmann (personal communication, 1959) called my attention to the fact that Exner (1894) used the same terminology in his *Outline of an Explanation of Mental Phenomena*, published a year before Freud wrote the Project and almost certainly known by him. In discussing the sexual desires of young men, Exner wrote that the cortical center of energy from sexual sources "has at times an increased tonus, and only a small impulse is required to establish an association between certain cortical events and this center. The tonus can be so high that it almost appears not to matter which girl the youth encounters in this condition" (quoted and translated by Amacher, 1965, p. 53). The idea that nerve cells had such tonic, nontransmitted excitations which facilitated the passage of neural currents seems, therefore, to have been very much in the air and not Breuer's original idea. Perhaps this accounts for the fact that when Freud was writing so soon after Breuer's theoretical chapter had been completed, he felt no need to attribute this conception from the "common domain" to his friend and colleague. Or perhaps the explanation is a more emotional one,[8] for Freud had written to Fliess that he specifically disassociated himself from Breuer's theoretical contribution to their *Studies on Hysteria*. In any event, Freud emphasized the conception when he wrote that a quantity "passes more easily from a neurone to a cathected neurone than to an uncathected one . . . *cathexis is here shown to be equivalent, as regards the passage of* Qἠ, *to facilitation*" (1950 [1895], p. 319).

Freud used this conception to account for sleep, in the same way that Breuer had done: "the precondition of sleep is a *lowering of the endogenous load in the nucleus*" (1950 [1895], p. 336; a little further down the page he makes it clear that this means a partial draining or discharging of the nontransmitted cathexis of the ego). "Thus, by an automatic mechanism, the counterpart of the mechanism of attention, Ψ excludes the Φ impressions [those arising from the senses] so long as it itself is uncathected" (p. 337). "Dreams are devoid of motor discharge and, for the most part, of motor elements. We are paralyzed in dreams . . . The motor excitation cannot pass over the barrier when a neurone is uncathected" (p. 338).

Incidentally, in several later treatments of sleep Freud used this same explanatory principle. I have not found it in *The Interpretation of Dreams*, but in "A Metapsychological Supplement to the Theory of Dreams," a good deal is made of "the principle of the insusceptibility to excitation of uncathected systems" (1917d [1915] p. 234 n.). He used this "hint that a complete emptying of a system renders it little susceptible to instigation" (p. 227) to account for the fact that motor discharge is ordinarily excluded in dreaming; later (p. 234) he used it to account for the fact that "the possibility of reality testing is abandoned."

Again, in *Beyond the Pleasure Principle* (1920g), Freud made brief reference to the same idea, just this one time linking it to binding: "The higher the systems's own quiescent cathexis [cf. tonic excitation], the greater seems to be its binding force; conversely, therefore, the lower its cathexis, the less capacity will it have for taking up inflowing energy and the more violent must be the consequences of such a breach in the protective shield against stimuli" (1920g, p. 30). Strachey footnotes the phrase that ". . . inflowing energy" as an instance of "the principle of the insusceptibility to excitation of uncathected systems" (1920g, p. 30 n.). In this context, it is interesting to see that Freud is clearly emphasizing the binding rather than bound nature of such a system.

The last instance of this usage I found is in Freud's little paper on the mystic writing pad. At the end of that paper, he wrote:

> My theory was that cathectic innervations are sent out and withdrawn in rapid periodic impulses from within into the completely pervious system *Pcpt.* [*perceptual*]-*Cs.* So long as that system is cathected in this manner, it receives perceptions (which are accompanied by consciousness) and passes the excitation on to the unconscious mnemic systems; but as soon as the cathexis is withdrawn, consciousness is extinguished and the functioning of the system comes to a standstill. [1925a, p. 231]

Thus, there is a "periodic nonexcitability of the perceptual system," which is apparently due to its not being cathected; again, Strachey cites the "principle of insusceptibility" (1925a, p. 231 n.).

To return to the Project: From the beginning, Freud was concerned with the restraint of the passions. He saw the importance of violent impulses and affect-laden memories; he saw that in normal behavior they were restrained and in neurosis severely inhibited. A constant theme in his theorizing is to provide some way to account for this inhibition of impulse. Just as the whole conception of defense was as late as 1915 considered in dynamic terms as a vicissitude of the drives, so with the problem of controls generally. In its beginnings, psychoanalysis was a thoroughgoing dynamic-economic theory. Ultimately, Freud developed structural concepts to take care of most of these problems he was wrestling with in the 1890s, when economic, energic concepts seemed to offer a solution.

By means of a clever assumption, Freud made the facilitative effect of (tonic) cathexis account for inhibition. This was the assumption of lateral cathexes or side-cathexes: statically charged (cathected) neurones branching off from the main channel, which are thus in a state of enhanced readiness for the transmission of current. A lateral neurone thus defends by serving as a kind of safety valve; it drains off the current that would otherwise have proceeded through the apparatus, since that current is offered less resistance in the facilitated lateral pathway. Such a network of cathected lateral neurones is the ego: "Now the ego itself is a mass like this of neurones which hold fast to their cathexis—are, that is, in a bound state; and this, surely, can only happen as a result of the effect they have on one another" (1950 [1895], p. 368).

In this passage, Freud seems to equate the bound condition of the nerve cell with its retention of a (tonic) cathexis, so that this meaning is indeed quite close to Breuer's. Note, however, that a slight shift in emphasis is occurring: The bound neurones still facilitate the flow of the current of quantity, but because of their lateral position have the effect of *inhibiting* the flow toward discharge. Since *binden* and *hemmen* are quite close in meaning, it should not be surprising that Freud gradually seemed to forget that the bound (i.e., cathected) neurone primarily facilitates the quantitative flow, and that the inhibiting effect is attributable to the lateral placement of the ego neurones, not to their being bound.

Shortly after introducing the ego, Freud described how its inhibitory defense could be used against the arousal of hostile memories and the unpleasant affect entailed.

> . . . with the help of a mechanism which draws the ego's *attention* to the imminent fresh cathexis of the hostile mnemic image, the ego can succeed in inhibiting the passage of quantity from a mnemic image to a release of unplea- sure by a copious side-cathexis which can be strengthened according to need. Indeed, if we suppose that the original $Q\eta$ release of unpleasure is taken up by the ego itself, we shall have in it itself the source of the expenditure which is required by the inhibiting side-cathexis from the ego. (1950 [1895], p. 324)

Parenthetically, it is interesting to see here a precursor of the signal theory of anxiety, and also Freud's characteristic economy—the use of the energy of the anxiety signal to accomplish the lateral cathexis that draws off the charge from the unpleasant memory and prevents the process that would release unpleasure.

Somewhat later on, Freud came back to this same problem, control of memories that tend to be accompanied by unpleasant affect. He noted, first, that

> . . . in time they lose this capacity. . . . What is it, then, that happens to *memories* capable of affect till they are *tamed*? It cannot be supposed that 'time,' repetition, weakens their capacity for affect, since ordinarily that factor [repetition] actually contributes to strengthening an association. Something must no doubt happen in [the course of] 'time,' during the repetitions, which brings about this subjugation [of the memories]; and this can be nothing other than that a relation to the ego or to ego-cathexes obtains power over the memories. . . . [This happens even with certain memories which] have acquired an excessively strong facilitation to the release of unpleasure and affect. Particularly large and repeated binding from the ego is required be- fore this facilitation to unpleasure can be counterbalanced. (1950 [1895], pp. 380–381)

And a couple of paragraphs later he referred to "the inhibiting effect of binding by the ego . . . ." In these passages, it seems clear that what was first described as lateral cathexis ends up being called binding. Moreover, in explaining the "fact" that memory is hallucinatory at first and later becomes a thought process, Freud remarked that "a bound neurone does not admit of such a flow" (p. 381)—in the terminology of 1900, regression backward to perception.

If "binding" were used only as a shorthand expression for "inhibition by means of the institution of a lateral cathexis," there would be little problem. But in the course of this long, quickly written manuscript (unrevised because never intended for publication), we should hardly be surprised to find that Freud used the term "bound" a few more times in ways that do not seem entirely consistent.

Discussing the secondary process, he argued that it must operate with small amounts of quantity, then asked:

> How can it be arranged that such small $Q\acute{\eta}$ shall have open to them pathways which, after all, are only traversable by larger ones than Ψ as a rule receives? The only possible reply is that this must be a mechanical result of the side-cathexes. We must conclude that matters stand in such a way that when there is a side-cathexis small $Q\eta$ flow through facilitations which would ordinarily be traversed only by large ones. The side-cathexis as it were '*binds*' a quota of the $Q\eta$ flowing through the neurone. (1950 [1895], pp. 334–335)

This usage looks, at first sight, much like the ones just discussed: Binding is done by lateral cathexis. Note, however, that this would be a strange answer to the question he set out to answer—how small quantities can get through paths ordinarily impassable even to larger ones. Rather, it seems to be an answer to another, unasked question: How is it that secondary processes operate with small quantities? Moreover, it appears puzzling that Freud should say that the side-cathexis binds part of the quantity, when we might have expected just the opposite characterization (if it is enabled to flow despite being small, the enabling lateral cathexis might be said to free, not bind it). Yet despite the reference in his letter of October 20, 1895 (quoted above), to "the free and bound states of [quantity]," the Project nowhere contains any reference to a *free* state of quantity [and "unbound" occurs only once]. (To be sure, the letter was written *after* the sections of the Project that have come down to us.) There is nothing about the concept of lateral cathexis that explains how the impoverished current is enabled to penetrate better than before; indeed, to postulate this property would seem to undo the defensive function of lateral cathexis. For if the effect were to enable the diminished quantity to traverse the neural pathways just as well as ever (or even better, as we shall see in a moment), then most of the effects that defense is needed for would take place anyway—unless the small quantities have a diminished capacity to activate memory traces and otherwise to cause trouble.

In a later discussion of the secondary process, however, Freud noted that although small quantities are involved, "perception and memory during the process of thinking must be hypercathected, and more intensely than in simple perception" (1950 [1895], p. 368). He was aware that these assumptions created problems:

> Here we have two apparently opposing requirements: strong cathexis and weak displacement. If we want to reconcile the two, we arrive at the hypothesis of what is, as it were, a *bound state* in the neurone, *which, though there is a high cathexis, permits only a small current.* This hypothesis can be made more plausible if we reflect that the current in a neurone is obviously influenced by the cathexes surrounding it. Now the ego itself is a mass like this of neurones which hold fast to their cathexis—are, that is, in a bound state; and this, surely, can only happen as a result of the effect they have on one another. (p. 368)

This passage helps to clear up the preceding one, though not entirely. I am able to make sense of this conception only by introducing some assumptions that may have been implicit in Freud's mind. The critical paradox here is the sequence of ideas: (Tonic or bound) cathexis makes a neurone more permeable because the pre-existing excitation puts it on hairtrigger, so to speak; therefore, binding allows even a small current to flow; but through the influence of the adjacent mass of (bound) ego neurones, the neurone is able to "hold fast to its cathexis" and large currents can*not* pass. If a small current can excite a neurone and get transmitted, one would expect that a larger one would be able to *a fortiori*. How, then, to understand the non-transmissibility of the large currents? If we assume that a neurone has only a finite capacity of excitation, E, and that part of this amount is taken up by a nontransmitted cathexis, C, to which the neurone is enabled to "hold fast" by the aid of its neighbors (mechanism unspecified), then only the difference, $E-C$, can be transmitted. The presence of C makes the cell easily excited even by a small current and certainly by a large one; but it also acts like a bottleneck or sieve, so that only a small current *or a small quotient* of a larger one can get through. What remains unexplained is the means by which the neurone is enabled to retain its cathexis instead of discharging to its full capacity, which my hairtrigger image would suggest. All we know is Freud's hypothesis that the mutual influence of the cathected ego neurones has this effect. It is a kind of inhibition, as was the original explanation of defense by means of lateral cathexis, but there has been a subtle change in the type and means of interference with the passage of current, and it does not appear that the neighboring neurones are laterally connected, being merely described as "surrounding."

Freud continued:

We can therefore imagine that a perceptual [neurone] which is cathected with attention is as a result temporarily, as it were, [taken up] into the ego and is now subject to the same binding of its $Q\eta$ as are all the ego neurones. If it is cathected more strongly, then the quantity of current may in consequence be diminished, not necessarily increased. We may perhaps suppose that as a result of this binding precisely the external Q remains free to flow while the cathexis of attention is bound[9]; a relation which need not, of course, be an invariable one.

This bound state, which combines high cathexis with small current, would thus characterize processes of thought mechanically. It is possible to conceive of other processes in which the current runs parallel with the cathexis—processes with uninhibited discharge. (1950 [1895], pp. 368–369)

Freud here went further with the new line of thought: Absorption into the ego accomplishes binding (by mutual influence). When a bound perceptual (W) neurone's cathexis is heightened, the current flowing through it is diminished; only the quantity derived from the sense organs is transmitted, while the "cathexis of attention" (hypercathexis) is temporarily bound, presumably meaning that it stays put. Freud did not explain, however, what the behavioral or phenomenal correlate of flowing quantity and bound hypercathexis would be. But it is contrasted to "processes with an uninhibited discharge," the current of which runs parallel to the cathected ego neurones. This last stipulation harkens back to the inhibiting effect of *lateral* (side-branching) ego neurones, suggesting that perhaps all the ego neurones are lateral to one another after all, which would be topologically possible, granted sufficient arborization of dendrites. But we are left with the contradiction that some of the time side-cathexis inhibits the passage of large currents, and some of the time it facilitates the passage of small currents.

The sentence that immediately follows the last-quoted passage suggests that Freud was aware of some difficulties in the concept: "I hope the hypothesis of a bound state of this kind will turn out to be mechanically tenable" (p. 369). He went on, also, to say that this hypothesis "appears at first to suffer under an internal contradiction. If the [bound] state consists in only small Qs being left for displacement when there is a fresh cathexis of this kind, how can it . . . draw fresh neurones into it—that is, cause large Qs to travel into fresh neurones?" (p. 369). Despite the apparent promise to carry the argument further in the words "appears at first," Freud did not explain away the contradiction, and was back at the question he had raised on p. 334.

Let us not lose sight of the fact that, in all of the above, Freud was trying to explain delayed, adaptive, purposive thinking. In essentially the same way that he treated it in 1900, he tried to conceptualize a temporary inhibition of discharge, which would still allow the trial activity of thought to go on. So he tried to create an account of the way much work could be done with small quantities, and used the idea of the cathectic level as a facilitator: "when the level [of cathexis] is high, small quantities can be displaced more easily than when it is low" (p. 372). Finally, when the route to the goal object has been found and action is initiated, "The 'bound' state is renounced and the cathexes of attention are withdrawn. What no doubt happens . . . is that at the first passage [of Q] from the motor neurones the level in the ego falls irresistibly" (p. 386–387).[10] In this, his last use of the concept at the end of the Project, Freud again attributed binding to the stable cathexes of the ego neurones, and linked it to the inhibition of action that makes secondary-process thought possible.

Thus, even though in this first approximation to a complete theory Freud did not clarify his own thinking about the complexly related issues of inhibition, facilitation, and the binding of neurones, he came close enough to making the whole thing work so that when he next tried, in 1900, he achieved a great deal more success.

THE CONCEPT IN CHAPTER VII OF
THE INTERPRETATION OF DREAMS

Chapter VII of *The Interpretation of Dreams*, that extraordinary theoretical achievement, contains five slightly differing usages of our concept, all of them showing a family likeness to passages in the Project.

1. After setting forth in full detail his idea that the dream involves a backward flow of cathexis to the system *Pcpt.*, Freud says that changes in the cathexes of energy make possible this regression, "changes which increase or decrease the facility with which these systems can be passed through by the excitatory process" (1900a, p. 544). Here the context makes it clear that he was speaking about the only kind of change in cathexes that he had proposed, modifications in the degree of binding.

2. Freud used the term "quiescent [*ruhende*] cathexis" (which Strachey explicitly though perhaps unfortunately equates with "bound" [p. 601 n.]) in a brief passage describing one fate of "the energy attaching to a train of thought": It "sets the whole network of thoughts in a state of excitation which lasts for a certain time and then dies away as the excitation in search of discharge becomes transformed into a quiescent cathexis" (p. 594). Here is a survival of the original (Breuer-like, tonic) meaning of cathexis.

3. The principal and most explicit discussion of bound and free cathexes in Chapter VII is in his introduction of the concepts of primary and secondary processes. After describing the dream-work mechanisms of condensation and displacement, Freud wrote: " . . . the chief characteristic of these processes is that the whole stress is laid upon making the cathecting

energy mobile [*beweglich*] and capable of discharge" (p. 597). [A little later, he said that the irrational primary processes] "appear wherever ideas are abandoned by the preconscious cathexis [hypercathexis?], are left to themselves and can become charged with the uninhibited [*ungehemmten*] energy from the unconscious which is striving to find an outlet" (p. 605). It is not clear to me whether Freud meant that since the energy of unconscious wishes is itself free, condensation and displacement come about, or whether he thought that these mechanisms are used to make the cathexes free, as in the former of these passages. At any rate, it is obvious that freedom of cathexis in the primary process refers to an unstable relationship between ideas and their drive cathexes.

In the secondary process, by contrast, drive energies are bound— apparently through the offices of hypercathexis (see the quotation above from p. 605).

> [Speaking of the *Pcs.*, he said that the activity of this system] constantly feeling its way, and alternately sending out and withdrawing cathexes, needs on the one hand to have the whole of the material of memory freely at its command; but on the other hand it would be an unnecessary expenditure of energy if it sent our large quantities of cathexis along the various paths of thought and thus caused them to drain away to no useful purpose and diminish the quantity available for altering the external world. I therefore postulate that for the sake of efficiency the second system [i.e., the *Pcs.*] succeeds in retaining the major part of its cathexes of energy in a state of quiescence [*in Ruhe*] and in employing only a small part on displacement. (p. 599)

Recall his statement, in the Project, that the ego's energies are stable and bound. In this passage, "binding" is used in the sense of conserving and operating with small quantities, delaying what would otherwise be a rash and wasteful discharge. The passage quoted continues:

> The activity of the first Ψ-system is directed towards securing the *free discharge* of the quantities of excitation, while the *second* system, by means of the cathexes emanating from it, succeeds in inhibiting this *discharge* and in transforming the cathexis into a quiescent [*ruhende*] one, perhaps with a simultaneous raising of its potential . . . When once the second system has concluded its exploratory thought-activity, it releases the inhibition and damming-up of the excitations and allows them to discharge themselves in movement. (pp. 599–601)[11]

In this same part of Chapter VII, Freud goes on to talk about the problem of how the *Pcs.* deals with unpleasant ideas. It must be able to use them, to cathect the corresponding memory traces, and to bring an unpleasant but necessary idea to mind without its automatic banishment by the pleasure principle. To do so, it must have some way "to avoid releasing the unpleasure"; therefore, it cathects memories in such a way that there is an inhibition of their discharge . . . in the direction of the development of unpleasure. [Cf. his earlier concern with binding the dynamic memories of traumatic experience.] We have therefore been led from two directions [the first was the last passage quoted] to the hypothesis that cathexis by the second system implies a simultaneous inhibition of the discharge of excitation.

[Soon after, Freud added:] I propose to describe the psychical process of which the first system [the *Ucs.*] alone admits as the 'primary psychical process,' and the process which results from the inhibition imposed by the second system [the *Pcs.-Cs.*] as the 'secondary process.' (p. 601)

It is noteworthy, I think, that in these important pages, Freud used the words "inhibition" and "binding" almost interchangeably. This fact keeps us from losing sight of the fact that Freud had several considerations in mind, several related but different properties of the primary and secondary process. In the primary process, cathexes shift easily from idea to idea and [are said to] press for immediate discharge; in the secondary process, they are more stable (bound) and are prevented from discharge (inhibited).[12] Since "inhibition" has clear structural connotations in German (*Hemmung* is the catch of a gun, or the escapement of a watch—both of them restraining apparatuses), it is perhaps surprising that Freud did not introduce an avowedly structural concept to account for inhibition of discharge. He was quite explicit about his preference, however:

What we are doing here is once again to replace a topographical way of representing things by a dynamic one [replacing "structural" by "economic," in Rapaport and Gill's (1959) terminology]. What we regard as mobile (*das Bewegliche*) is not the psychical structure itself but its innervation [i.e., the energy flowing through it]. (pp. 610–611)

Since the only structural concept he had at the time was the topographic, with its often inconvenient implications of states of consciousness, it is understandable that he turned to energic concepts instead—overlooking the fact that, in physics, transformations of energy are brought about through changes in structural conditions.

4. After stating that free energies are used in the construction of the dream, Freud provided for their control through the proposition that these unconscious cathexes are

bound by the preconscious . . . The cathexis from the *Pcs.* which goes halfway to meet the dream after it has become perceptual, having been directed on to it by the excitation in consciousness [which makes it amply clear that Freud meant hypercathexis], binds the dream's unconscious excitation and makes it powerless to act as a disturbance. (p. 578)

Dreaming thus allows a partial discharge of the *Ucs.* impulse and "serves it as a safety valve and at the same time preserves the sleep of the preconscious in return for a small expenditure of waking activity" (p. 579), which keeps the discharge down to the small amounts that a hallucination can release, preventing access to the motor system and thus the discharge of massive amounts of cathexis.

5. Finally, hypercathexis, the easily shifted energy corresponding to attention, is spoken of several times as "mobile[13] cathectic energy" (e.g., p. 615). It is plain, in these contexts, that Freud in no way identified attention cathexis with the free drive energies of the primary process. Indeed, because of this special kind of hypercathectic mobility, it is apparent that there would be difficulties in the way of a purely economic explanation of the *way* that this preconscious cathexis brings about binding of drive cathexis. Later, we shall see that Freud returned to the same problem.

THE CONCEPT IN MIDLIFE WORKS
AND THE METAPSYCHOLOGICAL PAPERS

Freud's book of 1905 on jokes contains a relevant section analyzing the economics of laughter.[14] In it, the concept of bound and free cathexis plays an important part.

> In laughter, therefore, on our hypothesis, the conditions are present under which a sum of psychical energy which has hitherto been used for cathexis is allowed free discharge. [Note the contrast, in the fashion of the Project, between cathexis and energy.] And since . . . laughter at a joke . . . is an indication of pleasure, we shall be inclined to relate this pleasure to the liftng of the cathexis which has previously been present. If we see that the hearer of a joke laughs but that its creater cannot laugh, this may amount to telling us that in the hearer a cathectic expenditure has been lifted and discharged, while in the construction of the joke there have been obstacles either to the lifting or to the possibility of discharge . . . the cathectic energy used for the inhibition [of a "proscribed idea"] has now suddenly become superfluous and has been lifted, and is therefore now ready to be discharged by laughter . . . the hearer of the joke laughs with the quota of psychical energy which has become free through the lifting of the inhibitory cathexis . . . (1905c, pp. 148–149)

Here is an interesting passage, with a number of links to the Project and to later papers. Freud was saying now that inhibitory energy is released and is discharged as free energy in laughter at a joke. While Freud was not specific about it, there is every reason to suppose that this "cathexis used for the inhibition" is hypercathexis being used for anticathexis, not drive cathexis. Here, then, without using the term "binding," Freud used the concept or something like it in a way we shall see several times again, in what may be called a structure-building usage. When hypercathexis is used for anticathexis (i.e., to inhibit), it is in one sense bound, unavailable for other employment; and when the defensive task is over, it is released and becomes free again.

Just before he entered his second great phase of theoretical work, Freud wrote a short but pithy paper, in which he said, discussing the consequences for action of the institution of the reality principle:

> Restraint upon motor discharge (upon action), which then became necessary, was provided by means of the process of *thinking*, which was developed from the presentation of ideas. Thought was endowed with characteristics which made it possible for the mental apparatus to tolerate an increased tension of stimulus while the process of discharge was postponed. It is essentially an experimental kind of acting, accompanied by displacement of relatively small quantities of cathexis together with less expenditure (discharge) of them. For this purpose the conversion of freely displaceable cathexes into 'bound' cathexes was necessary, and this was brought about by means of raising the level of the whole cathectic process. (1911b, p. 221)

Here is a succinct restatement of a number of ideas from the Project, virtually unchanged except for being made clearer and more explicit.

In the metapsychological papers, Freud came back to the theory of the primary and secondary processes, and wrote the passages quoted above (see p. 75). They are quite similar to statements I have quoted from 1900; indeed, the dream book and "The Unconscious" are more alike than different in the way they link free versus bound energy to primary versus secondary process.[15] Yet the new emphasis on ideas as having their quotas of cathexis marks the emergence of the concept of binding in a very important form.

The hallmark of the primary process, the hypothetical operation underlying all the forms of the dream work, is the free shiftability of the cathexis that is attached to ideas and is discharged in affects or action. It is implied that every mental presentation must have a (drive) cathexis, and that it is necessary to the logical orderliness of secondary-process thinking that each cathexis (or sum of cathexes) stay with its own thought. Contrasting the primary and secondary processes, Freud said that an idea's cathectic charge passes easily from one to another in the primary process, and that all of such a charge may be displaced or condensed. In the secondary process, however, these latter operations are largely excluded, and only small amounts of cathexis pass from one thought to another. It is clear that binding is a relative matter as presented here: Various degrees of displacement are considered possible in the *Pcs.*, implicitly connoting different degrees of binding.

In another important passage, Freud again linked binding (which was not explicitly mentioned) with hypercathexis. He referred to the idea (introduced in the Project) that consciousness is related to verbal ideas, so that

. . . the conscious presentation of the object can now be split up into the presentation of the *word* and the presentation of the *thing* . . . the unconscious presentation is the presentation of the thing alone. The system *Ucs.* contains the thing-cathexes of the objects, the first and true object-cathexes; the system *Pcs.* comes about by this thing-presentation's being hypercathected through being linked with the word-presentations corresponding to it. It is these hypercathexes, we may suppose, that bring about a higher psychical organization and make it possible for the primary process to be succeeded by the secondary process which is dominant in the *Pcs.* (1915e, pp. 201–202)

Although this attempt to explain consciousness in terms of verbal ideas will not hold up, the passage gives a clearer hint than we have seen before of the way that binding may be conceptualized as being effected by the use of hypercathexis (see below).

In another metapsychological paper, "Mourning and Melancholia," written in 1915 but not published until 1917, Freud used the concept of bound energies in a slightly different way. Reviving an old image, which the editor of the *Standard Edition* notes had been in his (otherwise quite dissimilar) early unpublished note on melancholia in the Fliess correspondence, Freud wrote:

The complex of melancholia behaves like an open wound, drawing to itself cathectic energies—which in the transference neuroses we have called 'anticathexes' [*Gegenbesetzungen*, sometimes translated as "countercathexes"]—from all directions, and emptying the ego until it is totally impoverished. (1917e, [1915] p. 253)

In mania, the ego must have got over the loss of the object (or its mourning over the loss, or perhaps the object itself), and thereupon the whole quota of anticathexis which the painful suffering of melancholia had drawn to itself from the ego and 'bound' will have become available. (p. 255)[16]

The accumulation of cathexis which is at first bound and then, after the work of melancholia is finished, becomes free [*frei*] and makes mania possible must be linked with regression of the libido to narcissism. The conflict within the ego, which melancholia substitutes for the struggle over the object, must act like a painful wound which calls for an extraordinarily high anticathexis. (p. 258)

The image of the wound, which recurs in *Beyond the Pleasure Principle* (1920g), may have brought to Freud's mind the gathering of leucocytes, those tiny defenders of the bloodstream, around such a lesion. This configuration may have suggested the novel idea that the injury inflicted by the loss of a loved person draws the defensive units of psychoanalytic theory, anticathexes, and *binds* them (i.e., holds them to the task, pre-empting them from other uses).

The underlying observation here seems to be the impoverishment of the ego—the inability of the depressed person to do intellectual work, for example. We do not ordinarily think of such operations as being carried on by anticathexes, but the preceding seems to be one of the passages in which Freud suggested an identity of the defensively used energies and hypercathexis, the energy freely available to the ego for work in the conflict-free sphere.[17] To restate it in Hartmann's terms, in depression we see a narrowing of the conflict-free sphere of the ego as the hypercathectic energies of an (only relatively) autonomous ego are drawn by the emergency into defensive use.

If we follow Rapaport's interpretation of the binding concept (1959, pp. 92, 126–128), this passage is Freud's clearest statement of binding as structure formation. Note, however, that here *hypercathexes*, clearly not drive cathexes, are spoken of as bound. Rapaport suggested (in a personal communication, 1960) that "the melancholia centers on an identification, which *is* a structure." On this supposition, it is reasonable to interpret Freud as saying that the illness consists in the erection of a structure, in which hypercathexes are immobilized, but may be released again if the structure is demolished. I shall come back to this new meaning of binding later on.

THE CONCEPT IN *BEYOND THE*
PLEASURE PRINCIPLE

In the second paragraph of *Beyond the Pleasure Principle*, Freud rather diffidently introduced a new hypothesis and a new usage of binding:

> . . . the least rigid hypothesis, it seems to me, will be the best. We have decided to relate pleasure and unpleasure to the quantity of excitation that is present in the mind but is not in any way 'bound'; and to relate them in such a manner that unpleasure corresponds to an *increase* in the quantity of excitation and *pleasure* to a diminution. (1920g, pp. 7–8)

Here is a surprising new usage of *gebunden* in the context of the pleasure principle, which Freud had discussed a number of times before, but never in this way.

In line with the general character of this, Freud's most speculative work, we find that in its later pages he returned to the problem of pleasure and unpleasure in a rather different way, with no backward glance at this preliminary formulation, and at the end broke off the paper as a whole rather abruptly, noting that the issue "raises a host of other questions to which we can at present find no answer" (pp. 63–64). A few paragraphs before those words, he had said:

> . . . there seems to be no doubt whatever that the unbound or primary processes give rise to far more intense feelings in both directions than the bound or

secondary ones . . . whatever it is that causes the appearance of feelings of pleasure and unpleasure in processes of excitation must be present in the secondary process just as it is in the primary one. (p. 63)[18]

In this formulation, he retains the idea that the most intense pleasures are those of the unbound energies, but concedes that affects exist when energies are bound. The earlier statement, then, was a first approximation, which is made more tenable by these later restrictions. [As we saw in Chapter 3,] it was characteristic of Freud to think aloud this way, and to retain his unqualified preliminary formulations—which can sound so outrageous when quoted out of context.

Much of this work is concerned with the concept of a "compulsion to repeat" and the closely related death instinct, which together constitute what lies "beyond the pleasure principle." They are assumed to be primordial antagonists to the pleasure principle and Eros: "there really does exist in the mind a compulsion to repeat which overrides the pleasure principle" (p. 22). How, then, can the pleasure principle attain its characteristic predominance?

It will perhaps not be thought too rash to suppose that the impulses arising from the instincts do not belong to the type of *bound* nervous processes but of *freely mobile* processes which press towards discharge . . .

Since all instinctual impulses have the unconscious systems as their point of impact, it is hardly an innovation to say that they obey the primary process. Again, it is easy to identify the primary psychical process with Breuer's freely mobile cathexis and the secondary process with changes in his bound or tonic cathexis. If so, it would be the task of the higher strata of the mental apparatus to bind the instinctual excitation reaching the primary process. A failure to effect this binding would provoke a disturbance analogous to a traumatic neurosis; and only after the binding had been accomplished would it be possible for the dominance of the pleasure principle (and of its modification, the reality principle) to proceed unhindered. Till then the other task of the mental apparatus, the task of mastering or binding excitations, would have precedence—not, indeed in *opposition* to the pleasure principle, but independently of it and to some extent in disregard of it. (pp. 34–35)

A little further on, he describes further what he has in mind:

We have found that one of the earliest and most important functions of the mental apparatus is to bind the instinctual impulses which impinge on it, to replace the primary process prevailing in them by the secondary process and convert their freely mobile cathectic energy into a mainly quiescent (tonic) cathexis. While this transformation is taking place no attention can be paid to the development of unpleasure; but . . . the transformation occurs on *behalf* of the pleasure principle; the binding is a preparatory act which introduces and assures the dominance of the pleasure principle. . . . The binding of an instinctual impulse would be a preliminary function designed to prepare the excitation for its final elimination in the pleasure of discharge. (p. 62)

In this formulation, binding is given a most basic task, that of mastering unruly and dangerous forces and making them manageable enough so that the pleasure principle can begin to operate. If the idea that the primary process operates with unbound energies were retained, then the paradoxical (and surely unintended) conclusion would be that the pleasure principle operated only in the secondary process! But the primary process is the true home of the pleasure principle, and to deny this basic proposition would overthrow much of the structure of the whole theory. Therefore, it seems probable that Freud meant to assume two quantitative stages or degrees of binding: a minimal one which would contain the instinctual energy enough to make the pleasure principle (and thus the primary process) possible, and then increasing degrees corresponding to transitional stages between the logical extremes of primary and secondary process. Perhaps Freud got himself into this difficulty through an attempt to make the distinction between bound and free cathexis correspond to that between the energies of Eros and the death instinct. This was, after all, his first introduction of the latter concept, and he did not say at this time that there might be separate energies for each of the instincts, though later on (when he made extensive use of the concept of instinctual fusion), he made this assumption explicit and abandoned the attempt to make binding the critical point of differentiation.

The other principal way in which the concept of binding appears in *Beyond the Pleasure Principle* is in connection with a figure of speech that is strikingly reminiscent of the one quoted from "Mourning and Melancholia." In this passage, Freud introduced the concept of the "protective shield" against stimuli (the *Reizschutz*, sometimes translated as "stimulus barrier"). He started with the hypothesis of a unicellular organism whose periphery is sensitive and unprotected against a surround of dangerously intense physical energies. The very effect of these impacts, in killing the outer layer, is to create a protection for the layers beneath, since Freud assumed that the dead layer of protoplasm would be more impervious to entering energies. Then, by a bold leap, Freud applied this conception to man, only gradually making it clear that when he spoke about "the protective shield's having been broken through" he did not mean the skin or any other somatic element.

This conception turns out to be basic to his explanation of traumatic neurosis:

> We describe as 'traumatic' any excitations from outside which are powerful enough to break through the protective shield. . . . such an event . . . is bound to provoke a disturbance on a large scale in the functioning of the organism's energy and to set in motion every possible defensive measure. At the same time, the pleasure principle is for the moment put out of action. There is no longer any possibility of preventing the mental apparatus from being flooded with larger amounts of stimulus, and another problem arises instead—the problem of mastering the amounts of stimulus which have broken in and of binding

them, in the psychical sense, so that they can then be disposed of. . . . Cathectic energy is summoned from all sides to provide sufficiently high cathexes of energy in the environs of the breach. An 'anticathexis' on a grand scale is set up, for whose benefit all the other psychical systems are impoverished, so that the remaining psychical functions are extensively paralyzed or reduced. (pp. 29–30)

In this last passage, Freud harkened back to the "open wound" of melancholia. Note that here, however, the anticathexes are not bound by the painful suffering, but they themselves do the binding of the free energy that is hypothetically pouring into the organism through the breach in the protective shield. Nevertheless, both are structure-building conceptions.

[Freud continued:] . . . we infer that a system which is itself highly cathected is capable of taking up an additional stream of fresh, inflowing energy and converting it into quiescent cathexis, that is of binding it psychically . . . As a new factor we have taken into consideration Breuer's hypothesis that charges of energy occur in two forms; so that we have to distinguish between two kinds of cathexis of the psychical systems or their elements—a freely flowing cathexis that presses on towards discharge and a quiescent cathexis. We may perhaps suspect that the binding of the energy that streams into the mental apparatus consists in its change from a freely flowing into a quiescent state. (pp. 30–31)

In these passages from the 1920 work, most of the time Freud used the concept of psychic energy without regard to its relation to specific ideas, though in the penultimate sentence just quoted he did speak of "kinds of cathexis of the psychical systems or their elements," by which last term I take it he means thoughts and ideas. For the most part, he used it to account for different degrees of quiescence versus pressure for discharge.

Freud next considered the role of sexual excitations in trauma and the fact that traumatic neuroses are more likely to occur when there has been no physical injury.

Thus, on the one hand, the mechanical violence of the trauma would liberate a quantity of sexual excitation which, owing to the lack of preparation for anxiety, would have a traumatic effect; but, on the other hand, the simultaneous physical injury, by calling for a narcissistic[19] hypercathexis of the injured organ, would bind the excess of excitation. (p. 33)

In these pages Freud suggested that the mechanism of binding is to be sought in the fact that additional (hypercathectic) energies are brought to bear. What remains unclear is how the first binding of cathexis could take place in the infant, before the development of the first anticathexes. Possibly it implies that there is a primordial and autonomous source of hypercathexis, something that Freud hinted at in several places and Hartmann (1950) treats more specifically.

Several other usages of the concept under scrutiny appear in *Beyond the Pleasure Principle*. For example:

> The patient behaves in a purely infantile fashion and thus shows us that the repressed memory-traces of his primeval experience are not present in him in a bound state and are indeed in a sense incapable of obeying the secondary process. It is to this fact of not being bound, moreover, that they owe their capacity for forming, in conjunction with the residues of the previous day, a wishful phantasy that emerges in a dream. (p. 36)

Here it is the memory trace that is bound or not bound, not the cathexis of an idea or the stream of energy. Indeed, Freud seems to imply that only certain traces (the bound ones) are available to the secondary process—a conception quite at variance with the one implied in his usual treatment of primary and secondary process. This sounds very much like a momentary throwback to his first theory of neurosis, in which it was the traumatic memory that caused the trouble. With the shift of responsibility to the drive that pushes memories into consciousness, the concept of binding is applied to the energy that cathects the traces—which Freud may have really meant here.

In another passage, Freud raised, but did not answer a rhetorical question: "Should the difference between these findings ['feelings . . . of a peculiar tension which in its turn can be either pleasurable or unpleasurable'] enable us to distinguish between bound and unbound processes of energy?" (p. 63). This is very close to Breuer's notion that binding could be directly sensed as a subjective state of tension. In both cases, however, we seem to be dealing with what Whitehead (1925) called "the fallacy of misplaced concreteness." A process like the binding of hypothetical psychic energy is on far too high a level of conceptual abstraction to be directly coordinated to a quality of experience. Besides, a little reflection reminds us that states of tension often accompany primary-process thinking, and states of relaxation do not rule out the possibility of effective secondary-process thinking, as would be implied by this proposition.

In one other place, Freud used the concept of bound and free energies in a way much more like Breuer's than his own (cf. also p. 84 above). In the context of his speculations about the origins of the protective shield against stimuli, Freud tried to derive one of his favorite ideas (one which, incidentally, appears in Breuer's theoretical chapter and in the Project)—that the system *Cs.* has no power of retention but can merely pass along excitations, adding to them the quality of consciousness.

> It may be supposed that, in passing from one element [of the psychic apparatus] to another, an excitation has to overcome a resistance, and that the diminution of resistance thus effected is what lays down a permanent trace of the excitation, that is, a facilitation. In the system *Cs.*, then, resistance of this kind to

passage from one element to another would no longer exist. This picture can be brought into relation with Breuer's distinction between quiescent (or bound) and mobile cathectic energy in the elements of the psychical systems; the elements of the system *Cs.* would carry no bound energy but only energy capable of free discharge. (pp. 26–27)

Recall that in Breuer's theory, tonic (i.e., bound) excitations—like cathexes in the Project—were not "carried" or transmitted from one neurone to another in any part of the apparatus. But with the idea that conscious thought involved mobile energy, Freud again approached his former friend's views. He attributed the failure of the system *Cs.* to form memory traces to a presumed lack of resistance to the passage of excitation, and apparently in doing so reverted to the conception (last encountered in the Project) that the contact barriers resist the passage of a current only in the Ψ system. Yet the idea that the system *Cs.* is *unable* to transmit bound cathexes seems glaringly out of keeping with the many statements elsewhere that bound energies *are* used in the *Pcs.* and *Cs.* An intimation of such a discrepancy may account for the sentence that immediately follows the above-quoted ones: "It seems best, however, to express oneself as cautiously as possible on these points" (p. 27).

In this one long paper, written directly after the war in an attempt to account for phenomena that threw doubt on the most basic premises of Freud's system, we have seen that there are several differing and indeed partly incompatible usages of the concept of binding. Jones (1957) has written about this book:

> In dealing with such ultimate problems as the origin of life and the nature of death Freud displayed a boldness of speculation which was unique in all his writings. . . . It is somewhat discursively written, almost as if by free associations, and there are therefore occasional gaps in the reasoning. . . . This mode of writing in itself indicates that the ideas propounded must be transmuted from some personal and profound source . . . (p. 266)

Jones comments further that it differed from Freud's previous work in giving evidence that Freud had at long last unleashed his penchant for philosophic speculation, about which he had on a number of occasions said that he feared it and tried to check it firmly.

Once he did release his long inhibition and came to grips with the problem of death, which had haunted his thoughts for at least 20 years, Freud left behind much of his accustomed rigor and clarity of thought and writing. The confusions in the applications of the concept of binding seem like symptomatic expressions that something unusual was going on. And that something was the genesis of his most controversial (and among other analysts least accepted) doctrine, that of the death instinct.

THE CONCEPT IN LATER WORKS

In Freud's major work of 1923, *The Ego and the Id*, binding and related concepts are referred to several times. In speaking about the ego's energy, he wrote: "We have reckoned as though there existed in the mind—whether in the ego or in the id—a displaceable energy, which, neutral [indifferent] in itself, can be added to a qualitatively differentiated erotic or destructive impulse, and augment its total cathexis" (1923b, p. 44). He spoke about this displaceable energy [*Verschiebungsenergie*] frequently in the next four pages. Another significant passage reads:

> . . . this displaceable libido is employed in the service of the pleasure principle to obviate blockages and to facilitate discharge. . . . If this displaceable energy is desexualized libido, it may also be described as *sublimated* energy; for it would still retain the main purpose of Eros—that of uniting and binding—in so far as it helps towards establishing the unity, or tendency to unity, which is particularly characteristic of the ego. (p. 45)

The displaceable energy in question seems to be the same as the *mobil* energy of Chapter VII, or hypercathexis. As before, here the suggestion is that binding is accomplished by means of hypercathexis.

There is some doubt, however, that in these passages Freud meant the binding of cathexis; it sounds as if he was using *binden* in a general literary sense as a synonym of *vereinigen*. Indeed it is probable that Freud was discussing here the synthetic function, not binding in the narrow sense. In the spirit of these passages, Nunberg (1931) speaks about the synthetic function as being synonymous with binding, and as having the characteristics of Eros.

Very shortly thereafter, Freud used the term in a somewhat different way: ". . . the ego deals with the first object-cathexes of the id . . . by taking over the libido from them into itself and binding it to the alteration of the ego produced by means of identification" (pp. 45–46). Here he was clearly speaking of the process by which the ego captures cathectic energy by offering itself to the id as a love object. It is an interesting introduction of identification into this obscure process, but the usage seems again nontechnical.

There are a number of other passages in *The Ego and the Id*, however, that imply a new technical meaning. Freud started with a discussion of a condition in which love has been transformed into hate of the object:

> Here again the instinct of destruction has been set free [*frei*] and it seeks to destroy the object. (p. 53)

> After sublimation the erotic component no longer has the power to bind the whole of the destructiveness that was combined with it, and this is released in

the form of an inclination to aggression and destruction. This defusion . . .
(pp. 54–55)

A few pages later, discussing sublimation further, he said that it produces a defusion of instincts and a setting free of the aggressive drive in the super-ego. So here, free and bound are contrasted, but they are now assimilated to the new concept of defused and fused instinctual drives.

A very similar usage occurs in an important paper of the next year. He wrote of the death instinct that part of it "remains inside the organism and, with the help of the accompanying sexual excitation . . . , becomes libidi-nally 'bound' there" (1924c, pp. 163–164).[20]

Freud was apparently taken at this time with the idea that the two drives existed simultaneously (even in the single cell) in a kind of relation-ship whereby Eros held in check the destructiveness of the death drive when they were fused, and released this destructiveness on defusion. This is an interesting return of the early attempt to explain defense and control in dynamic–economic terms (e.g., as instinctual vicissitudes). How ironic that in the monograph wherein Freud introduced his principal structural con-cepts, he made a partial retreat from a structural view of control and defense! Nothing is said about what brings about or maintains a condition of fusion or defusion; and it gets Freud into the curious position of saying that whenever there is sublimation, there must be an increase in "inclinations to aggression and destruction."

Freud's next great theoretical work, *Inhibitions, Symptoms and Anx-iety*, contains several passages that seem to be relevant, but only two of them clearly bear on binding of cathexis, in relation to anxiety. In the ninth section of the book, Freud wrote that "symptoms are formed only in order to avoid anxiety: they bind the psychical energy which would otherwise be discharged as anxiety" (1926d, p. 144).[21]

Here we seem to have a revival of the old inhibitory meaning: Binding is a process that prevents discharge. On the other hand, this may well be interpreted as a structure-building usage: Here the symptoms would be the structures into which cathexes are bound. The case is not entirely clear, since this latter usage usually means that *anticathexes* are bound into the structure, whereas here Freud was probably speaking about drive cathexis.

On the last page of the Addenda to *Inhibitions, Symptoms and Anxiety*, there appears a rather obscure sentence that *seems* to say that psychic pain involves high bound cathexis. Freud was speaking about the state in which a person has lost a loved object:

If the feeling of unpleasure that then arises has the specific character of pain . . . instead of manifesting itself in the reactive form of anxiety, we may plausibly attribute this to a factor which we have not sufficiently made use of in our explanations—the high level of cathexis and 'binding' that prevails while these processes that lead to a feeling of unpleasure take place. (p. 172)

Parenthetically, this last passage is noteworthy for the explicit way in which it makes binding a quantitatively varying concept, rather than being all-or-none as it frequently sounded before. Rapaport pointed out (personal communication, 1960) that here Freud may mean again the binding of anticathexes into a defensive structure—the identification with the lost, mourned-for object. In such a case, the resulting hypercathectic shortage should produce a sensation of emptiness, the peculiarly unpleasant or painful affect of depression (or depersonalization). The painful affect would then be an indirect, not a direct, effect of "the high level of cathexis and 'binding' that prevails."

To deal with the other usages quickly: In one, Freud used binding in the sense of the synthetic function as in *The Ego and the Id* ("Its desexualized energy still shows traces of its origins in its impulsion to bind together and unify, and this necessity to synthesize grows stronger in proportion as the strength of the ego increases"—1926d, p. 98); and in one[22] he applied the term "freely mobile"—hitherto reserved for cathexis in the nonbound state—to an ego function. This last passage is a discussion of the compulsion to repeat, and Freud was simply saying that it is opposed by a kind of flexibility. Despite the verbal coincidence, he was clearly not talking about energic cathexes.

In the *New Introductory Lectures on Psycho-Analysis* (1933a), I found six passages in which Freud used the concept, but no new usages. [First he attributes to id energy "a state different from that in the other regions of the mind, far more mobile and capable of discharge" (p. 74). Then come the ideas that "masochistic impulses" bind "destructive trends" (p. 116) and that] free aggression is bound by the superego (p. 150); that anxiety is "psychically bound" by symptoms (p. 118) [just as "the fear of demons" undergoes "psychical binding" by religion (p. 166)]; and that repressed impulses are bound by "defensive acts" (p. 125).

Again, in "Analysis Terminable and Interminable," Freud referred obliquely to the destructive drive or one component of it ("the sense of guilt and need for punishment") as being "psychically bound by the superego" while other portions may exist elsewhere, "bound or free" (1937c, p. 242).

In all the works of this period of ego psychology, we find that the concept is usually applied to drive energy at large, not in its relation to ideas. Doubtless that was because of the fact that Freud had made no major additions to his theory of thinking; rather, he was trying to work out the implications of his new dual-instinct theory, his final theory of anxiety, and the idea of ego synthesis.

)

THE CONCEPT IN *AN OUTLINE OF PSYCHO-ANALYSIS*

When Freud came to write his last major work, **An Outline of Psycho-Analysis** (1940a), in which he stated his ideas "in the most concise form and in the most positive terms," there are three major statements about binding, two of them in relation to the theory of thinking. After introducing the idea of mental qualities (conscious, preconscious, unconscious), Freud asked:

> [What] is the true nature of the state which is revealed in the id by the quality of being unconscious and in the ego by that of being preconscious and in what does the differences between them consist? But of that we know nothing. . . . We assume, as the other natural sciences have led us to expect, that in mental life some kind of energy is at work; but we have nothing to go upon which will enable us to come nearer to a knowledge of it by analogies with other forms of energy. We seem to recognize that nervous or psychical energy exists in two forms, one freely mobile[23] and another, by comparison, bound; we speak of cathexes and hypercathexes of psychical material, and even venture to suppose that a hypercathexis brings about a kind of synthesis of different processes—a synthesis in the course of which free [*freie*] energy is transformed into bound [*gebundene*] energy. . . . we hold firmly to the view that the distinction between the unconscious and the preconscious state lies in dynamic relations of this kind. (1940a, pp. 163–164)

He went on to say that one new fact lies behind all these uncertainties: the knowledge that the laws of primary process govern "processes in the unconscious or in the id" while those of the secondary regulate "events in the preconscious, in the ego" (p. 164).

In this passage, Freud came full circle to his first writings on binding in the Project and in *The Interpretation of Dreams*, where the concept was closely connected with that of the primary and secondary processes. The basic observation underlying this association he restated a little later on in this last work: "From the evidence of the existence of these two tendencies to condensation and displacement our theory infers that in the unconscious id the energy is in a freely mobile state [*freier beweglichkeit*]" (p. 168). To understand the cognitive transformation of the dream, one must assume the mechanisms of the dream work, and the theory of cathectic mobility restates these operations in terms of the energy language with elegant simplicity. And the idea that first appeared in the Project, then in various other contexts, makes a final appearance: Hypercathexes accomplish binding by means of a "synthesis of different processes."

The last reference is as follows: "Its [the ego's] psychological function consists in raising the passage [of events] in the id to a higher dynamic level (perhaps by transforming freely mobile [*frei bewegliche*] energy into bound energy, such as corresponds to the preconscious state)" (p. 199). At the end of his life, Freud thus still maintained the proposition that a distinction between bound and free energies explained something about the difference between the secondary process and the primary process, and that between the unconscious and the preconscious condition of processes, even though he never made wholly clear in much detail what he meant, nor how ego functions involving hypercathexes and synthesis can bind the originally fluid energies. Moreover, he applied the concept to the energies of the id and the preconscious ego generally, as well as to the specific relation of cathexes to ideas and thoughts. In it, he dropped most of the different usages that had occurred to him at earlier times, and left us with a relatively unitary conception with which to work in trying to establish a satisfactory definition.

DISCUSSION OF THE VARIOUS DEFINITIONS

In the accompanying exhibit [Table 4.1], I have tried to summarize all the various definitions of binding versus freedom and their subvarieties. Besides Breuer's original concept, Freud contributed 14 different usages of these terms, only two minor ones of them (usages 2 and 13, plus his original concept of cathexis) having much in common with Breuer's. In a way, this table exemplifies a good deal of the development of psychoanalytic theory. As Freud's ideas and his conception of man grew, earlier meanings became obsolete. Thus, for example, the first three of the senses in which he used the term are intimately tied to his early neurophysiological models. When he adopted a purely psychological theory, they dropped by the wayside. Nevertheless, it is interesting to reflect that two of them were structural attempts to solve what today [i.e., in 1962] would be considered structural problems: control, delay, and the development of thought.

    Similarly, four of the other usages are basically attempts to solve structural problems of control and defense by means of a dynamic–economic concept. After the introduction of the structural point of view in 1923 (and especially after its elaboration by Rapaport; e.g., Rapaport, 1957, 1958a; Rapaport & Gill, 1959; Rapaport, Gill, & Schafer, 1945–1946), psychoanalysis has had concepts of psychic structure that made usages 4, 5, 6, 7, 8, and 11 unnecessary. (In addition, usage 8 is little more than a curiosity, since it deals with the pseudo problem of *physical* energies, which do *not* pour into the human organism when the latter is injured.)

    Sense 11 is required by and useful only in connection with the theory of life and death instincts, which has not found wide acceptance among analysts. The psychological issue dealt with (the control of destructiveness) is better handled by means of structural concepts (e.g., defense).

    Sense 13 is another curiosity, a throwback to Breuer, which may be contradictory to and inconsistent with most of the other usages (especially

#4, 5, and 6). Again, the issue involved can be dealt with simply by means of structural concepts.

Sense 12 is a general descriptive statement which seems to have little essential theoretical content.

Sense 10, which links affects and the degree to which cathexis is bound, raises the question of the relation of binding to neutralization. Hartmann (1950) has been reluctant to equate these two concepts; although Rapaport did explicitly say (1951a) that they meant the same thing, or that binding was the means by which neutralization came about, both he and Gill as well as G. S. Klein (personal communications, 1961) agree that the two processes are theoretically quite separate. It seems fairly clear that the qualitative change in cathectic energy brought about by the new structural conditions of the defenses, controls, and other apparatuses of primary and secondary autonomy is best called "neutralization." Since, as we have seen, Freud once used binding to describe just such consequences of delay and inhibition[24] (especially sense 5), there was good precedent for considering binding to be closely related to neutralization. The latter concept is now firmly established, and has pre-empted the meaning of sense 5; moreover, it can only clarify the concept of binding to give up this sense and strive for a single definition that is clearly differentiated from neutralization.

Therefore, let us assume that the processes of binding and neutralization are distinguishable but proceed more or less coordinately, as two relatively independent consequences of maturation. Sense 10 then becomes unnecessary (as does #2). To the degree that the "taming of affects" (Fenichel, 1934) implies a change in the cathexes involved, that change should be considered to be neutralization, not binding.

What remain, unsupplanted by later developments of the theory, are two concepts: #9, binding as a kind of relation between cathectic quanta and ideas, the contents or material of the mind; and #14, mobility as a special property of hypercathexis. Moreover, the first of these concepts is an essential part of the theory of primary and secondary process. So let us examine conception #9 once more.

The sense of Freud's discussions in 1900 and 1915 is that in the most primitive kind of thinking, ideas are cathected with psychic energy that has an unstable and irregular relation to them. It is easily displaced or lost by condensation; thus, it is called "freely moving" [*frei bewegende*]. As Gill (1963) points out, in the primary process cathectic freedom is never complete, but always relative: The primary process is not the chaos that absolute freedom of drive cathexis would imply, with an incessant shifting, fragmentation, and recombination of ideas. When we speak of condensation and displacement as mechanisms, we imply structures that regulate free cathexis, use it in specific ways, and set limits to its fluidity. Freud hinted at one such structural condition that brought a purposive order to the potential

TABLE 4.1   Summary of Definitions and Definition-like Propositions
Concerning Binding and Free Mobility in the Writings of Freud
and Breuer

a. Tonic (or, sometimes, quiescent) excitation [N.B.: *not* tonic binding], or
   cathexis, is a state of neurones of a slight continuous excitation, which facilitates the transmission of the current required for thought (Breuer, in Breuer &
   Freud, 1985; Freud, 1950 [1895], 1917d, 1925a).
   Referent: the neurone, its physiological excitation. A dynamic concept of
   facilitation. (Freud's original concept of cathexis, vs. the insusceptibility to
   excitation of uncathected systems.)

1. Tonic (bound) energies can be subjectively felt, corresponding to states of
   phenomenal tension or affect (Breuer, in Breuer & Freud, 1985; Freud, 1920g
   [cf. #10, below]).
   Referent: physiological or psychic energy. A phenomenological concept.

2. Binding is the channeling of excitation into usual channels of instinctual discharge, preventing its transformation into anxiety (Freud, 1894a, [1911c,
   1933a; or into grandiosity, 1911c]).
   Referent: the stream of neural energy [or libido]. A protostructural concept.

3. Binding enables the ego neurones (or neighboring neurones) to accumulate
   and retain much Quantity (cathexis) and to let only a small amount of it flow
   on to other neurones (Freud, 1950 [1895]).
   Referent: neurones; their physiological excitation. A structural (neurohisto-
   logical) concept.

4. Binding is a process carried on by the ego on memory traces, preventing them
   from giving rise to unpleasure (Freud, 1950 [1895]).
   Referent: memory traces. A concept of defense (structural).

4a. Binding is a way of cathecting memory traces to inhibit their discharge
    (Freud, 1900a; cf. #4, almost identical).

4b. When not bound, a memory trace is available to the primary process for dream
    formation; when bound, it is available to the secondary process (Freud, 1920g).

5. Bound energy (or quiescent cathexis) is inhibited from the immediate discharge that free cathexis seeks, delayed until the appropriate need-satisfying
   object can be found; the process of binding raises the potential of psychic
   energy (enabling small amounts to do much thought work) (Freud, 1950
   [1895], 1900a, 1911b, 1926d, 1933a).
   Referent: the stream of cathectic (psychic) energy. A structural–economic
   concept.

6. Binding is a process that prevents the regressive flow of cathexis to *Pcpt.*, by
   causing neurones to hold fast to their cathexes (Freud, 1950 [1895], 1900a).
   Referent: neurones; cathectic charges. A structural concept.

7. Binding is a process in which anticathexes are held to one controlling or
   defensive task (e.g., the work of mourning) and thus are unavailable for other
   work (Freud, 1917d).
   Referent: anticathexes (hypercathexes). A structure-building concept.

8. Binding is a process carried out by anticathexes to master dangerous breakthroughs of physical energy rupturing the *Reizschutz* (Freud, 1920g).
   Referent: physical energies. A structural (structure-building) concept.

TABLE 4.1 (*Continued*)

8a. Binding is a process of converting traumatically inflowing physical energy into quiescent cathexis by the operation of a narcissistic hypercathexis of the injured organ (i.e., by bringing to bear additional libidinal energies) (Freud, 1920g).

9. The free energies of the primary process are easily condensed or displaced from one idea to another; when energy is bound in the secondary process, only part of it can be displaced from its idea (Freud, 1950 [1895], 1900a, 1911b, 1915e).

    Referent: cathexes of ideas. An economic concept.

9a. Binding of the cathexes of the "material of the mind" occurs through the operation of hypercathexes and the synthetic function (Freud, 1940a; cf. #5 and 9).

10. Free (unbound) excitation is the energy construct corresponding to affect; when it increases in quantity, pain results; when it decreases (i.e., is bound), pleasure results. Binding corresponds to stability, free mobility to instability (Freud, 1920g; see also 1950 [1895], bound quantity is stable; and 1900a, p. 594).

    Referent: cathectic energy (generally). An economic–phenomenological concept.

10a. Binding is a process which, when applied to cathexis to a high degree, gives rise not to anxiety but to psychic pain (Freud, 1926d).

11. Destructive freedom is the original condition of drive energy; the ego binds it and, by curbing its destructiveness, makes possible the operation of the pleasure principle (Freud, 1920g).

    Referent: cathectic energy in general. An economic–structural concept.

11a. Binding is the controlling of destructiveness accomplished by the fusion of the energies of the life and death instincts (Freud, 1923b, 1924c, 1926d, 1933a).

11b. The superego binds the energy of the death instinct (Freud, 1933a, 1937c).

12. The ego binds energy, thereby raising id processes to a higher dynamic level (Freud, 1919g, 1923b, 1940a [cf. #3, 4, 5]).

    Referent: cathectic energy (id processes). An economic–structural concept.

[12a. The ego ideal binds narcissistic and homosexual libido, making it available to the ego (Freud, 1914c).]

13. Bound energy cannot be carried by elements of the system *Cs.*, only mobile energy; otherwise memory traces would be laid down in the *Cs.*, which cannot be (Freud, 1920g; cf. definition a).

    Referent: drive cathexis (bound) versus hypercathectic energy (mobile). An economic–structural concept.

14. Hypercathexis, the neutral energy freely available to the ego for use in defense (anticathexis) and consciousness (attention cathexis) is mobile (*mobil*) or displaceable (*vershiebend*) (Freud, 1950 [1895], 1900a, 1923b).

    Referent: hypercathexes of the *Cs.* or *Pcs.* ego. Not to be confused with free drive cathexes. An economic concept.

chaos of the primary process when he noted repeatedly that the censorship (or, more generally, defenses) makes use of condensation and displacement to disguise threatening material. The effective limitation of the primary process to the drive organization of memories (see below) is another structural condition setting limits to the possible scope of cathectic freedom. Other such conditions remain to be specified [see Chapter 10, this volume].

Be that as it may, a kind of change takes place, the result of which is that the cathectic charge becomes increasingly more difficult to separate from its idea—a state that is aptly called "bound." A bound cathexis stays with a content, at least for the most part, contributing to the sustained identity of thoughts.

Freud was always convinced that it made a good deal of difference whether a process was conscious or not; in recent years, a number of researchers from the Research Center for Mental Health (Bach, 1960; Klein, 1959; Klein & Holt, 1960; Klein, Spence, Holt, & Gourevitch, 1958; Pine, 1960) and elsewhere (e.g., Fisher, 1960a) have shown some of the differences that focal awareness contributes to a perceptual or other thought process. In general, it has turned out that the hypercathexis of attention produces secondary-process thought operations; and without hypercathexis, the way is opened for the primary process to operate on the cognitive materials. This is, of course, what Freud was saying many years ago! The relation is not an entirely simple one, however. Freud pointed out both of the following exceptions: Sometimes a process occurs entirely outside of awareness yet with perfect accuracy, so that the secondary process clearly does not require consciousness to operate. And it does occasionally happen that the primary process shows itself unmistakably in waking, conscious thought—regression in the service of the ego (Kris, 1952). The state of consciousness, and specifically the deployment of hypercathexes (Klein, 1959), are not the only determinants of the degree to which thought processes are primary or secondary.

Nevertheless, let us consider for a moment how hypercathexis may be used in binding (sense 9a). One possibility might be that it takes energy to do the work of binding a drive cathexis to an idea so that it stays put; in that case, it would be reasonable to assume the use of the all-purpose neutral energy used by the ego for all such tasks, hypercathexis. This would be a kind of synthesis, as Freud mentioned in *An Outline of Psycho-Analysis*.

Another possibility (the two are not mutually exclusive) derives from the proposition that states of consciousness are related to the kind of organization of memories that is accessible (Rapaport, 1951a, 1957). For reasons that have not been fully elucidated, consciousness brings about the registration of experience in the conceptual organization of memories and permits access to past experience only via that organization, instead of the drive organization of memories, which is all that unconscious thinking can use. This is a structural explanation of the order that results in thought as a result of hypercathexis: Consciousness brings into play organizing structures which prevent the irrationality and fluidity of the primary process. There are exceptions, of course, to the exclusiveness just described, yet the general tendencies are marked.

Perhaps the key to this relation of state of consciousness to the different types of memory organization is to be sought in a closer consideration of the way we get access to our memory traces. We know, for example, that a subliminal stimulus gets into the psychic apparatus and primes the trace aggregates (or memory schemes), so that they have subsequent effects on dreams, imagery, and the like (see, e.g., Fisher & Paul, 1959; Klein & Holt, 1960). The content of what is registered subliminally may be quite innocuous, so that there is no question of repression, yet the subject has no direct access to the primed schemes—he sees nothing, and thus can recall nothing. It seems, therefore, that if an experience is fully hypercathected, its trace is laid down in the conceptual organization of memories, and a channel is opened for its direct recall (unless such channels are closed by defense). If a stimulus is not hypercathected, or if the experience occurs during a moment when the psychic apparatus is dominated by free drive cathexis—consider the difficulty of remembering the moment of orgasm—channels for voluntary recall (a process that must use hypercathexis to do the work of remembering) are not opened.

One important source of the confusion that arises in the mind of the student of Freud's works when he looks over the usages of free and bound cathexis is that Freud often failed to make explicit whether he was speaking about drive cathexis or hypercathexis. From the beginning he distinguished these two kinds of energy, and rather consistently used them in contrasting ways. It is late to try to introduce terminological distinctions, yet it seems to me that some clarity would be gained if we would not speak of both drive cathexis and hypercathexis as "mobile"; this English word is cognate with *mobil*, the German word Freud most often applied to hypercathexis, so it might make most sense to restrict it that way, and speak of drive energy as "free" (cognate with Freud's *frei*, a word he often applied to id energy).

By the same token, the term "bound" has been applied to both of these kinds of energy with unfortunate ambiguity. As early as the Fliess letters, Freud suggested that hypercathexis could be bound or "riveted" to a particular organ; as we have seen, the conception of usage 7—the binding of hypercathexes into defensive structures—occurred a number of times later on. In his last major work, Rapaport (1959) defined binding in this sense, as structure building. Since the process and the effect are so different for hypercathexis and for drive cathexis, and since in the vast majority of Freud's usages of *binden* he referred to the latter, I suggest that when hypercathexes are immobilized in their structure-building function, we call them "immobile" or "fixed." Thus, only drive cathexes could be "bound," and hypercathexes alone would be called "immobile" when used anticathectically.

Likewise, the distinction between binding and neutralization should make it apparent that drive energies can be either bound or free regardless of their degree of neutralization (or virtually so). Even the highly neutralized cathexes of ego interests can occasionally shift, according to the rules of the primary process, from one mental presentation to another so long as these ideas or images are not hypercathected. These operations should not be confused with the quick but orderly transfers of attention cathexis in conscious secondary-process thinking.

Note that the secondary process does not lose the flexibility that might seem to be implied by the binding of its drive cathexes. We have only to keep in mind that an image or other mental presentation may have drive cathexis and also hypercathexis, and that the former may be bound while the latter is mobile. Primary-process thinking is fluid, and the free displaceability of drive cathexes can give rise to extraordinary originality of its undisciplined products. But the *flexibility* of secondary-process thinking is given by the fact that its drive cathexes are bound (so that thoughts retain their identities and can be freely manipulated without changing), yet the hypercathexes that do the manipulative work are mobile, easily transferred from one thought to another.

The way should now be clear for a definition of binding. Two definitions seem defensible, in light of the preceding considerations—a more inclusive and a less inclusive one. The more inclusive definition would be as follows: Binding is a synthetic process by means of which psychic entities are combined into new organizations. But this seems indistinguishable from the definition of the synthetic function. The less inclusive definition, which I prefer, is a special case of the one just cited: Binding is a synthetic process, carried out by hypercathexes, wherein drive cathexes are stably linked to mental representations. It is a quantitative, not an all-or-none, concept, so that free energy can be thought of as becoming increasingly bound, as we go from the primary-process pole along the continuum of thought toward the secondary-process pole.

But perhaps the time has not come even yet when the concepts of bound versus free cathexis and mobile versus immobile hypercathexis should be "confined in definition" (Freud, 1915c, p. 117). They stand or fall with Freud's controversial decision to abandon his early psychological theorizing and to create a bold new concept of psychic (cathectic) energy. As long as psychoanalysis retains that concept, however, there should be value in restricting the concepts to the core meanings suggested here.

SUMMARY AND CONCLUSIONS

1. Freud used binding (and its opposites, freedom or mobility of cathexis) in over a dozen different ways as his thery developed. The major usages are (a) to describe the inhibition and delay of discharge, the diminution of peremptoriness; (b) to describe the close union of cathexis and mental presentation; (c) to describe the building of structures.

2. Any discussion of binding and mobility must distinguish two kinds of energy: that of the instinctual drives (of whatever degree of neutralization) or drive cathexis, and neutral energy (hypercathexis). One can make this distinction without taking a stand on the question whether neutral energy is wholly, partly, or not at all derived from drive energy.

3. Various usages of binding by Freud refer to these different energies: Inhibition and delay, and the binding of cathexis to idea, refer to drive energy; structure building refers to hypercathexis. Corresponding terminological innovations are proposed, to clarify such distinctions as that between the slippery freedom of drive cathexis and the useful mobility of hypercathexis.

4. Defense (including inhibition) and delay are now handled by means of structural concepts and the energic concept of neutralization. Hence binding should not be used in such senses.

5. Binding of drive cathexis to idea is a conceptual usage essential to explain (in part) the distinction between primary and secondary processes, and this meaning should be retained.

6. Binding of hypercathexes, as in the formation of a structure, is an essentially different idea than the binding of drive cathexis, so the term "immobilization" is proposed for it.

7. At the extreme primary-process end of a continuous series of thought processes, drive energy is both free and not neutralized; at the secondary-process pole, it is both bound and neutralized. Nevertheless, binding and neutralization are independent (if partly correlated) processes, the degree of binding being coordinated to formal properties of thought, the degree of neutralization to its content. Both binding and neutralization are continuous and quantitative concepts, not dichotomies.

8. The binding of cathexis to idea is brought about by hypercathexis. An unsolved theoretical problem is how to conceptualize the three different effects hypercathexis may have on a presentation: It may bind its drive cathexis to it; it may make it focally conscious (attention-cathectic use); or it may inhibit its discharge or access to consciousness (anticathectic use).

9. The relation of primary and secondary processes to consciousness is therefore not a simple one; it does not necessarily happen that the drive energy of a conscious thought is highly bound. There does, however, seem to be a partial relation, in that consciousness brings about the recording of experience in the conceptual organization of memories, from which it is recoverable at will.

10. In the secondary process, ideas have both drive cathexes and hypercathexes; the bound state of the former provides the stability, the mobility of the latter provides the flexibility of this type of thinking.

AFTERWORD

It would not say much for the effectiveness of my theoretical reflections and labors of the past two and a half decades if, on returning to the topic of my first effort at theoretical critique, I felt that no substantial changes needed to be made. To be sure, if I judged that the paper had little lasting merit, I would not bother to reprint it. Taken on its original terms, it makes a few points that are still worth reiterating, and it needed only a few corrections and supplementation to do so.

Nevertheless, with the notoriously cheap wisdom of aftersight, I feel that much of this chapter suffers from a common error made by beginners in the realm of theory: looking for complicated explanations of matters that are actually rather simple. Like many another Freudian scholar, I assumed that Freud had something far more complex in mind than he probably did. It seemed to me that he had thought out a vast and intricate theoretical design, only parts of which he ever put down in one place; hence, our task was to integrate the scattered pieces of the theory and to reconstruct that master plan, making it explicit. The truth, I now believe, is simpler and more human. Freud did the best he could, in some respects not taking his theoretical efforts as seriously as we tend to do; he made it up as he went along without any organized and conscientious effort at consistency. As a result, any one paper or chapter is more internally coherent than the larger works, and when one goes from the output of one year to that of another, the more separated in time they are the more inconsistency one must expect to find, even to the point of direct self-contradiction.

A second general reflection: When it comes to interpreting the meaning of technical terms, we should apply common sense before laborious scholarship. After only a little effort to find the antecedents of the technical terminology of psychoanalysis, one becomes aware that most of it consists of ordinary German words pressed into service where a specialized vocabulary did not exist. As Bettelheim (1983) has argued, the reader of Freud in German does not get as much of an impression that the theory is written in a technical jargon as those of us who rely on the various English translations, including the Standard Edition. *It is highly doubtful that Freud often (if ever) said to himself, as it were, "Come, let us create a concept; let there be [for example] 'cathexis' where before there was but a theoretical void." Instead, he wrote freely and un-self-consciously, drawing on the ample resources of a rich literary vocabulary and shaping words to new metaphorical uses as any creative writer or scientist does constantly.*

Usages in Other Sciences. *It was that way, surely, with respect to most of the terms with which this chapter is preoccupied—the German originals of "free" and "bound," "tonic" and "mobile," and the rest of them. They had been used by scientists for quite some years, also in a variety of more or less metaphorical senses. Spalding (1956) remarks that "the use of binden for non-physical 'bringing together' goes back at least to the 16th century" (p. 317). As indicated, its root meaning is very similar to that of its English cognate—to tie together, to cause to become firmly associated. Chemistry dealt from its beginning with combination, and for centuries to combine anything chemically was etwas binden. Likewise in English:* The Compact Edition of the Oxford English Dictionary *(1971) quotes one Grew as writing in 1674, "Their Alkaly binds in with some preternatural Acid in the Stomach" (Vol. 1, p. 217). The state opposite to combined or bound was uncombined or free, as in "free acid." With the advent of modern atomism, chemists spoke often of binding elements together, and when it became desirable to have a term for hypothetical entities with the aid of which such stable associations between atoms took place, it was natural to speak of* Bunden—bonds.

Likewise, a number of parallel usages existed in physics. As early as 1838 (in the Proceedings of the American Philosophical Society*), power or energy was spoken of as free when "disengaged, available for 'work'" (Compact OED, 1971, Vol. 1, p. 1075). What English calls "latent heat," German made* gebundene Waerme. *Since the latent heat of boiling is the amount of heat that must be added to water once it reaches $100\,°C$ to convert it into steam at $100\,°C$, the accompanying image is that the added heat, which mysteriously does not result in any rise of temperature, is forcibly restricted in some way—bound. Similarly, there is a concept of* gebundene Elektrizitaet, *latent electricity (T. Jones, 1963; Spalding, 1952).[25] In Freud's own time, Helmholtz made the following distinction:* $F = E - TS$, *where E is the total energy of a system, T is its temperature, and S stands for entropy. The quantity F is called "Helmholtz free energy," the amount that is available to do work. I have been unable to find out whether Freud knew this concept, though I have never seen a context in which he refers to it— surely not in the* Standard Edition. *We should keep in mind the fact that when he came to write theoretical works in psychoanalysis, his studies of physics were long behind him, and though he shared with Fliess a great respect for Helmholtz, that was not because the latter's contributions to physics seemed directly usable in the new discipline. So, when Freud used the term* Spannung *(usually translated as "tension"), it is most doubtful that he bore in mind that it was the German word for potential energy. It is seductive to conclude that since the words cited had various scientific connotations, and since Freud had a scientific education, he deliberately incorporated those into his own usages; however, one could thereby easily fall into serious error.*

Viewed in the light of the shifting meanings of the terms in the hard sciences, there should be no wonder that it is possible to find over a dozen kinds of ways in which Freud used the same term with slightly varying meanings. It is necessary only not to take his theorizing more seriously than it was meant, and surely to avoid the fallacy of assuming that wherever the same word appears it must refer to an identical process or entity, as it plainly did not in physics and chemistry. Freud did err that way sometimes; if we wish to learn from his mistakes as well as his insights, we must stay alert to the ever-present danger of reification—treating abstractions as if they refer to concrete entities or things.

In retrospect, my effort to distinguish between "technical" and "non-technical" usages looks misguided. No sharp boundary can be drawn. In one sense, no usages by Freud are technical if that term is restricted to the precisely controlled coinage of words for specific and rigidly defined employment in theory. Not many scientists are that compulsive; Freud surely was not. Instead of "technical," I should have written "economic," for it seems that I was looking for instances when "bound," "free," and the like were used within the economic point of view of metapsychology. This chapter was the first skirmish of what was to be a continuing battle with metapsychology, in which I initially concentrated almost entirely on what I took to be its most vulnerable aspect. So I was concentrating, somewhat artificially, on the instances when Freud was talking about the confinement, constraint, or degree of stable association of some form of (predominantly, psychic) energy with something else, such as ideas or other "presentations."

Usage #15. Here I must record my one new find, an additional type of usage that can be distinguished from its 14 predecessors in Table 4.1. The following seems to be the type instance. Freud is speaking about the patient's libido: "we look for the object-presentations to which it is bound and free it from them, so as to place it at the disposal of the ego" (1917a, p. 138). At first sight, I took it to be a variant of #9, the binding of cathexis to presentation that is said to make possible the secondary process. Yet the state of being free, in the latter context, would seem to relegate the energy to the id rather than the ego, since it is coordinated with primary-process functioning. For the most part, when talking about the status of libidinal attachments to "objects," Freud used "fixated" instead of "bound," with the same antithesis—"mobile." Thus,

> A particularly close attachment of the instinct to its object is distinguished by the term 'fixation.' This frequently occurs at very early periods of the development of an instinct and puts an end to its mobility through its intense opposition to detachment. (1915c, p. 123. Other similar usages occur in 1916–1917, pp. 346, 455; 1937c, p. 241; and 1940a, p. 151.)

What at times he called the "adhesiveness of libido" he also referred to as "sluggishness," as in the following passage concerning the Wolf Man's fixations, written in 1914 though not published for four years:

> Great mobility or sluggishness of libidinal cathexes (as well as of other[26] kinds of energic cathexes) are special characteristics which attach to many normal people. . . . the mobility of the mental cathexes is a quality which shows striking diminution with the advance of age. . . . some people . . . retain this mental

plasticity . . . others . . . lose it very prematurely. If the latter are neurotics, we make the unwelcome discovery that it is impossible to undo developments in them which, in apparently similar circumstances, have been easily dealt with in other people. So that in considering the conversion of psychical energy no less than of physical, we must make use of the concept of an entropy, *which opposes the undoing of what has already occurred. (1918b, p. 116)*

In a footnote at this point, Strachey repeats Freud's error in an effort to be helpful, explaining that "Entropy is the force which, according to the Second Law of Thermodynamics, tends to make certain physical changes irreversible." Entropy is, of course, not a force at all, but an abstract quantity referring to the nonavailability of energy to do work—the complement of Helmholtz free energy. For better or for worse, Freud did not take his own advice; very rarely thereafter did he speak about either entropy or the conversion of energy. Indeed, the word "entropy" appears only one other time in his published works, in a similar discussion of rigidity in his last great paper:

One finds the same thing ["all the mental processes, relationships and distributions of force are unchangeable, fixed and rigid"] in very old people, in which case it is explained as being due to what is described as force of habit or an exhaustion of receptivity—a kind of psychical entropy. (1937c, p. 242)

I have been able to find only one reference to anything like conversion of energy in works subsequent to 1914: "a system which itself is highly cathected is capable of taking up an additional stream of fresh inflowing energy and of converting it into quiescent cathexes, that is of binding it psychically" (1920g, p. 30). So far as I know, Freud's only references to the conversion of anything like energy allude to binding, in just this way.

Free and Bound Anxiety. Several colleagues expressed disappointment with or criticism of my original paper for its virtual silence on the question of what bound anxiety might be and how it is (or is not) related to bound energy. The question is easily answered: Fundamentally, when Freud distinguished bound and free forms of anxiety, he meant to imply a basic distinction between degrees of control. The typical example of bound anxiety is a phobia; its opposite he variously called "free anxiety" (1918b, p. 113), "freely floating anxiety which is ready to attach itself to any idea that is in any way suitable" (1916-1917, p. 398), and once "unbound anxiety" (1916-1917, p. 403). Though I doubt that anything much should be made of them, it is possible to find transitional passages that seem to serve as "missing links" between this and the economic usage. For example, when renouncing the "fermentation theory" of anxiety and partly undoing the retraction, Freud said that sometimes

anxiety arises directly out of libido. . . . though the matter is of little importance, it is very possible that what finds discharge in the generating of anxiety is precisely the surplus of unutilized libido. . . . This looks as though the ego were *attempting to save itself from anxiety, . . . and to bind it by the formation of symptoms. (1926d, p. 141)*

To fill in speculatively: Since, in definition #10, all affects are the discharge of free energy, anxiety too is the discharge of the "unutilized libido" of the actual neurotic. So, when anxiety is bound by symptom formation, that is a kind of binding of free energy, a preventing of an affect discharge. Another passage from the same work, quoted in the text, is supportive: "symptoms . . . bind the psychical energy which would otherwise be discharged as anxiety" (1926d, p. 144).

Most of the time, when Freud speaks about anxiety, he leaves one uncertain whether he means that affect in a phenomenological sense (the experienced emotion), more organismically (the entire psychological and physiological process), or metapsychologically with an emphasis on the psychic energies involved. In this connection, see the passage (1900a, p. 578) quoted on p. 86. There, as here, he was casual about distinctions among phenomenological, psychological, and physiological terms. Apparently he did not even notice that he was mixing together into a single formulation elements from three incommensurate frames of reference.

In retrospect, we can see a better way of proceeding: first, establishing the observations about clinical phenomena, such as dreams, which he wanted to conceptualize and explain; constructing a psychological theory of dreaming (the dream process); and then developing a model of the latter (e.g., in anatomical and physiological terms; on the distinction between model and theory, see Chapter 12, this volume). It may be that our knowledge of the structure and functioning of the brain is still not sufficient to permit a complete realization of the psychological (psychoanalytic) theory of dreaming. In addition, we have today a much more extensive factual base of observations about dreaming that must be incorporated into an adequate theory, though in some respects they contradict some of Freud's assumptions (Breger, 1967; McCarley & Hobson, 1977). Anyway, the point I wish to stress is that we can all too easily lose sight of the prime importance of maintaining and respecting these distinctions.

Consider, for example, another passage in this chapter—the second and third sentences of the large paragraph on p. 104. I let this bit of embarrassing naivete stand, much as I would prefer to conceal it, because it is such a good example of the same faults I am criticizing in Freud, and also because it nicely exemplifies the way many of us have persuaded ourselves that Freud was remarkably prescient. In the first of these sentences I mixed, in a single proposition, observational terms ("attention"), clinical–theoretical ones ("secondary process"), and metapsychological terms ("hypercathexis"), in a way that implies a statement of fact. Actually, the original clinical observation restated something known for centuries: that the most logical and clearest thinking takes place in states of full awareness, with active attention to (or concentration upon) the subject matter; and that thinking becomes most magical and bizarre in dreams, fantasies, and other nonvigilant states of consciousness. It is embarrassing to realize how little any available theories add to these observations.

Similar methodological errors flaw the entire final section of the chapter following the list of usages, but it has been retained for whatever didactic value it may have. I did, however, omit the quotation of the page-long first paragraph of "Instincts and Their Vicissitudes" preceding my final, hesitant implication that the concept of psychic energy might not be a permanently valuable contribution to psychoanalytic theory. It was not long before I began to voice such doubts more openly.

CHAPTER 5

A Review of Some of Freud's Biological Assumptions and Their Influence on His Theories[1]

Shortly after the original publication of Chapter 4, Robert W. White asked me to contribute to a book he was assembling in honor of our dear friend and mentor, Henry A. Murray (White, 1963b). The paper I put together for it (Holt, 1963) was my first attempt to psychologize Freud and his works, much influenced by Bernfeld's (1944) notions about the "School of Helmholtz." Its naivete was properly scolded shortly thereafter (Cranefield, 1966, 1970)—an unpleasant learning experience from which I nevertheless profited. I set myself a higher standard of scholarship and continued to try to figure Freud out.

During the whole decade of the 1960s, I immersed myself in the study of Freud and his works. The year I spent in Palo Alto was a real turning point; the leisure to read and get deeply into topics that interested me made it possible for me to get started on a kind of methodological and historical scholarship for which I had never had the time before. When, at David Rapaport's suggestion, Peter Amacher sent me his doctoral dissertation (later published as a monograph; see Amacher, 1965), I was able to plunge into it and follow up some of its implications.

Again, an invitation from a friend catalyzed a paper (Holt, 1965a). William C. Lewis, a psychiatrist at the University of Wisconsin Medical School whom I had gotten to know and admire when he was a resident at the Menninger School of Psychiatry and a subject in our Selection Project (Holt & Luborsky, 1958), asked me to participate in a symposium on Psychoanalysis and Current Biological Thought. The symposium proceedings were published a couple of years later as a book by the same title (Greenfield & Lewis, 1965).

Once again, Professor Cranefield wrote me a long and scholarly letter, correcting some points in the history of medicine, on which he is an outstanding authority. I have resisted the temptation to change the text extensively, but have included his correctives in footnotes.

After reading Sulloway's (1979) brilliant revelations of many other biological assumptions in Freud's work besides those discussed here, particularly the influences of 19th-century evolutionary biology, I was tempted to *add a good deal to my 1965 paper. I believe, however, that I can not do better than strongly recommend a reading of Sulloway's book to anyone who may have missed it.*

———

To the contemporary student, many aspects of Freud's theories seem only partly plausible and difficult to grasp with any sense of secure understanding. Those who are predisposed to rebellion often react by rejecting psychoanalysis as a whole, or turn to a more "modern" form of it, without ever knowing just what it is they are discarding, and on the basis of some stereotyped formula like "unscientific" or "too biological." Those who are predisposed to uncritical admiration of an authentic genius, as Freud unquestionably was, accept those obscure parts of the psychoanalytic canon as the truly profound passages which are simply beyond their own capacity to follow.

To one who finds neither of these styles of reaction ego-syntonic, there remains one principal course of action: to undertake a close study of the texts themselves under light from whatever historical windows he can find open to the intellectual ambience of Freud's formative years. My own struggles for understanding have been aided first by the teaching of David Rapaport, from whom I learned how to read Freud with some structural understanding, and then by some historical readings.[2] Of these, I would single out the brilliant series of papers by Bernfeld (in particular, 1944 and 1951) and a recent doctoral dissertation by M. Peter Amacher (1962) entitled *The Influence of the Neuroanatomy, Neurophysiology and Psychiatry of Freud's Teachers on His Psychoanalytic Theories.* I will present a brief résumé of its main points as part of the development of my argument.

From these historical studies, the following summary formulation has forced itself on me: Many of the most puzzling and seemingly arbitrary turns of psychoanalytic theory, involving propositions that are false to the extent that they are testable at all, are either hidden biological assumptions or result directly from such assumptions, which Freud learned from his teachers in medical school.[3] They became a basic part of his intellectual equipment, as unquestioned as the assumption of universal determinism, were probably not always recognized by him as biological, and thus were retained as necessary ingredients when he attempted to turn away from neurologizing to the construction of an abstract, psychological model.

To buttress this conclusion, I shall present, first, a summary of Amacher's findings on the doctrines of Freud's teachers, then a demonstration that their conceptions of the structure and functioning of the nervous system were incorporated into "the Project." I shall adduce evidence that, when

Freud replaced the explicitly physicalistic theory of the Project with a psychological one, he did so only partially and inconsistently. Next, I want to show how the same biological propositions were retained as fundamental assumptions in Freud's post-1900 theories, with only some terminological changes; and, finally, I shall indicate the paradoxes, inconsistencies, and other difficulties created by this set of assumptions and by Freud's ambivalence regarding the nature of the fundamental ideas with which he was working.

THE DOCTRINES OF FREUD'S TEACHERS

From Bernfeld's inquiries, we know that Freud received most of his education about the nervous system, its structure and functioning, during the years 1874–1878 from Ernst Brücke and Theodor Meynert, who were outstanding professors at the University of Vienna medical school and were internationally known authorities; in addition, he worked in the laboratories of both men and spoke in terms of the highest admiration about each of them (Bernfeld, 1951). He was more competitive with the younger Sigmund Exner, who was more nearly his contemporary, but who nevertheless was his instructor in physiology and his senior in Brücke's laboratory.

All three of these men wrote books between 1875 and 1894, setting forth either the actual lectures Freud attended or their essential substance. The historian Amacher has read these German tomes, informed by an acquaintance with psychoanalytic theory, and has excerpted and translated many passages that have a surprisingly familiar ring to the Freudian student. All three give an account of the structure and function of the central nervous system that is essentially the same and is similar to the theoretical chapter by their friend Josef Breuer in *Studies on Hysteria* (Breuer & Freud, 1895), which sketches a neuropsychology. All four of these men were admirers and followers of Helmholtz, zealously preaching the doctrine of physicalistic physiology, which Bernfeld (1944) portrayed as an attempt to overthrow the preceding *Naturphilosophie* and vitalism by a rigorous attempt to treat the organism as a mechanical system.

Freud's teachers, Amacher demonstrates, shared

> the idea that the nervous system functioned by transmitting a quantitatively variable phenomenon which was the mechanism of the nerve impulse from the afferent nerve endings to the efferent nerve endings. The entire quantity of this "excitation" . . . originated at the afferent nerve endings [i.e., at the sensory organs]. (Amacher, 1962, Chapt. 1)

There was no general agreement on the nature of this excitation; Brücke believed it was electrical, though he never referred to it as "energy."

They had advanced beyond the ancient idea that nervous excitation was transmitted by the movement of some sort of fluid or spirit through the [assumedly] hollow nerves, but it was still possible to think of the transmission of excitation in the nerves as analogous in many ways to the transmission of a fluid in a pipe. (Amacher, 1965, p. 14)

Amacher makes the interesting observation that Brücke did not explicitly discuss the mind–body problem, but everywhere wrote as if he assumed that all mental processes were simultaneously paralleled by physical ones. This tacit assumption "allowed him . . . to describe a process partly in physical and partly psychological terms." "This unrestrained shifting from descriptions in terms of mind to descriptions in physical terms is characteristic of the work of Freud's teachers and of Freud," Amacher (1965, p. 17) notes.

As part of his rejection of the vitalism of his own teacher, Johannes Müller, Brücke introduced the idea that there was no spontaneous central activity of the brain, but explicitly declared that the functioning of the entire brain followed the model of the reflex arc: "voluntary movements . . . too are originated by centripetal impulses; however, from them the conduction goes through parts of the cortex which serve consciousness, ideas, and will" (Brücke, 1876, p. 25; translated by Amacher). The result was an implicit conception of the whole nervous system as a passive instrument which remained in a state of rest until stimulated, when it functioned so as to rid itself of the incoming exogenous energies.

One other statement of Brücke's (quoted in paraphrase not by Amacher but by Jones, 1953, p. 42) is worthy of note: "The physical energies alone cause effects." Brücke's lectures on physiology contained a great deal about forces and energies (concepts he did not clearly differentiate), and he dwelled on the doctrine of the conservation of energy, elegantly promulgated by his friend and colleague Helmholtz with the "purpose of giving a sound foundation to the new physiology" (Bernfeld, 1944, p. 349). It remained an act of faith, but symbolically a very important one, to believe that the concept of energy was just what physiology needed to put it on a quantitative and thus rigorously scientific basis.

Meynert's conceptions of the nervous system were, in the respects with which we are concerned here, similar to Brücke's. Actions, the ultimate effects of consciousness, "are not the result of force innate in the brain. The brain does not, like a fixed star, radiate its own heat; it obtains all the force underlying all cerebral phenomena from outside" (Meynert, 1884, p. 146; translated by Amacher). He sometimes used the term "energy" for neural impulse, but his reference to "synthetic chemical events" accompanying its passage may imply a recognition that not all the energy involved originated at the afferent nerve endings.

Exner's book is of interest largely because it contains a synthesis of the same set of ideas and appeared in 1894, when Freud was beginning to flex his own theoretical muscles and just before he wrote the Project. Exner wrote: "The excited condition of a nerve fiber appears to have no quality . . . [but] it is to the highest degree variable quantitatively" (1894, p. 37). When this excitation reached a large enough quantity through being accumulated in a "summation center," it would be transmitted to a hypothetical "pain center." The latter could also be set in action from the activation of unpleasant memories or other cortical events. Something virtually identical with what Breuer called "tonic excitation" of a nerve center appears in Exner's discussion of sex in "every normal young man"—his cerebral "center for sexual instincts . . . has at times an increased tonus, and only a small impulse is required to establish an association between certain cortical events and this center" (1894, p. 345). [In the previous Chapter,] I demonstrated that this concept and Breuer's version of it, tonic excitation, were adopted by Freud as the original meaning of "cathexis," and lingered on in the doctrine of "the insusceptibility to excitation of uncathected systems" (Freud, 1917d [1915], p. 234 n.). I shall therefore spend no further time on this bit of conceptual inheritance.

For convenience of exposition, I shall refer to the foregoing set of interrelated propositions about the nervous system and its functioning in relation to external inputs as "the passive reflex model."

In the preceding brief and highly selective summary, I have not cited Amacher's detailed documentation of the presence of similar ideas in the works of these three of Freud's teachers, nor his presentation of certain other doctrines such as Freud's theory of learning by association (which was not very specifically psychoanalytic); nor have I brought out the qualifications and reservations with which these physiologists stated the essentials of the passive reflex model, which indicate that it was more implicit than explicit in their teachings and was probably considered a rough first approximation. Yet it is easy to see how it was inculcated in Freud, who digested these various sources, extracted what was latent in them with brilliant clarity, and stated the implicit model with elegant economy of exposition in 1895.

BIOLOGICAL ASSUMPTIONS IN THE PROJECT

A year after Exner's book, and only a few months after their mutual elder friend and colleague Breuer's similar neuropsychological essay, Freud turned his hand to the ambitious task of putting together the existing knowledge about the nervous system in a detailed neurological model, the psychology for neurologists that is now familiarly known as "the Project." The commitment to physicalistic physiology is obvious in its opening lines and throughout: It is an ambitious attempt to be as scientific in the 19th-century Helmholtzian sense as possible, which meant to be rigorously materialistic and mechanistic: ". . . to represent psychical processes as quantitatively determinate states of specifiable material particles" (Freud, 1950 [1895], p. 295). Indeed, so thoroughgoing was Freud's attempt at materialism that he adopted the Hartleyan position that the nerve impulse was a mechanical vibration of "the material particles in question . . . the neurones."[4]

He then launches into an admirably clear formulation of "the principle of neuronic inertia: that neurones tend to divest themselves of Q"—his shorthand term for the neural impulse conceived of as purely quantitative *à la* Exner (p. 296). Consequently, the nervous system as a whole strives to keep itself "free from stimulus. This discharge represents the primary function of the nervous system" (p. 357). This was the "constancy principle," which, we have seen, was the prevailing, antivitalist neurological dogma of Freud's time.[5]

How did quantity get into the nervous system, then, if the latter did not generate any of its own? From two sources, Freud said: from external reality via the sensory organs, and "from the somatic element itself—endogenous stimuli, which have equally to be discharged. These have their origin in the cells of the body and give rise to the major needs: hunger, respiration, sexuality" (Freud, 1950 [1895], p. 297). In these few words are contained both a theory of reality and a theory of motivation as tension reduction. With defiantly materialistic overtones, Freud (p. 308) declares that "in the external world . . . there are only masses in motion and nothing else."[6] If the nerve cells, too, consisted of material particles that vibrated in accordance with the laws of motion, it is easy to see how Freud was led to the complementary assumption that external physical energies enter and traverse the nervous system almost as directly as light does a transparent body—or at least the portion (or quotient) that is not screened out by the surface of the body.

The consequence of such a conception of the nervous system as a passive conductor was that it could be disrupted or burned out by the passage of too great a current of energy without a protective system of resistors. To take care of this problem, Freud adapted his teachers' views, which were not exactly that external energies entered the nervous system untransformed, but that the system's excitation was directly *proportional* to the amount of stimulation. In Freud's simpler conception, the impinging

> amounts of excitation . . . from outside . . . first come up against the nerve-ending apparatuses and are broken up by them into quotients. . . . Here there is a first threshold: below a certain quantity no effective quotient at all comes into being, so that the effective capacity of the *stimuli* is to some extent restricted to *medium* quantities. (1950 [1895], p. 313)

This is what he later (Freud, 1920g) called the stimulus barrier or protective shield against stimulation.[7]

In these contexts, where Freud affirms the quantitative nature of reality, he echoes Exner's concern with the "problem of quality," which is really a major chunk of the mind–body problem: the existence of conscious phenomena, or qualities, in a material world. "Consciousness gives us what are called *qualities*," he wrote; "It may be asked *how* qualities originate and *where* qualities originate. . . . Not in the external world" (Freud, 1950 [1895], p. 308). He decided, after considering various possibilities, that there had to be a special system of perceptual neurones "whose states of excitation give rise to the various qualities—are, that is to say, *conscious sensations*" (p. 309). And the vehicle of quality was the frequency of the vibratory energy, which he called "period." This was an allowable hypothesis, "for the mechanics of the physicists has allowed this temporal attribute to the motions of masses in the external world as well" (p. 310).

Turning back to the impingements of energy from within the organism, we should take notice of the fact that, although Freud's concept was essentially the same as that of his teachers, there is one major difference. They made no distinction as to relative odiousness between the stimuli arising from the two sources, but Freud noted one critical difference: "From these [endogenous stimuli] the organism cannot withdraw as it does from external stimuli" (p. 297). This fact upsets the principle of inertia "from the first," for they cease only if "particular conditions [are] . . . realized in the external world." Because of the "exigencies of life," to do so usually requires more energy than the endogenous qualities themselves provide, so the system "must put up with [maintaining] a store of [quantity] sufficient to meet the demand for a specific action" (p. 297). Brücke had postulated a superficially similar central summation of excitations, but of Freud's elders only Exner had what we can recognize as a central theory of motivation or a concept of drive.[8] From the beginning,[9] however, motivation was for Freud a matter of the reduction of tensions or energic inputs.

As we shall see in Chapter 6, Freud came up against an inability to furnish a satisfactory account of defense or of consciousness, because in both cases he got into a kind of regress in which he did not know when to stop. Something more like a person or a knower had to "notice" the danger signal or the indication of quality, he felt; he did not recognize that the model he had constructed was so well supplied with feedback loops (no fewer than five may be distinguished) that it was adequately self-regulating, in this respect at least. Though Freud was many decades ahead of his time, he was too much its prisoner to see that the informational return provided by a feedback loop could obviate any hypothetical nonconscious process of attention; ironically, he concluded that he had failed to provide a "mechanical (automatic) explanation" (p. 360) and committed his first great infidelity to the antivitalism of his teachers: He postulated an observing ego. True, they used the same term (*"Ich"*), and Meynert had a rather elaborate and Freudian-sounding ego theory; but they used *Ich* in the same way that

Freud did at first in the Project, when it was merely "the totality of ca-thected neurones." In the end, however, he was forced to revive an essen-tially philosophical conception in which the ego is a prime mover, the willer, and ultimate knower, and thus a vitalistic homunculus with some degree of autonomy.

This was one respect in which the Project failed. Despite Freud's great ingenuity and inventive resourcefulness, it also failed in a number of other ways: For example, concepts underwent such changes from one section to another as to be contradictory, as he molded them to the needs of the problem under discussion at the moment. It is worth noticing, however, that Freud simply went ahead and did the best he could, letting the contradic-tions stand and introducing nonphysicalistic concepts when he could see no other way out. Paradoxical as it may sound, this was to be one of his saving traits as a scientist—his way of enabling his theory to grow and new ideas to emerge before he was ready to fit them smoothly into the existing corpus.

Amacher points out a number of other points made in the Project that were obviously foreshadowed by one or more of Freud's teachers, but I shall not review them here. I am deliberately focusing attention on a limited range of propositions about the nature of external reality and about the passive reflex nature of the nervous system, because these determine the characteristics of the theoretical model and shape a great many subsequent assumptions and propositions. Moreover, these are the parts of the theory that have become testable and have been overthrown.

RETENTION OF BIOLOGICAL DOCTRINES
IN POST-1900 WORKS

Only a few months after Freud had sent the first sections of the Project to Fliess, he became increasingly dissatisfied with it. For several years there-after he blew hot and cold, at times rejecting the whole enterprise as "philosophical stammering," at other times making fresh efforts to rear-range its parts in a hope that it might begin to work. Finally, he turned his back on the attempt to work with an anatomical–physiological model and produced his first great work, *The Interpretation of Dreams* (1900a). It was not an isolated decision, but was part of a major turn in Freud's whole life—changes in his type of professional practice, the nature of his research, his friendships, his self-understanding, his very sense of identity. It is not easy to appraise these changes accurately. In many respects Freud seems to have undergone a profound reorientation as he turned from being a neuroana-tomical researcher to a clinical neurologist who experimented with psycho-therapy, finally becoming the first psychoanalyst (Erikson, 1956). We would be poor psychologists, however, if we imagined that there was not at least as much continuity as change in this development. Twenty years of passionate investment in the study of the nervous system were not easily tossed aside by Freud's decision to become a psychologist instead and to work with a purely abstract theory.

Yet this is the usual assumption—that, beginning with 1900, Freud rejected all physiologizing and all attempts to localize the parts of the "psychic apparatus" within the substance of the brain.[10] It would be tedious, however, to give a full documentation for my contention that Freud did not succeed in making a clean break with his past theoretical position (some of the most relevant passages are cited in Chapter 6; see also below). Let me here merely assert (a) that he never gave up the hope to "find the solid ground on which I can cease to give psychological explanations and begin to find a physiological foundation!" (Freud, 1985 [1887–1904], p. 193), as he wrote to Fliess in 1896, after his first disillusionment with the Project; (2) that he continued to use neurological terminology and propositions from the Project in Chapter VII of *The Interpretation of Dreams* even after explicitly disclaiming the attempt to do, despite the fact that the new theory had no place for these elements; (3) that he did not attain methodological clarity about the nature and status of the non-neurological theory he ostensibly was building, particularly with respect to the mind–body problem (Rubinstein, 1965); and (4) that, whenever the nature of his data demanded it, he lapsed into the silent assumption that the psychic apparatus was the brain, that the "pathways" in it were nerve tracts, and that the energy it used was physical in nature, located in and affecting the corporeal substance of the organs. I hope that some of the evidence for these points will become apparent later, as I discuss some of the theoretical difficulties occasioned by this ambivalence.

It may be appropriate also to say a few words about theoretical models[11] and the ways in which Freud used them. A model is a formal structure the parts of which are manipulable to generate consequences, and which in one or more important ways is isomorphic with observed reality. It may be a physical replica or mock-up in which the isomorphy is visual resemblance (a model car); it may be a physical system in which the emphasis is on one or more modes of functioning (the iron wire model of neural conduction or an analog computer); it may be a purely formal and abstract set of symbols and rules for their manipulation (mathematical models of various types of learning). Implicitly, Freud always worked with some type of theoretical model, though he rarely used the term, and for all I know never heard of it in today's sense—certainly it did not become familiar to most of us until well after Freud's death. Yet a *bourgeois gentilhomme* may speak prose all his life without realizing it; and Molière's quip contains something very apposite, for naive speakers of a highly inflected language may scrupulously observe all its complicated rules—which can be extracted as a functioning formal system, a model—without ever being able to formulate one of them.

When a theory has as many difficulties as psychoanalysis does, a useful way of trying to understand and order it is to inquire into the nature of the model of man that it involves. Let us then examine some of Freud's major theoretical works from this standpoint. Our task is made easier by virtue of the fact that he spoke often about the psychic apparatus and even provided a few diagrams of this conceptual structure, indicating that he was thinking in terms of a theoretical model whatever his terminology.

Freud proposed two principal versions of the psychic apparatus: the topographic systems of Chapter VII of *The Interpretation of Dreams*, and the so-called "structural hypothesis" or tripartite theory of the ego, id, and superego. He began his description of the topographic model by stating: "All our psychical activity starts from stimuli (whether internal or external) and ends in innervations" (1900a, p. 537). Note, as Strachey does, the ambiguity of this last anatomical term, which is also used "to mean the transmission of energy *into a system of nerves*" (emphasis added). This is only one page after the famous statement: "I shall remain upon psychological ground." Freud then mentions in passing as if it were almost too obvious to dwell on, "a requirement with which we have long been familiar, namely that the psychical apparatus must be constructed like a reflex apparatus. Reflex processes remain the model of every psychical function" (1900a, p. 538). So faithfully did he follow this assumed requirement that the diagrams accompanying this part of the text are one-track affairs, perfect examples of the stimulus–(intervening variables)–response type of model, without even an input channel for drive impulses. A little later, Freud expands on his conception of the psychic apparatus:

> Hypotheses, whose justification must be looked for in other directions, tell us that at first the apparatus's efforts were directed towards keeping itself so far as possible free from stimuli; consequently its first structure followed the plan of a reflex apparatus, so that any sensory excitation impinging on it could be promptly discharged along a motor path. (1900a, p. 565)

"The exigencies of life," he goes on, first in the form of "the major somatic needs," impel the apparatus to further development; whereupon he repeats the essence of the passage already quoted from the Project describing the development of ideation and thought, and of roundabout methods to the ultimate discharge of tension.

Recapitulating a little later (p. 598), Freud makes it virtually explicit that he is thinking in terms of a model:

> We have already explored the fiction of a primitive psychical apparatus whose activities are regulated by an effort to avoid an accumulation of excitation and to maintain itself so far as possible without excitation. . . . We went on . . . to add a second hypothesis, to the effect that the accumulation of excitation

(brought about in various ways that need not concern us) is felt as unpleasure and that it sets the apparatus in action with a view to repeating the experience of satisfaction, which involved a diminution of excitation and was felt as pleasure.

Here Freud adds his basic proposition about the affects of pleasure and unpleasure, closely following the formulations of Exner. It is an appealingly simple and logical assumption: If the fundamental tendency of the human being is to seek pleasure and avoid unpleasure (the pleasure principle), and if the basic property of its psychic apparatus is to rid itself of "excitation" (note the lack of specification of just what is meant by that term), why not equate them? He had done so explicitly in the Project (Freud, 1950 [1895], p. 312): "Since we have certain knowledge of a trend in psychical life towards *avoiding unpleasure*, we are tempted to identify that trend with the primary trend towards inertia."

In 1915, Freud restated these ideas, referring to the first as "the most important" of his postulates:

This postulate is of a biological nature, and makes use of the concept of 'purpose' . . . : the nervous system [N.B.: here he slips back into neurology and does not speak about the 'psychical apparatus'] is an apparatus which has the function of getting rid of the stimuli that reach it, or of reducing them to the lowest possible level; or which, if it were feasible, would maintain itself in an altogether unstimulated condition. (1915c, p. 120)

After discussing the complications and developments introduced by the presence of "an incessant and unavoidable afflux of stimulation" from the drives, Freud continues:

When we further find that the activity of even the most highly developed mental apparatus is subject to the pleasure principle, i.e., is automatically regulated by feelings belonging to the pleasure–unpleasure series, we can hardly reject the further hypothesis that these feelings reflect the manner in which the process of mastering stimuli takes place . . . unpleasurable feelings are connected with an increase and pleasurable feelings with a decrease of stimulus. (pp. 120–121)

He added a note of caution, indicating an awareness that this was too simple a picture, concluding: "It is certain that many very various relations of this kind, and not very simple ones, are possible" (p. 121).

In 1920 came the best known and perhaps most clearly formulated statement of the principle of constancy. In the first pages of *Beyond the Pleasure Principle* (1920g), he quotes Fechner (1873): "Every psychophysical motion rising above the threshold of consciousness is attended by pleasure in proportion as, beyond a certain limit, it approximates to complete stability, and is attended by unpleasure in proportion as . . . it deviates from complete stability." Freud continued immediately after:

> The facts which have caused us to believe in the dominance of the pleasure principle in mental life also find expression in the hypothesis that the mental apparatus endeavors to keep the quantity of excitation present in it as low as possible or at least to keep it constant . . . the pleasure principle follows from the principle of constancy. (1920g, p. 9)

In 1924, Freud returned to these same ideas:

> The principle which governs all mental processes is a special case of Fechner's 'tendency toward stability,' and [I] have accordingly attributed to the mental apparatus the purpose of reducing to nothing, or at least of keeping as low as possible, the sums of excitation which flow in upon it. Barbara Low [1920, p. 73] has suggested the name of 'Nirvana Principle' for this supposed tendency, and we have accepted the term. But we have unhesitatingly identified the pleasure–unpleasure principle with this Nirvana principle. Every unpleasure ought thus to coincide with a heightening, and every pleasure with a lowering, of mental tension due to stimulus. . . . But such a view cannot be correct. It seems that in the series of feelings of tension we have a direct sense of the increase and decrease of amounts of stimulus, and it cannot be doubted that there are pleasurable tensions and unpleasurable relaxations of tension. . . . It appears that they [pleasure and unpleasure] depend, not on this quantitative factor, but on some characteristic of it which we can only describe as a qualitative one . . . Perhaps it is the rhythm . . . We do not know. (1924c, p. 160; see also 1940a, p. 146 where the same points are repeated)

Note that, even after the introduction of the new tripartite structural model, Freud still treats it as a passive reflex apparatus, even though he provides no circuitry in his diagrams (either the one in *The Ego and the Id* [1923b] or that in the *New Introductory Lectures* [1933a]) to represent a sequential course from input to output.

In his published works, Freud was never as explicit as he was in the Project about the nature of reality. Whenever he discusses it, however, the emphasis is more often on dangers than on beneficent qualities or opportunities, though of course one of the principal contexts in which he treats of reality is as a source of need-satisfying objects. In 1914, for example, he wrote, "We have recognized our mental apparatus as being first and foremost a device designed for mastering excitations which would otherwise be felt as distressing or would have pathogenic effects" (1914c, p. 85). This harsh picture of reality is repeated in *Instincts and Their Vicissitudes*.

> Let us imagine ourselves in the situation of an almost entirely helpless living organism . . . which is receiving stimuli in its nervous substance . . . On the one hand, it will be aware of stimuli which can be avoided by muscular action (flight); these it ascribes to an external world. On the other hand, it will also be

aware of stimuli against which such action is of no avail . . . instinctual needs. (1915c, p. 119)

In both of these works, reality is treated as primarily a source of disturbances which must be escaped or wrestled with.

This last passage foreshadows the famous introduction, in 1920, of the protective shield against stimuli:

> Let us picture a living organism in its most simplified possible form as an undifferentiated vesicle of a substance that is susceptible to stimulation. . . . It would be easy to suppose, then, that as a result of the ceaseless impact of external stimuli on the surface of the vesicle, its substance to a certain depth may have become permanently modified, so that . . . it would present the most favorable possible conditions for the reception of stimuli. . . . This little fragment of living substance is suspended in the middle of an external world charged with the most powerful energies; and it would be killed by the stimulation emanating from these if it were not provided with a protective shield against stimuli . . . its outermost surface . . . becomes to some degree inorganic and . . . resistant to stimuli. . . . *Protection against* stimuli is an almost more important function for the living organism than reception of stimuli. (1920g, pp. 26–27)

This picture of an organism as a helpless creature "threatened by the enormous energies at work in the external world" makes it amply explicit that Freud conceived of external reality as primarily a source of dangerous energies directly penetrating the organism, except for the screening effects of its protective shield.

An obvious corollary of the passive reflex model, the conception of motivation as the reduction of tension, is perhaps too familiar to require elaborate documentation. The following passage from *Instincts and Their Vicissitudes* is typical:

> An instinctual stimulus does not arise from the external world but from within the organism itself. For this reason it operates differently upon the mind and different actions are necessary in order to remove it. . . . Since it impinges not from without but from within the organism, no flight can avail against it. A better term for an instinctual stimulus is a 'need.' What does away with a need is 'satisfaction.' This can be obtained only by an appropriate ('adequate') alteration of the internal source of stimulation. (1915c, pp. 118–119)

Thus, the assumption of endogenously arising instinctual needs ingeniously provides an explanation for the kind of behavior that the vitalists had called "spontaneous," and therefore Rapaport (1958a) could write that the instinctual drives are the ultimate guarantees of the ego's autonomy from the environment. As Miller (1962) points out, however, behavior that is dominated by instinctual drives can hardly be considered autonomous, even with respect to the environment. (He gives the example of the way the attention and efforts of starving men are captured by putatively need-satisfying objects.) Therefore, it remains exceedingly difficult to account for ego autonomy as long as the assumption of a basically passive psychic apparatus is retained.

The final basic characteristic of psychoanalytic theory in its mature form that shows an obvious continuity with and indebtedness to the doctrines of Freud's teachers is the heavy emphasis on forces and energies as explanatory concepts. Again, it is by no stretch of the imagination necessary to demonstrate by painstaking documentation that psychoanalysis is a dynamic psychology. Gill (1959) has convincingly argued that a principal fault of psychoanalytic theory has been an overemphasis upon dynamic and economic considerations to the neglect of structural ones, a state of affairs he calls "reductionism to motivation."[12]

DIFFICULTIES CREATED BY FREUD'S BIOLOGICAL ASSUMPTIONS

I have attempted to demonstrate so far that the prevailing conception of the nervous system during Freud's years as a student and budding scientist was that of a passive reflex apparatus; that Freud unhesitatingly adopted it as a set of necessary starting points in his own neuropsychological theorizing; and that the ostensibly nonphysiological models of his later years still incorporated these same assumptions.

Let us now go back briefly to the question of what I have called Freud's ambivalence about the nature of his model. Recall that the change in theoretical stance and terminology that took place between the Project and *The Interpretation of Dreams* coincided with a set of far-reaching changes in Freud's personality: his change in professional identity, his self-analysis, his withdrawal from the medical community, and other correlated changes (which I have summarized elsewhere; Holt, 1963). It left him isolated not just personally but conceptually; before, he had been able to build on a sizable body of fact and accepted theory. In the Project, he did not create his theory from scratch, but simplified and extended what was standard doctrine. Later, with the declared intention of striking out on his own theoretically as well as professionally, he was in the exposed position of a frontiersman, forging ahead into the darkness without familiar landmarks, precedents, or findings—a prospect that would have daunted a lesser man! Small wonder, then, that he used the basic pattern of many familiar neurological concepts, with largely terminological changes.

Another less noticed change took place at the same time. The Project had been an ambitious attempt to account for normal psychological processes and also for dreams and psychopathology. He decided afterward to work with a minimum of assumptions and concepts, to explain one phenomenon at a time, and to proceed as modestly and cautiously as he could.

The aim of Chapter VII is, accordingly, much smaller in scale, being primarily an attempt to provide a psychology of the dream process. With each successive work the scope of the theory expanded in another way, so that ultimately psychoanalysis dealt with a virtually unparalleled breadth of topics. Yet even in the two sets of introductory lectures (1916–1917, 1933a) and the final *Outline of Psycho-Analysis* (1940a), Freud did not go back to the attempt to write a psychology of normal thought and action. He was not confronted by the necessity to conceptualize more than he felt he could handle at any one time, and thus did not have to face the inconsistencies in his theories.

When I look closely at the various passages in which Freud discussed the nature of the psychic apparatus, the realization is forced on me that it was something very much like what Hebb (1955) calls the CNS—a conceptual nervous system or a "brain model." True, Freud at times made characteristically hyperbolic statements about its freedom from any anatomical implications; but when we see how often he lapsed into neurological terminology, we may be tempted to interpret the repeated protestations in the way he taught us to do in his paper "Negation" (1925h). It is certain, at any rate, that Freud hoped for an eventual integration of his theory with neurology (1915e, p. 175) and that he always considered the biological facts to be quite relevant to his decisions about his own model.[13]

I believe, therefore, that Freud would have considered it of great significance if he had known the following five biological facts (most of which, to be sure, have become familiar to us only since his death).[14] Taken together, they decisively refute and contraindicate the model of a passive reflex mechanism.

1. The nervous system is perpetually *active*. Electroencephalographic [EEG] data have shown that even in the deepest sleep and in coma the brain does not cease its activity; at these times of minimal input and behavioral output, hypersynchrony seems to produce the most massive discharges. The resting nerve cell periodically fires (produces a spike potential), and its nontransmitted activity waxes and wanes, all without any outside stimulation.

2. Thus, the effect of stimulation is primarily to *modulate* the activity of the nervous system. It may step up the frequency of discharge but mainly imposes an order and patterning on it; that is to say, encodes it.[15]

3. The nervous system does not *conduct* energy; the nervous impulse is rather propagated. An appropriate physical analogy is not current running along a wired circuit, but the traveling flame of an ignited train of gunpowder.[16]

4. The energies of the nervous system, whether or not triggered by the sensory organs, are *different in kind* from the impinging external stimuli. The sensory surface is thus not a conductor but a transducer.[17]

5. The tiny energies of the nerves bear encoded information and are *quantitatively negligible*; their amount bears no relation to the motivational state of the person. The electrical phenomena associated with the neuron are accessible to quantitative study today, but this work offers no basis for the economic point of view—the assumption that mental events might be meaningfully examined from the standpoint of the "volumes of excitation" involved. Rather than this kind of "power engineering," "information engineering" seems to be the relevant discipline.[18]

Freud was wrong, therefore, as his teachers had been before him, or else he misunderstood them: The nervous system is not passive, does not take in and conduct out again the energies of the environment, and shows no tendency to "divest itself of" its own impulses. The principle of constancy is quite without any biological basis. The notion of homeostasis, which is more a point of view than a working concept in physiology today, is only a vague analogy and cannot be used to prop up this hoary anachronism.

If we follow Rapaport (1959) in his attempt to order psychoanalytic theory and make it what Freud called a "pure psychology," it may be argued that these biological facts have no relevance to the fundamental assumptions of such a psychology. May one not, with Strachey (1957b), even maintain that "much of what Freud had written in the 'Project' in terms of the nervous system now turned out to be valid and far more intelligible when translated into mental terms" (p. 164)?

On the contrary, I believe that *many of the obscurities, fallacies, and internal contradictions of psychoanalytic theory are rather direct derivatives of its neurological inheritance.* In the space remaining, I want to sketch out these dark areas of the theory, indicating what some of their principal difficulties are and their conflicts with the facts.

Problems in the Psychoanalytic Theory of Motivation and Affect[19]

From preceding sections, it should be obvious how the nature of the model results in a tension reduction conception of motivation and the pleasure principle. If it is the nature of the psychic apparatus to rid itself of tension, then behavior will be driven and organized by this necessity. The pleasure principle is the conceptual link between this viewpoint and the theory of pleasure and unpleasure as falls and rises in the amount of this inherently noxious quantity. Similar theories of motivation as tension reduction have been widespread in academic psychology.

Yet there are a number of logical difficulties with this conception. The term tension is conveniently ambiguous, to begin with; at least three types of meanings for it can be distinguished:

1. *Phenomenological*—tension is the subjective, conscious feeling of being tense. Freud espoused this definition in a passage quoted above

(1924c, p. 160): "In the series of feelings of tension we have a direct sense of the increase and decrease of amounts of stimulus," presumably meaning both exogenous and endogenous types of stimulation. This theory owes its tenacity to a number of supportive observations, which it fits neatly: If you sit on a tack, you jump up; if you get hunger pangs, you eat. Freud took these two types of motive, I believe, as paradigmatic in his conception of drives in general. Yet psychoanalysis is characteristically preoccupied with precisely the sorts of motive that operate silently, without identifiable conscious feelings of tension—which introspection does not turn up most of the time anyway, despite the assumption that *all* behavior is motivated. In general, then, conscious feelings of tension or unpleasure do not operate in the required ways often enough to serve as a satisfactory definition.

2. *Physiological*—tension is an objectively measurable disequilibrium in the body. This in turn might be of three principal types: muscular tonus or strain; a state of biochemical imbalance in the blood (glandular hyper- or hyposecretion, too little blood sugar, too much CO_2, etc.); or an "alerted" or "activated" state of the brain as indicated by the EEG or other electrical measurement. These three do not have any simple pattern of relations, and each subtype is actually so complex that it would be a hopeless and meaningless task to try to cast up a sum of all physiological tensions at any one time and then follow its fate. This biological meaning is hardly suitable, moreover, to be a motivational concept in pure psychology.

3. The final possibility is *abstract*—tension is a hypothetical disequilibrium of purely conceptual forces. This is the way Rapaport (1959) defined it; it is the logically implied definition if the psychic apparatus involved is itself an abstract, conceptual fiction. Tension so defined is a redundant concept, however, formally equivalent to "cathexis," "quantity," "psychic energy," or whatever else one assumes is the economic factor in psychoanalytic theory—the excitation that traverses the model's structural pathways. By this interpretation, also, it becomes so remote from any conceivable operations as to be scientifically trivial, a redundancy defined as what gets reduced when motivated behavior occurs. For a concept like tension to have scientific value, it must be measurable (at least crudely) in some way that is *independent* of the behavior it is invoked to explain.

Some years ago, Murphy (1947, pp. 996-997) argued cogently for a group of activity drives and sensory drives ("drives manifested in a need for specific sensory experiences") and collected a good deal of evidence in their support. Since then, empirical evidence against the theory of tension reduction has been mounting steadily (see, e.g., Cofer, 1959; Harlow, 1953; Hebb, 1955; Morgan, 1959; Stellar, 1954; White, 1963a). Experiments with rats have shown that the sweet taste of saccharine in water will be accepted as rewarding—hungry animals will work and learn for it, despite the fact that this substance cannot reduce any known psychological tension (Sheffield & Roby, 1950). Male rats will similarly exert themselves considerably to get access to a receptive female, even though the experimenter removes them after they have mounted and penetrated but before ejaculation, so that the "sexual tension" is never allowed to be discharged (Sheffield, Wulff, & Backer, 1951). In a notable series of studies done at the University of Wisconsin, Harlow (Butler & Harlow, 1957; Harlow, 1953, 1958) has shown that monkeys will work for the stimulus-increasing reward of getting to look out of a box into the laboratory room; will work at mechanical puzzles for no reward other than the fun of doing them; and—as infants—have a strong need for the contact stimulation provided by a mother-substitute.

To revert to the human level, a number of investigators (e.g., Duffy, 1957; Hebb, 1955; Lindsley, 1957), working with the concept of cortical activation as a result of volleys from the reticular formations, have shown that there is an optimal, midrange level of activation (which might be taken as a physiological definition of tension) for most kinds of behavior, and that people tend to seek mild to moderate levels of stimulation which maintain cortical activation.

A logical implication of the tension-reduction theory is that a state of affairs in which all stimulus inputs, both external and internal, are reduced to a minimum should be a blissful Nirvana. Experimental attempts to achieve this kind of situation for periods of time ranging from a few hours to a few days—in the wake of the pioneering experiments of Lilly (1956) and the McGill investigators (Bexton, Heron, & Scott, 1954)—have not been in complete agreement, but none of them has reported that people find the state of undistracted perceptual deprivation combined with rest and gratification of tissue needs very blissful. Many subjects grow restless and feel a positive need for stimulation, counter to the requirements of the theory. It has been assumed by a number of psychoanalytic theorists that under such conditions there would be nothing (besides the internal barriers of defense) to prevent sexual and aggressive drives from dominating the typically wandering thought processes, since most subjects report an inability to think connectedly and purposefully for very long (see Solomon et al., 1961). In point of fact, however subjective reports reveal very little takeover by drive fantasies (Miller, 1962), pointing to the dependence of these motives on external incitements and releases [see Chapter 9, this volume].

The work of Olds (1958; Olds & Milner, 1954), Miller (1958), and others on the effects of direct electrical stimulation of subcortical structures in the brain has a number of major implications for the psychoanalytic theory of motivation and affect. These studies, by now too well known to require extensive review, have discovered septal areas which, when stimulated by appropriate pulse trains delivered by implanted electrodes, give rise to unmistakable aversive behavioral signs of intense unpleasure or distress. By itself, this finding would seem consistent with Exner's and Freud's hypotheses; but it turns out that the quantity of stimulation (above a certain threshold) is unimportant, whereas the location of the stimulated site is vital. In some instances, a shift of a few millimeters will put the electrode in a spot which, when given the same quantity of electrical stimulation, yields exactly opposite results. Rats trained to press a lever for brief pulses of stimulation will do so uninterruptedly for hours—indeed, until they drop with exhaustion—when the intracranial electrodes have been implanted in one of these rewarding or pleasure centers. In studies with human subjects (e.g., Bishop, Elder, & Heath, 1963), the result of such stimulation is subjective reports of intense pleasure or unpleasure. Any further attempts to link pleasure with a drop in some kind of physiological tension, or other such economic theories of affect, are decisively refuted—unless a retreat is made into the untestability of the tautological concept of abstract, purely conceptual tension.

We know now from the data cited that motivation is *not* a matter of reducing either a physiological or a phenomenological tension and that pleasure is a valid and separate phenomenon in its own right, not merely the absence or reduction of pain or unpleasure. Thus, it seems clearly established that there are both positive and negative motivations, not merely negative ones. Observation surely suggests that there are adient, or approaching, as well as abient, or stimulus-reducing, motives, and we need no longer go through theoretical gymnastics to make it appear that what looks like approach and stimulus hunger is actually a way of fleeing from even stronger, internal tensions.

Aggression was always a problem for Freudian theory. For many years, Freud maintained a curious kind of blind spot concerning it; he saw and worked with it clinically, but when it came to theoretical statements tried to get rid of it as a special kind of self-preservative manifestation of ego instinct or a sadomasochistic form of sexuality (Freud, 1905d). When he finally came to grips with the necessity to postulate a separate hostile or destructive motive, he produced the theory of the death instinct. Freud's shaky logic in developing his case, the questionable and speculative nature of the facts he adduced, and the general lack of evidential support for this theory are well known. I believe, therefore, that I need not do more here than show the linkage of this concept to the reflex-arc model.

Freud introduced the argument for the death instinct by a kind of generalization of the principle of constancy into the conception of the conservative nature of instincts. It is a logical enough extension of the notion that the nervous system tends to rid itself of stimuli and restore its previous state of rest, to assume that all drives "tend toward the restoration of an earlier state of things" (1920g, pp. 37–38). Then, since all living matter can be assumed to have once been lifeless, it should have a drive to return to a nonliving condition. "The attributes of life were at some time evoked in inanimate matter by the action of a force of whose nature we can have no conception. . . . The tension which then arose in what had hitherto been an inanimate substance endeavoured to cancel itself out. In this way the first instinct came into being" (p. 38)—the death drive. This is truly tension reduction carried to its bitter end!

In a passage from *The Economic Problem of Masochism* which I have cited repeatedly, Freud made the linkage between the principle of constancy and the death instinct explicit by clarifying the relationship between the pleasure principle and the Nirvana principle. The Nirvana principle is the tendency to reduce stimuli to the absolute minimum and thus "expresses the trend of the death instinct" (1924c, p. 160).

In summary, the extensions and applications of his passive reflex model to problems of motivation and affect led Freud's theory into many conflicts with fact and to little of lasting value.

Problems of the Energy Doctrine
(the Economic Point of View)

The propositions I have been criticizing are largely energic, despite the fact that references to a reflex-arc model may sound structural. In line with the tradition of the school of Helmholtz, however, Freud consistently followed the assumption that scientific explanation had to rely primarily on forces and energies, and devoted a great part of his theorizing to dynamic and economic propositions. At the beginning of the final section of Chapter VII of *The Interpretation of Dreams*, for example, after summarizing part of his argument, which had been partly in structural terms, he said:

> Let us replace these metaphors by something that seems to correspond better to the real state of affairs, and let us say instead that some particular mental grouping has had a cathexis of energy attached to it or withdrawn from it. . . . What we are doing here is once again to replace a topographical way of representing things by a dynamic one. (1900a, p. 610)

It is apparent that he felt on sounder ground and closer to reality with the cathectic language than with his structural concepts, which he recognized were metaphors. What he did not see was that psychic energy was just as metaphorical a concept [see Chapter 3, this volume].

Even if one wished to work with the concept of psychic energy, it is difficult to see how this hypothetical entity could exist outside of some kind of structures to accumulate, transmit, and discharge it. Once one accepts the need to work with structural concepts, it begins to seem unnecessary to try to account for the delay of inhibition in energic discharge by the postulation of qualitative changes in the energy itself, when a structural conception of defense and control can do the job with a minimum of new assumptions. In this respect, however, Freud was unable to change the habits of thought he had learned from his physicalistic mentors and seems not to have questioned the assumption that a dynamic or economic concept is always preferable to any other, even if it involves the successive postulation of a bewildering variety of types and modes of psychic energy (e.g., bound, fused, neutralized, aim-inhibited, etc.).

The classic laws of thermodynamics were taken by Helmholtz's colleagues and followers as directly and definitively applicable to all matters pertaining to energy in physiology. These laws apply to any Newtonian system within which all quantities of energy involved can be specified, thus in principle to organisms as well as solar systems; the simplest example of such a system, however, is an artificially closed system with a fixed amount of energy. Brücke understood the basic facts about the energy exchanges carried on by organisms (in nutrition, respiration, etc), which had been clearly enunciated by the 1860s, as his lectures show.[20] Nevertheless, the didactic value that was lent to the closed system by its very oversimplification made it play an important role as a paradigm for the post-Helmholtzians, shaping their thought even when they were aware of its deficiencies. Hence, it was natural for Freud to adopt as a first approximation the assumption of a fixed amount of libido, reverberating around within a closed system so that the fate of quantities could be traced (at least in principle, for in practice no operations were ever adduced to make the measurement of psychic energy possible). Thus, if a certain amount of libido were withdrawn from objects, it had to cathect some part of the body, the ego, or another psychic structure. Within these assumptions, the economic point of view seems appealingly rigorous and scientific, apparently opening up explanatory possibilities unique to psychoanalysis. The inexorable law of entropy seems also to support the postulation of a death instinct (see also Szasz, 1952).

The work of Bertalanffy (1950) has brought sharply to our attention the facts that a human being or any other living organism is very far indeed from being a closed system and that there are rigorous and lawful ways of dealing with open systems. The very concept of an equilibrium of forces is inappropriate to a living system, which tends to maintain steady states in which inputs are in balance with outputs (cf. Pumpian-Mindlin, 1959). Such a system can show the characteristics of negative entropy as it grows and develops, which was inconceivable in a closed physical system.

With the advent of open-system conceptions, the main arguments for the predominance of the economic point of view (the quantitative treatment of energies) collapse, as does the entropic argument for the death drive.

Problems in Psychoanalytic Psychopathology

For the most part, Freud's clinical theories about the nature of neurosis and its genesis stayed rather close to his clinical observation, remaining a solid and permanent contribution. Yet in a few matters, the assumptions of the passive reflex model led him into clinical *culs-de-sac*. I have in mind the early theory of anxiety and the related conception of "actual neurosis," and the theory of traumatic neurosis.

In the 1890s, let us recall, much of Freud's psychopathology was built on a conception that, at some point, physical phenomena became psychic. Thus, his first account of sexuality includes the assertion that, after the neural impulses generated by the distinction of the seminal vesicles in an abstinent man reach a certain threshold level, they became a psychical stimulus. That was the normal state of affairs; in hysteria, the constitutional capacity for conversion permitted the transmutation of affect charge back into somatic excitation (1894a). At this time, the "fermentation" or "toxic" theory of anxiety appeared: "the mechanism of anxiety neurosis is to be looked for in a deflection of somatic sexual excitation from the psychical sphere, and in a consequent abnormal employment of that excitation" (1895b [1894], p. 108). The other actual neurosis was given a similarly somatic explanation:

> Neurasthenia develops whenever the adequate unloading [of somatic sexual tension] (the adequate action) is replaced by a less adequate one—thus, when normal coition, carried out in most favorable conditions, is replaced by masturbation or spontaneous emission. Anxiety neurosis, on the other hand, is the product of all those factors which prevent the somatic sexual excitation from being worked over psychically. The manifestations of anxiety neurosis appear when the somatic excitation which has been deflected from the psyche is expanded subcortically in totally inadequate reactions. (1895b [1894], p. 109)

In his paper on "wild" psychoanalysis, Freud (1910k) admitted that he had seen few cases of such actual neurosis, but he did not cease believing in it, and continued to classify neurasthenia and anxiety neurosis under this heading. In an encyclopedia article (1923a, p. 243) he said that the actual neurosis "could be traced to contemporary abuses in the patients' sexual life and could be removed if these were brought to an end," adding that they occurred "by chemical agency."

Looking back on his early psychoanalytic work (1925d, pp. 25-26), Freud told about his "discovery" of the actual neurosis and confidently described the different types of abnormal sexual practice found in each. He added: "Since that time [the 1890s] I have had no opportunity of returning to the investigation of the 'actual neuroses'; nor has this part of my work been continued by anyone else." He speaks of these "early findings" slightly apologetically, maintaining, however, that

> they seem to me still to hold good. . . . I am far from denying the existence of mental conflicts and of neurotic complexes in neurasthenia. All that I am asserting is that the symptoms of these patients are not mentally determined or removable by analysis, but that they must be regarded as direct toxic consequences of disturbed sexual chemical processes.

The connection of this theory to the biological notions we have under consideration here is directly pointed out by Strachey (1959, p. 78):

> Following Fechner, he had taken as a fundamental postulate the "principle of constancy," according to which there was an inherent tendency in the nervous system to reduce, or at least to keep constant, the amount of excitation present in it. When, therefore, he made the clinical discovery that in cases of anxiety neurosis it was always possible to discover some interference with the discharge of sexual tension, it was natural for him to conclude that the accumulated excitation was finding its way out in the transformed shape of anxiety.

The signal theory of anxiety had existed side by side with the toxic theory almost from the beginning, and Freud had expressed doubts about the latter in a letter to Fliess in 1897 (as Strachey points out; 1959, p. 79). In 1926 he gave up all but a small vestige of the toxic theory, and in the *New Introductory Lectures* finally abandoned it even as an explanation of anxiety neurosis. Today very few clinicians indeed can be found whose experience confirms the etiological sequences Freud thought he saw in actual neurosis, so that one wonders whether the whole concept was not based on the coincidence of a few chance clinical observations with an obvious derivation from the passive reflex model.

Freud's conception of traumatic neurosis is closely linked to his "protective shield against stimuli," the relation of which to the physicalistic view of reality we have already reviewed. In *Beyond the Pleasure Principle*, he wrote:

> We may . . . tentatively venture to regard the comon traumatic neurosis as a consequence of an extensive breach . . . in the protective shield against stimuli. . . . Because of lack of any preparedness for anxiety, including lack of hypercathexis of the systems that would be the first to receive the stimulus . . . those systems are not in a good position for binding the inflowing amounts of excitation. (1920g, p. 31)

What is the effect of "this invasion" of physical energies?

> Cathectic energy is summoned from all sides to provide sufficiently high cathexes of energy in the environs of the breach. An 'anticathexis' on a grand scale is set up, for whose benefit all the other psychical systems are impoverished, so that the remaining psychical functions are extensively paralysed or reduced. (p. 31)

Freud concluded his explanation by invoking the compulsion to repeat.

This theory has a number of esthetically pleasing ingenuities, as Freud's constructions almost always do, but it also has such serious inconsistencies that it cannot be considered tenable. The central concept of the protective shield is tantalizingly elusive, an excellent example of Freud's ambivalence about mental versus physiological models. When he first introduces it, he is plainly talking about a physical feature, an external anatomical layer. Yet [as detailed in Chapter 3 of this volume], he soon switched, without warning, to a metaphorical/psychological meaning. If Freud had consistently kept to the anatomical/physiological realm, he would never have been able to make his concept perform such gymnastics and would not have approached an explanation in this way at all. If he had kept to a consistently "pure psychology," he would have had to eschew the attempt to explain *any* condition marked by somatic symptoms. Fortunately for the development of clinical psychoanalysis, he did not take this last course, but faced up to psychosomatic complications wherever he met them (in affects, sexuality, organ neuroses, conversion symptoms, etc.), sacrificing the internal consistency and clarity of his system rather than deny clinical reality.

Problems in the Theory of Object Relations

In *Instincts and Their Vicissitudes*, Freud advances the rather startling doctrine of the primary hate of objects: "It cannot be denied that hating . . . originally characterized the relation of the ego to the alien external world with the stimuli it introduces. . . . At the very beginning, it seems, the external world, objects, and what is hated are identical" (1915c, p. 136). "Hate, in relation to objects, is older than love. It derives from the narcissistic ego's primordial repudiation of the external world with its outpouring of stimuli" (p. 139). This conception is sharply at variance with direct observation of infants, with their delight in new experience, their fascinated staring at freshly presented objects, their pleasure in bringing about "pleasing spectacles" (Piaget, 1936). Yet it is directly consequent from the passive model: If the apparatus has as its basic principle the tendency to get rid of stimuli and if the increase in energy within it is unpleasant, then the approach of any object must be originally distressing and must arouse an emotional rejection that might be called hate. Only after the organism discovers from bitter experience that it is necessary to have traffic with this noxious world in order to escape the persistent and equally unpleasant tensions within does this model allow for the secondary development of any positive striving for persons, things, or experiences generally.

   This basic difficulty pervades the whole Freudian theory of object relations, which he never fully clarified. The basic paradigm of the analytic concept of objects and their interaction with drives seems to be food and food seeking. The hunger drive arises internally, causing discomfort and restlessness; the external object, a piece of food, which formerly was indifferent, now becomes attractive, so that we can say that the percept is cathected with oral libido. This energy is discharged in the act of eating; the drive subsides, and food objects are now indifferent at best, even disgusting. This common-sense account does not completely accord with modern studies of the nature of the hunger drive, but it is appealing and easy to fit in with the Brücke–Meynert model. With only slightly more difficulty, casual sexual encounters can be conceptualized in this way too; but this kind of interaction with objects is properly a matter of discharge rather than cathexis. Major difficulty begins when one considers *enduring* object relations. In 1921, Freud wrote:

> In one class of cases being in love is nothing more than object-cathexis on the part of the sexual instincts with a view to directly sexual satisfaction, a cathexis which expires, moreover, when this aim has been reached; this is what is called common, sensual love. But, as we know, the libidinal situation rarely remains so simple. It was possible to calculate with certainty upon the revival of the need which had just expired; and this must no doubt have been the first motive for directing a lasting cathexis upon the sexual object and for 'loving' it in the passionless intervals as well. (1921c, p. 111)

A brief digression on the concept of cathexis is in order at this point. In the basic reflex model, there is no provision for the delay of discharge; yet observation insists that there is such a phenomenon most of the time. Exner and Breuer were therefore forced to include what was a common neurophysiological assumption, that there could be a nontransmitted excitation of the nerve cell, which they called "tonic" in analogy to muscular tonus. When Freud incorporated this concept in the Project, he called it *Besetzung*, the "occupation" of a nerve cell by quantity; the conventional English rendition of this word as "cathexis" loses the static connotation of the German. As time went on, Freud began to use "cathexis" as a general term for the energy of the neural or psychic apparatus and (as we saw in Chapter 4) referred to this energy when in a sedentary, nontransmitted state as "bound." Nevertheless, the original connotation tended to cling to the concept of cathexis, particularly in usages like "object-cathexis." For example, in the just-quoted passage, note that the cathexis "expires" in the process of sexual gratification or discharge.

To account for lasting cathexes, which are more than temporary delays of discharge, Freud had therefore to introduce a further qualitative differentiation of energies, despite his vigorous rejection (in 1950 [1895] and again in 1915c) of the idea that drive energies could have any qualitative characteristic other than "period" (frequency—itself a quantitative characteristic). This innovation was aim inhibitedness: As a consequence of the Oedipus complex and its resolution, "the child still remains tied to his parents, but by instincts which must be described as being 'inhibited in their aim.' The emotions which he feels henceforward towards these objects of his love are characterized as 'affectionate'" (1921c, p. 111). "The depth to which anyone is in love, as contrasted with his purely sensual desire, may be measured by the size of the share taken by the aim-inhibited instincts of affection" (1921c, p. 112). This assumption nicely fits the requirement of an economic explanation for persisting attachment that does not die down after orgasm, as sexual desire proper does. The trouble is that it seems almost entirely *ad hoc*; Freud simply postulated that it takes place as a result of frustration, without explicating any mechanism or making it plausible in terms of the passive reflex model. Moreover, he does not account for the fact that as a person builds up many friendships, and consequently accumulates more aim-inhibited, undischargeable libido, there is not a general rise in the subjective sense of unpleasure. Actually, of course, the reverse tends to take place: The more affection we have for our friends, the better we feel, and surely not depleted of energy.

Freud argued just the opposite, however; and here is another respect in which his theory of object relations seems unsatisfactory and his reported observations at variance with what most of us see today. In the paper *On Narcissism*, Freud declared that "it is easy to observe that libidinal object-cathexis does not raise self-regard. The effect of dependence on the loved object is to lower that feeling: a person in love is humble" (1914c, p. 98). He does allow for the possibility of "a real happy love" through the complementary assumption: "Loving in itself . . . lowers self-regard; whereas being loved, having one's love returned, and possessing the loved object, raises it once more" (1914c, p. 99). Nevertheless, it remains a puzzle that Freud should have thought that loving lowered self-esteem, until one recalls that closed-system implication of his energetics: If there is just a limited supply of libido, and if a major part of it is committed to a love object, it must follow that less is left over for the self. This is indeed an economics of scarcity (Ghent, 1962) applied to love, whereas an open-system approach allows one to observe that loving tends to be a positive feedback system: The more we give, the more we have both for ourselves and for others (Fromm, 1939).

There are a number of related criticisms of Freud's theory of narcissism that might be added: the odd contention that schizophrenics have a great deal of self-esteem; unsolved economic problems in the relation of narcissism, identification, and sublimation; and the difficulty in comprehending how there can be "an internal draining away of excitations which are incapable of direct discharge outwards . . . by means of an internal process of working-over . . . carried out upon real or imaginary objects" (1914c, pp. 85–86). But I believe that I have probably cited enough examples of theoretical difficulties that follow quite directly from Freud's basic assumptions, which, as we have seen, derived directly from essentially biological propositions.

CONCLUSION

In one of his best-known declarations of independence from neurology, Freud wrote (1915e, p. 175):

Our psychical topography as *for the present* nothing to do with anatomy; it has reference not to anatomical localities, but to regions in the mental apparatus, wherever they may be situated in the body. In this respect, then, our work is untrammelled and may proceed according to its own requirements.

He hoped, therefore, that a shift to a kind of abstract brain model, without commitments to precise localization and even without explicit statement that it was a neuropsychology, would free him from the limitations of the biological disciplines within which he had labored so many years. Ironically, by this very shift he concealed the biological nature of his theoretical starting points and protected them from correction when at last neurophysiology and neuroanatomy began to make great strides. By taking his teachers' statements about the nature of the nervous system not as empirical propositions subject to verification or correction, but as unquestioned postulates, he put the whole theory further away from testability.

In bringing these hidden, and now clearly erroneous, biological propositions out into the open and showing their mischievous ramifications in psychoanalytic theory, Amacher and I have tried to remain true to the spirit of Freud's reiterated hopes that his science could someday be brought back into contact with biology. He wrote, for example: "we must recollect that all our provisional ideas in psychology will presumably some day be based on an organic substructure" (1914c, p. 78).

I believe that day is fast approaching. An organic substructure can be provided today, incorporating nearly a century of research, which has greatly changed our understanding of the brain's structures—both gross and fine—and its functions since the doctrines of post-Müllerian physiology were laid down. The breathtaking rapidity of advance in neuropsychology today is in the most instructive contrast to the hesitant pace of change in psychoanalysis. Yet by making some basic modifications, psychoanalysis can take itself out of its dangerously encapsulated position and get back into the mainstream of scientific advance. I get an irrational glow of gratification at the poetic justice in the prospect that psychoanalysis may at last become the kind of productive science Freud wanted it to be by a return to the disciplines in which he did his first scientific and professional work. Aside from sentiment, however, we owe it not only to Freud but to ourselves to protect the many and vitally important substantive contributions of psychoanalysis from the danger of wholesale rejection to which the general theory's vulnerability to methodological criticism exposes them.

CHAPTER 6

Beyond Vitalism and Mechanism: Freud's Concept of Psychic Energy

Over the years, I have had useful conversations about psychoanalytic theory with many friends and colleagues, most notably David Rapaport. Since his death, the most helpful and stimulating such friend I have had is Benjamin B. Rubinstein, M.D. In a conversation we were having about theoretical matters once in the summer of 1962, he remarked to me in passing that psychic energy was a vitalistic concept. At the time, I knew little about vitalism, but the term seemed to me to carry a pejorative connotation. I recall bridling and saying something to the effect that it was no good simply insulting psychic energy. My friend responded in some such way as to indicate that he was making a substantive characterization, not just decrying the concept; either then or shortly thereafter, he suggested that I read Schlick (1953). Thus, I am glad to acknowledge that the basic idea for the present chapter and its principal insight came from Ben Rubinstein. The interested reader can find a number of original and powerful arguments against the concept of psychic energy in his various papers, most notably his first two (Rubinstein, 1965, 1967a).

I presented the first draft of this paper as part of a panel on psychic energy at the December 1962 meetings of the American Psychoanalytic Association. In the original published version of the paper (Holt, 1967c), I indicated that my principal source for the history of science was the excellent book by Singer (1959). Since then, I have done a good deal more reading in the history of science generally and of the vitalism–mechanism controversy in particular. In fact, I have included a longer retelling of what is covered in the few pages of the section on "Vitalism and Mechanism: A Historical Review" in a chapter of another book, an intellectual biography of Freud on which I am still working. So as not to repeat myself, I have done little more than to correct and slightly amplify the present brief account.

The concept of psychic energy is central to Freud's metapsychology; in fact, it was the principal means he called upon to help him explain the events of clinical observation. In its development during the past 40 years, the concept has steadily ramified into a conceptual thicket that baffles some, impresses many, and greatly complicates the task of anyone who tries to form a clear idea of what the basic theory of psychoanalysis is. Up to a point, one can get a good deal of clarification by tracing its place in the development of Freud's ideas, but the thoughts of no man are a closed system. The search for historical understanding leads us past Freud's immediate intellectual ancestors, past the bounds of psychology, and into one of the major themes in the history of biology: the opposing views of vitalism and mechanism. Before considering the present methodological status of psychic energy, therefore, let us review the history of the theoretical antitheses out of which it grew.

VITALISM AND MECHANISM: A HISTORICAL REVIEW

First, some definitions. The term "mechanism" has a greater variety of meanings than "vitalism"; even as an abstraction, it can refer to a complete metaphysical system or to much narrower notions—here, to the mechanistic theory of life. A biological mechanist begins with the assumption that an organism is a machine, which we call "alive" when it functions properly. Therefore, it can be completely explained and understood by calling on no more theoretical resources than those of physics and chemistry. In its hardest, most reductionistic version, Newtonian mechanics (dynamics)—the laws of motion—allegedly will suffice.

For several centuries, there were two main alternatives, animism and vitalism, which may usefully be distinguished. The former (and older) doctrine distinguishes body and soul, identifying life with the state in which the two are in some kind of intimate association. The conceptions of mind, soul, and ghost are closely related. Obviously, both common sense and most religions are animistic in this sense, clearly opposed to the nonmystical, "nothing-but" hardheadedness of mechanism. Vitalistic theories substitute some other, secular concept—a vital principle or force—for the soul, but agree with animism in protesting that the animate and inanimate worlds are fundamentally different, and that there must be a separate and irreducible science of biology devoted to living things.

The first point to be made, in tracing the history of an idea like vitalism, is that we must not fall into the trap of thinking of it as a single, coherent doctrine to which many generations of writers adhered. Rather, the term alludes to a range of similar conceptions, related to one another largely through being parts of a genetic (historical) series.

As is true of so much of the history of ideas, this theme begins with the ancient Greeks. Before either vitalism or mechanism (yet eventually to be intertwined with them) came the opposed concepts of "being" and "becoming," which became ingrained in Western thought. Of the several thinkers whose work gave rise to this antithesis, there is space here to mention only two. Around 500 B.C., Heraclitus promulgated the idea that "all things are in flux"—everything is so constantly changing that becoming is the true reality and fire the ultimate substance. Democritus, 70 years his junior, is the most famous opposing atomist of antiquity. Far from admitting any reality to process, he taught that only atoms and the void are real. The qualities we perceive are produced by motion of the hard, indestructible bits of substance he conceived atoms to be, and all motion originates in previous movement of atoms.

Plato was enough influenced by Heraclitus to believe that the direct objects of observation were but transitory appearances; what persisted and was ultimately real, he thought, was the *idea*. In more modern terms, he rejected concrete particulars as of only passing and accidental importance and was much more impressed by the enduring abstract concept. It is easy to see how this point of view was favorable to the development of mathematics. Yet Plato's doctrine of ideas gives these abstractions a metaphysical status of a higher reality than that of sensory presentations.

It happens that the Greek word *idea* is equally well translated by the English words "form" and "idea." (Hence Pepper, 1942, calls Plato's philosophical system "formism.") This association of form with the transempirical *idea* may have been a subtle obstacle hindering empirical scientists of many later centuries from tackling structure and organization analytically.

[In Plato's time, the Greek word *psukhe* also had a variety of meanings: "breath," "life," "mind," "spirit," and "soul." Not surprisingly, these diverse concepts were not clearly differentiated in classic Greek thought. Thus, the idea that was to become first animism and then vitalism began as an undifferentiated matrix of partly concrete, partly abstract notions. Doubtless they were strongly influenced by the mystery of death, when breath, motion, warmth, and a person's humanity cease all at once in the end of life. By combining the wish to undo the loss of those we love and the wish to avoid a definitive end to our own existences, human beings have very widely produced concepts like *psukhe*, in which the mystery of life is thought of as a kind of spirit or essence that departs with a person's last breath, leaving the still, cold body and perhaps having an independent subsequent existence.]

Aristotle did not differ a great deal from Plato in his treatment of these issues; but where the teacher was a dualist, the great student held to a kind of monism, with the soul not conceptualized as existentially separate from the body. Many writers (e.g., Nagel, 1953; Rapoport, 1962; Schlick, 1953) stress the similarity with which Aristotle treated the physical and biological worlds. He viewed the motions of smoke and birds alike as a seeking after their "natural positions" in the sky; it was a thoroughgoing teleology, applied to all of nature (which is probably why Driesch repeatedly—e.g., in 1914 and 1929—hailed him as the first true vitalist).

Aristotle modified and qualified Plato's doctrine of ideas without rejecting what was fallacious in it, which Popper (1957) calls "essentialism":

taking universal or generalized terms as real. Indeed, Popper says that
Aristotle founded the school of methodological essentialism, which

> taught that scientific research must penetrate to the essence of things in order to
> explain them. Methodological essentialists are inclined to formulate scientific
> questions in such terms as "what is matter" . . . and they believe that a penetrat-
> ing answer to such questions, revealing the real or essential meaning of . . .
> terms and thereby the real or true nature of the essence denoted by them, is at
> least a necessary prerequisite of scientific research, if not its main task.
> *Methodological nominalists* . . . hold that the task of science is only to describe
> how things behave . . . they regard *words* merely as *useful instruments of
> description.* [Most people, Popper concludes,] will admit that methodological
> nominalism has been victorious in the natural sciences. (1957, p. 29)

But that is jumping far ahead in the story. For the moment, I wish only to
point out how essentialism characterized all of early Greek thought and how
such a doctrine as vitalism—the postulation of some kind of vital force,
entelechy, or the like as the ultimate explanation of the difference between
living and nonliving things—is an excellent example of essentialism.

Around 400 A.D., St. Augustine brought a good deal of Plato into
Christianity, and about 850 years later St. Thomas Aquinas integrated Aristotle with Christian theology. It did not prove difficult to fit the immortal
and transmaterial soul, the interventions of a personal God in a material
world, and other supernatural dogmas into the great Greek philosophies,
making a unified world view of enormous prestige and authority. It dominated the entire intellectual world for many centuries, and still controls
more of it than many of us realize.

Under the sway of Thomist scholasticism, vitalism and mechanism
could not very well emerge as opposing ideas—not until Galileo had promulgated modern mechanics in the early part of the 17th century and put to
rout the anthropomorphic view of force in the physical world.[1] But not only
there: "His conception of a mechanical universe swiftly reacted even on the
biological sciences," Singer (1959, pp. 250-251) notes. Rejecting the Aris-
totelean view, "biologists sought to explain the animal body as a machine.
The first important biological works of the seventeenth century—for example, those of Santorio . . . , of Harvey . . . , or Descartes . . . —all sought
thus to explain the body."

The first post-Galilean proponent of a widely influential unified theory
of the universe, René Descartes (1596-1650), did not break with religion but
kept God and the soul in a mechanical world of bodies by means of a
metaphysical dualism. He conceived of man's body as a machine animated
by a rational soul, a nonmaterial spirit that interacted with the world of
matter in only one locality, the pineal gland. It is particularly worthy of our
note that for Descartes, "the special prerogative of the soul is to originate
action" (Singer, 1959, p. 277). Since it was not part of the material world, it

did not obey natural laws, but was *free*. Lacking this free will, lower animals were capable only of automatic actions. To him they were machines, like the impressive hydromechanical[2] automata at the Austrian palace of Hellbrunn (dating from 1615) with which he was familiar (Culbertson, 1963). Although Descartes did not originate the concept of the reflex, he focused attention on it and gave it wide currency.

Was Descartes a mechanist, then, or an animist? The answer must be that he was both; his influence stimulated and supported both tendencies. Even though he did not himself focus on a gap between the living and the nonliving, his dualistic philosophy laid down a general model for the vitalist contention and helped provide a truce between religion (which could concern itself with the soul and spiritual matters) and science (to which was left the entire physical world). This Solomon's judgment split the previously prevailing unity of knowledge, however, into two great departments— natural philosophy and moral philosophy—a division that still survives.

With Newton (1642–1727), science proceeded to move in and take command over the material universe. One of the reasons Newton was so honored in his lifetime was that his elegant formulation of the laws of mechanics synthesized elements that were already familiar. Galileo had broken ground and made the rough sketches; Newton built a logically unassailable theoretic structure, which was, moreover, completely hospitable to empirical research. But even a mansion is not a lofty enough metaphor for his achievement; here was one of those grand syntheses, which so capture the imagination that they are easy to overextend.

The full extent and revolutionary character of the change that Newton was working in men's minds was not at first recognized even by himself, but it became apparent in the course of the eighteenth century. The essential revolutionary element was that Newton had conceived a working universe wholly independent of the spiritual order.[3] This was the profoundest break that had yet been made with all for which the Middle Ages stood. With Newton there set in an age of scientific determinism. (Singer, 1959, p. 294)

. . . the course of the new science, as a progression from the observation of a few phenomena to a world-outlook, was transmuted into a world-outlook imposed on those phenomena. . . . It had been the habit of philosophers to see all detailed things *sub specie aeternitatis* [that is, in terms of Platonic essentialism]. Hence, no sooner was the conception of inert bodies passively following the dictates of blind forces seen to be applicable to the motion of mass-points, than it was immediately generalized into a world-philosophy. Instead of being accepted as what it was—a generalized statement of certain particularly simple motions—it became a principle of universal determinism or materialism and to that principle phenomena and experiences quite unrelated to such motions were held to be subject. (Singer, 1959, pp. 419–420)

The central elements of this concept of the world were *forces* acting on material *bodies*. But as Singer points out,

There was still much vagueness as to the limits of the two. Thus, "phlogiston," which was supposed to go forth from a body on combustion, and "ether," which was at once agent and medium of light, no less than the electric and magnetic "fluids," remained ambiguous conceptions to the very end of the eighteenth century and even into the nineteenth. (1959, p. 347)

Some of them, like heat ("caloric") and electricity, were thought to be weightless substances, the "imponderables."

One result of the Newtonian revolution was a great impetus to a mechanistic conception of biology. It took such extreme forms as the following:

> Given the principle of least motion, animated bodies will have all that is necessary for moving, feeling, thinking, repenting, and in a word for conducting themselves in the physical realm, and in the moral realm which depends upon it. Let us then conclude boldly that man is a machine, and that in the whole universe there is but a single substance variously modified. (La Mettrie, 1748)

Note the phrase "but a single substance"; it negates the contemporaneous vitalistic doctrine that living things contained unique substances, or at least a special chemistry with compounds that required life to come into being. In the unitary world of Aristotle, there was no such dichotomy of substance; indeed, it was assumed that complex living beings could arise by spontaneous generation from dead matter. With the rise of microscopy in the second half of the 17th century, it was possible to trace the life cycle of insects and to see their previously invisible eggs, and thus to prove that it was not the sun that bred maggots in dead animals. Further technical advances made the microbiologists of the 18th century increasingly skeptical that spontaneous generation occurred even in the wholly microscopic world of the infusoria, but the doctrine was not laid to rest until the conclusive demonstrations of Pasteur and Tyndall in the second half of the 19th century. Long before, in 1828, Wöhler had struck a decisive blow at the vitalist conclusion that there must be special life-substances, by his synthesis of the organic compound urea. Thus the decisive evidence for a basic split between living and nonliving matter came after an impressive demonstration of continuity on the level of substance.

In the 18th century there was no dearth of vitalists to combat those biologists who adopted the prevailing mechanistic philosophy. The chemist G. E. Stahl (1660–1734), who gave the notion of phlogiston wide circulation, was one spokesman for the biological vitalists of his day. In obscure and mystical prose, he taught that the "sensitive soul" follows its own laws, which govern life. But even such men as Hoffman (1660–1742), Boerhaave (1668–1738), and von Haller (1708–1777), who had also held dualistic beliefs about the influences on the body of the mind or soul as a living principle or vital spirit, made their important contributions by applying the principles of mechanics to the physiological study of the body, treated essentially as a machine.

Not nearly so half-hearted was the reaction against universal mechanism of a new, largely philosophical school which arose around the middle of the 18th century, attained an enormous vogue in Germany particulary, and subsided slowly a hundred years later: *Naturphilosophie*, or naturephilosophy. Not a tightly knit school, it included many thinkers, from the logical rationalist Kant to wild and fantastic speculators such as Oken. In part, it was a return to Aristotle. It taught that dualism was an unstable equilibrium, which had been denied by a radical mechanism via the reduction of life and mind to atoms and their motions. *Naturphilosophie* also proclaimed a unity, but more by a blurring of distinctions than by a consistent idealistic monism in which mind might be the one true reality. All of Nature was viewed as an organic, evolving unity by Schelling (1775–1854), perhaps the central figure. His philosophy, says Schlick (1953, p. 523), "makes organic processes into fundamental explanatory principles, thus attempts to reduce nonliving nature to the living." Kant (1724–1804) was a great deal more sophisticated; it was an abstract unity that he postulated in nature uniting the mechanical and teleological. Yet he taught that the parts of living organisms could be understood only in terms of their functions for the whole. As Singer (1959, p. 385) summarizes and paraphrases: "The very existence of the whole implies an end. True, says Kant, Nature exhibits to us nothing in the way of purpose. Nevertheless we can only understand an organism if we regard it as though produced under the guidance of thought for the end."

Under Kant's influence, Goethe developed the Platonic implication of this guiding thought into the conception of "ideas" in the mind of God, which were manifested as a limited number of patterns for the structure of organisms. Oken (1779–1851) took up this notion and applied it with a combination of shrewd observation of animals' structure and rank speculation, developing such hypotheses as the essential similarity of the human head and trunk, or that of the vertebrae and the skull. To quote Singer once again:

> For these Nature Philosophers the repetition of organs, "segmentation," in many plant and animal types [for example, as in the earthworm] was a plan or "idea" (in the Platonic sense) in the mind of God. . . . Whence comes the continued fascination of thoughts so little related to the daily task of the scientific observer? The essence of the thought of such men is that the process of the mind reflect the processes of Nature. (1959, p. 389)

This is a well-known Kantian doctrine, with roots in Plato's conception of the macrocosm of nature as reflecting the microcosm of man.

By one of the choicest ironies in the history of psychology, one of its most suffocatingly rigorous branches is a direct offshoot of nature-philosophy, for Fechner (1801–1887) invented psychophysics as the great link between mind and matter that would prove their underlying unity. Taken ill in middle life, he turned from physics to religious philosophy. With his deepening interest in the immortal soul, "he was troubled by materialism" (Boring, 1929, p. 269) and in 1848 published a book arguing for the mental life of plants.

> His philosophical solution of the spiritual problem lay in his affirmation of the identity of mind and matter and in his assurance that the entire universe can be regarded as readily from the point of view of its consciousness . . . as it can be viewed as inert matter. (Boring, 1929, p. 269)

Consciousness, Fechner argued, is in all and through all. This scant selection of his views, which were set forth in a series of seven philosophical volumes, will, I hope, suffice to show that psychology's founding father, Fechner, was a true *Naturphilosoph*.

Nature-philosophy was, by its attempt at monism, not quite a vitalism, but it kept alive many of the same ancient ways of thought (both have the Heraclitean emphasis on becoming) and its influence is strongly felt in the work of Lamarck (1744–1829).[4] As Gillispie (1958) summarizes Lamarck's thought,

> In living nature inheres a plastic force—indeed living nature *is* a plastic force— forever producing all varieties of animals. . . . The dead hand of inorganic nature causes discontinuities in what the organic drive toward perfection would alone achieve. . . . In Lamarck, only life can act, for life and activity are ultimately one. . . . It was rather as a consequence than as a statement of his view of nature that Lamarck laid down two corollaries which he described as laws: that of the development or decay of organs through use or disuse, and that of the inheritance of the characteristics acquired by organisms in reacting to the environment. (p. 32)

In reacting *purposively*, that is, since Lamarck stresses the role of goal striving in the development of adaptive changes that are passed on to an organism's descendants.

The next great name among vitalists was Johannes Müller (1801–1858), who worked at the height of the German nature-philosophical rage. "It is significant," Singer (1959, p. 491) remarks, that Müller, "the most effective critic of mid-nineteenth-century mechanism . . . was himself an experimental physiologist of genius who is largely responsible for the picture of the body as a machine." He rejected the relevance of what many thought convincing antivitalistic evidence that urea could be synthesized, pointing out that it was after all only an excretory breakdown product of living tissue, not in itself a part of life.[5] Convinced that there was something about life that could not be measured physically and explained mechanically, he said in print that the velocity of the nervous impulse could not be determined—and in a few years, Helmholtz had measured it! Müller's respect for life did not keep him from studying it as objectively as possible; he achieved fame for his great and exhaustive *Handbook of Human Physiology* and is remembered today for his doctrine of the specific energies of nerves. A measure of his greatness is that most of the leading physiologists of the next generation were his pupils, notably Helmholtz, du Bois-Reymond, and Brücke. These young men, together with Emil Ludwig, formed a club which later became the Berlin Physical Society. The purpose of their association, Bernfeld (1944, p. 349) tells us, was "to destroy, once and for all, vitalism, the fundamental belief of their admired master."

In 1842, du Bois-Reymond had written the following rather melodramatic statement in a letter to a friend:

> Brücke and I pledged a solemn oath to put into effect this truth: "No other forces than the common physical–chemical ones are active within the organism. In those cases which cannot at the time be explained by these forces one has either to find the specific way or form of their action by means of the physical-mathematical method, or to assume new forces equal in dignity to the chemical–physical forces inherent in matter, reducible to the force of attraction and repulsion."' (Quoted by Bernfeld, 1944, p. 348)

In this brief text, notice first the great emphasis on forces; it is surely a dynamic commitment! Second, it is clearly an oath of fidelity to mechanism, the kind of prohibition law that is necessary only in the face of temptation—to invoke some kind of special nonphysical, vital energy. Third, take careful note of the strategy proposed for the difficult times the swearers saw ahead: If physical–chemical forces should prove insufficient, "new ones equal in dignity" might be assumed, but only as a temporary expedient and with the understanding that they should ultimately be *reducible*. Finally, it is an oath of loyalty to the scientific, or "physical-mathematical," *method*, which as A. Rapoport (1962) points out was always the most effective weapon of the antivitalists.

One wonders what must have been the excitement of a group so committed when at one of its meetings in 1847 Helmholtz presented his paper on the conservation of energy—interestingly enough, according to Bernfeld (1944), as a contribution to physiology. Singer writes,

> There are certain seminal scientific ideas, the appearance of which makes it possible for the historian to establish time boundaries. . . . Such a one is the doctrine that any form of measurable physical activity is convertible into any other form, and that the total amount of such activity in the world is limited and remains the same. (1959, p. 375)

Thus, "the fundamental doctrine of the nineteenth century, that of energy, was long in gestation but was developed in the decade before 1850" (Singer, 1959, pp. 417–418). The first of the two principal points of the doctrine was mainly the work of Joule, who discovered the mechanical equivalent of heat and made the bold generalization (also in 1847) that "Heat, living force and attraction through space (to which I might also add *light* . . .) are mutually convertible" (quoted by Singer, 1959, p. 377) For all its vitalistic ring, Joule meant by "living force" (or *vis viva*) nothing other than energy; there was also ambiguity in the German, for Helmholtz, like du Bois-Reymond, had used the word *Kraft* (now usually translated as "force"). Thomson (Lord Kelvin) supplied the clarifying term "energy" in 1852, besides making important substantive contributions to the theory and the precise measurement of energy.

Several of the great physicists of the 17th century, from Galileo to Huygens, had suggested that "all basic physical phenomena—heat, light, chemical action, electricity, and magnetism—were susceptible of mechanical explanation. It was believed that all were due to the movements on the part of small particles of the affected bodies" (Singer, 1959, p. 347), a theory that led to many important advances, even before the mutual convertibility of these forms of energy had been demonstrated. In 1831, Faraday had done extensive work on fields of electromagnetic force, and Maxwell's mathematization of Faraday's keen intuitions was published in 1856.

> [These] phenomena which appeared to involve action at a distance, such as gravitational attractions and electrical and magnetic attractions and repulsions, must, if everything had a mechanical explanation, be regarded as actions through a medium connecting the bodies concerned . . . this could be no other than the luminiferous ether. (Singer, 1959, p. 428)

Accordingly, the resulting mechanical conceptions of the ether had an extraordinary complexity, which by the end of the century was approaching that of the cycles and epicycles needed by the Ptolemaic theory to account for the movements of the planets before the Copernican revolution.

But the time did not become ripe for Einstein's new synthesis until after 1900. In the middle of the preceding century, Helmholtz was confidently writing:

> We discover the problem of physical material science to be to refer natural phenomena back to unchangeable attractive and repulsive forces whose intensity depends wholly upon distance. The solubility of this problem is the condition of the complete comprehensibility of nature. (Quoted in Einstein & Infeld, 1938, p. 58)[6]

Despite this mechanistic imperialism, there were still undaunted vitalists. The purposiveness of organisms was the key to their belief that living organisms were different in kind from anything nonliving. A well-known botanist of Freud's generation, Reinke (1849–1931), put it thus:

> Every biological process is determined by preceding events: this is causality. But such processes can also be determined by later conditions inasmuch as the preceding ones are indispensable preliminary stages for them; this is finalism. . . . While causal necessity characterizes all natural sciences alike, finalism prevails exclusively in the field of biology. . . . In the case of teleological phenomena, the essential conditions lie not in the past but in the future. (Quoted in Schlick, 1953, p. 530)

Darwin's theory of natural selection, the other great scientific event of the century, was like the theory of energy a major contribution to the ideal of a completely mechanical world. Heraclitean concepts of flux in the organic world were central to nature-philosophy, as we have seen, and to Lamarck. With Darwin, it became possible to explain the origin of species and their transformations without any guiding divine purpose, Platonic ideas, or life force "striving for perfection." Random inherited variations, the struggle for existence, and the resulting survival of the fittest could account for it all. Therefore, among Darwin's stubbornest opponents were the last of the nature-philosophers, Owen, Agassiz, and von Baer. Yet Darwin unintentionally contributed to the survival of teleology! Perhaps it was too much in the air; anyway, he did not succeed in getting it out of his masterpiece, *On the Origin of Species by Means of Natural Selection, or the Preservation of Favored Races in the Struggle for Life* (1859). As the title itself shows, he treated "natural selection as though it were an active and directive agent" (Singer, 1959, p. 509). Though he repudiated teleology, he constantly reverted to teleological metaphors, and surely many of his readers took his work as a confirmation of the earlier, purposive view of evolution.

"The teaching of Darwin," Singer (1959, p. 395) notes, "gave the effective stimulus" to comparative anatomy. "The alliance of comparative studies with evolutionary doctrine focused attention on structure as distinct from function. Comparative anatomy in its turn became largely a study of developmental stages, and embryology became the comparative study *par excellence*." These closely related developmental disciplines became the last strongholds of vitalists like von Baer (who around 1830 first compared slits that appear on the chick embryo to a fish's gill slits) and Driesch (1867–1941), the last major spokesman for vitalism within science. In the 1890s, however, vitalism had many highly capable proponents—for example, E. B. Wilson (1897; as quoted by Bergson, 1911, p. 330): "The study of the cell has, on the whole, seemed to widen rather than to narrow the enormous gap that separates even the lowest forms of life from the inorganic world." And:

> One of the most notable naturalists of our time has insisted on the opposition of two orders of phenomena observed in living tissues, anagenesis and katagene-

sis. The role of the anagenic energies is to raise the inferior energies to their own level by assimilating inorganic substances. . . . It is only with . . . facts of katagenetic order that physico-chemistry deals—that is, in short, with the dead and not with the living. (Bergson, 1911, p. 35)

Here Bergson is referring to E. D. Cope (1896), a well-known American paleontologist and evolutionist.[7]

THE INFLUENCE OF THE VITALISM CONTROVERSY ON FREUD'S WORK

In the preceding section, I hope to have demonstrated (1) that the issue of vitalism versus mechanism was a major focus of controversy in the development of science, which entailed many kinds of differences in approach to and use of concepts: (2) that Freud's teachers and many of his intellectual heroes (e.g., Goethe, Helmholtz, Fechner) were deeply involved in this controversy, so that he must have been thoroughly exposed to both sides of it; (3) that vitalism was an active and respectable doctrine throughout the years when Freud was getting his education and forming his basic theoretical ideas—that is, up to the turn of the century; and (4) that the only-recently differentiated concepts of force and energy were so important to the mechanistic world view that to use them was almost the hallmark of science. Let us look next at some of the evidences of direct impact of these issues on Freud's work.

We know from the pioneering researches of Bernfeld (1944, 1951) that the medical school Freud attended and the Physiological Institute of Brücke, where he obtained his scientific training, were centers of a mechanistic biology that had successfully revolted against vitalism with its mystical and nature-philosophical taint.[8] Freud (1925d) tells us that he came to medicine because of an attraction to the grandiose and romantic scientific visions of the *Fragment on Nature* attributed to Goethe. He served his apprenticeship working on comparative anatomy with an evolutionary aim and at times using embryological techniques, which probably exposed him to vitalism as the ever-waiting alternative against whose siren songs Brücke would most likely have warned him. Though he flirted for a time with philosophy, Freud became converted to the outlook of physicalistic physiology and worked within the framework of such ideas until the late 1890s, afterwards gradually swinging back in the direction of his speculative, philosophical leanings.

The high point of Freud's commitment to mechanism is the Project of 1895, written under the influence of Fliess, another admirer of that Helmholtz whom Freud once described as "one of my idols."[9] Yet even here, there are occasional passages in which Freud faltered a bit in his aim to explain normal and abnormal thought and behavior in a strictly mechanistic way. For example, he complains of an inability to give a "mechanical (automatic) explanation" (1950 [1895], p. 360), indicating that his goal was a mechanical model like an automaton which would not require the postulation of any psychic concepts (such as attention) except as *results* of its operation. Thus, he had described the process of primary defense as one in which the partial release of unpleasure resulting from the cathecting of a traumatic memory would serve as a signal, attracting the ego's attention so that it would institute a lateral cathexis and divert the current in question from the neurones embodying the memory, thus preventing the full release of unpleasure. Yet a few pages later, he indicates that this explanation, with its assumption of a homuncular ego capable of attending and acting, was not what he was after: "How *primary defence* . . . is to be represented mechanically—this, I confess, I am unable to say" (1950 [1895], p. 370). His attempts to cope with the problem of consciousness via the non-physico-chemical concept of *quality* involve a similar uncomfortable regress, and an apparent necessity to leave the realm of science: "our consciousness furnishes only *qualities*, whereas science recognizes only *quantities*" (p. 309). It was in this context that he gave his first definition of reality: "Where do qualities originate? Not in the external world. For out there, according to the view of our natural science, to which psychology too must be subjected here . . . there are only masses in motion and nothing else" (p. 308).[10] Ideally, then, quality should have been explained away or at least not used as a causal variable; yet despite a couple of efforts to show it redundant, he was unable to proceed without giving quality a central explanatory role.

In these important aspects, the Project failed in its central aim: "to furnish a psychology that shall be a natural science . . . [by representing] psychical process as quantitatively determinate states of specifiable material particles" (p. 295). Note well that accordingly, the only energies considered in it were physical ones, *not* psychic energy.

The usual account is that after recognizing the failure of the Project, Freud rejected the mechanistic doctrine of physicalistic physiology; turned resolutely to a pure psychology; and created an abstract, hypothetical psychic apparatus in place of the nervous system, in which the operative quantity was psychic, not physical energy. It is easy to get the impression that Freud gave up neurologizing and turned to pure psychology because, with characteristic overstatement, he said as much. Many writers, including Rapaport (1959), have been more impressed with Freud's announcement, "I shall remain upon psychological ground" (Freud, 1900a, p. 536) than with his many slips in the same work back into neurological terminology [see Chapters 3 and 5, this volume]. But through his years of constructing theories, whenever it was necessary to consider somatic events such as conversion symptoms, Freud unhesitatingly spoke as if cathectic energy was *not* psychic but physical (neural). It is to his everlasting credit, and to the huge benefit of psychoanalysis, that whenever the facts demanded it— even grubby facts involving the connection of the abstract mind with a heavy, smelly, affect-shaken, unruly body—Freud reverted to a psychosomatic view of the organism as a whole. If he had been consistent, if he had insisted on a pure psychology in which there *could* have been a consistent concept of psychic energy, psychoanalysis would have lost its principal claim to scientific interest: that it alone really takes into account all the facts about human beings, their secret desires, their somatic aches and lusts, the pervasively psychosomatic nature of behavior and thought.

Despite this historical justification, it is a valid criticism of the psychoanalytic energy concept that it fluctuates, depending on the context—at one point being a survival of Freud's original concept of a physical cathectic quantity traversing the fibers of a somatic nervous system, and then being a purely psychological, non-physico-chemical concept. In this inconsistency, it reflects Freud's inability to reach a satisfactory position in relation to the mind–body problem. For the most part, as Rubinstein (1965) has shown, he assumed that physical energy could somehow be converted into psychic energy, and vice versa—the interactionist solution, which today has relatively few adherents. [See, however, Popper and Eccles (1977).]

Interactionism is the prevailing conception of the common-sense psychology that talks about will power as "mind over matter." It assumes causal chains such as this: A physical event (e.g., a pattern of light) causes another physical event (a neural current from retina to brain), which then causes a psychological event (visual perception); this in turn causes a further psychological event (an intention to act), which causes a physical event (movement of the body). Sounds reasonable enough, doesn't it? Reflect, however, that if one were to follow this chain of events on the purely physical/physiological level, there would have to be puzzling and inexplicable lacunae. At the point where the ontological gap was jumped, and physical energy was transformed into psychic energy as Freud assumed (1895b, p. 108), there would be a deficit, and at the corresponding point when the psychic was transformed into the physical there would be a surplus. Presumably these two would cancel one another out, and thus might be hard to detect, though not when there is extensive "delay of discharge." But the fact is that no hint of any such gap in the application of the first law of thermodynamics has ever appeared, no matter how the precision of measurement has been refined; the physical causal sequences flow without a ripple and with complete conservation of physical energy.[11] If you ask why psychoanalysts are not troubled by this glaring incompatibility with facts of their theory's dualistic stand on the mind–body problem, I can only answer that so far as I know, they are almost all of them totally unaware of it. Yet it is a necessary consequence of the doctrine of psychic energy.

When Freud turned away from mechanism, did he opt for vitalism? Before attempting an answer to that question, I shall discuss the parallels between psychic energy and the active principles postulated by vitalism. First, it will be necessary to review the major characteristics of vital force; in doing so, I shall make principal reference to the two vitalistic theorists who were most nearly Freud's contemporaries, the embryologist Driesch and the philosopher Bergson.

1. *Vitalistic theories are dualistic, and the vital principle is accordingly something ontologically quite unlike and even antithetical to the world of matter.*

The fundamental dualism Bergson sees between life and "inert matter" is evident throughout his work, but it is difficult to find a succinct avowal of metaphysical dualism. He makes many such statements as "In reality, life is no more made of physiochemical elements than a curve is composed of straight lines" (1911, p. 31).

According to Driesch, ". . . Absolute Reality has also a dualistic structure. There is a permanent struggle between wholeness and non-wholeness in Reality, a struggle between *form* and *matter*" (1929, p. 327). "Life . . . is not a specialized arrangement of inorganic events: life is something apart; and biology is an independent science" (1929, p. 105).

2. *The vital principle is therefore not localized in space.*

"In reality, life is of the psychological order, and it is of the essence of the psychical to enfold a confused plurality of interpenetrating terms. . . . What is of psychical nature cannot entirely correspond with space" (Bergson, 1911, p. 257).

"An agent which is of a non-spatial nature cannot be said to have a definite localization in space. Entelechy [his term for vital force] therefore cannot possess a 'seat'" (Driesch, 1929, p. 299).

3. *The vital principle is like, and at times is described as, energy, but it is not physical energy.*

"Our philosophy represents the organized world as a harmonious whole. But . . . it admits of much discord, because each species, each individual even, retains only a certain impetus from the universal vital impulsion and tends to use *this energy* in its own interest" (Bergson, 1911, p. 50; my emphasis). Note the Lamarckian, nature-philosophical tone. This "vital impulsion" is the translation of his famous *élan vital*.

According to Driesch,

Ostwald, and many others following him, have admitted that, in cases of morphogenesis, and probably in nervous phenomena too, some unknown potential forms of energy may be at work, and that the specificity of vital phenomena and their autonomy is due to the peculiarities which that unknown energy possesses. . . . In other words: that entelechy is *itself* a peculiar form of energy. . . . *But entelechy lacks all the characteristics of quantity:* . . . Thus I decline most decidedly any kind of 'energetical' vitalism whatever. (1929, pp. 256–257)

Note, however, that in his view entelechy causes animal movements and has the kinetic if not the quantitative property of energy.

4. *It is directional: It steers and organizes, impels toward goals.*

"An *original impetus* of life . . . is the fundamental cause of variations . . . that accumulate and create new species" (Bergson, 1911, p. 87). "The force which is evolving throughout the organized world . . . is always seeking to transcend itself and always remains inadequate to the work it would fain produce" (p. 126).

Driesch (1929) asks, "Why then occurs all that folding . . . and all the other [embryological] processes we have described? There must be something that drives them out, so to say" (p. 32). He answers: "We have shown that there is at work a something in life phenomena 'which bears the end in itself,' the entelechy" (p. 106).

5. *It is treated anthropomorphically: It has powers of decision, does things.*

"The profound cause [of evolution] is the impulse which thrust life into the world, which made it divide into vegetables and animals, which shunted the animal on to suppleness of form, and which . . . secured that . . . it should rouse itself up and move forward" (Bergson, 1911, p. 132).

"There was a natural factor at work, *autonomous* and *not* resulting from a combination of other agents, but elemental in itself; this factor, then, may be called a factor of dynamical teleology—on analogy. There is something teleological *within* its acting. If . . . we allow ourselves still a little more of it [analogy], we may say that it is *as if* our entelechy is endowed with *knowing and willing*" (Driesch, 1929, p. 244). "Super-entelechy, bound into matter, *wants to know* what is has done . . . suffering from its own products" (p. 244; emphasis in the last sentence is mine).

6. *It is closely related to the psychic.*

"Life, that is to say, consciousness launched into matter. . . ." (Bergson, 1911, p. 181). See also quotation above under point 2.

"The 'acting something' . . . which *directs* the body" Driesch calls "the psychoid" (1929, p. 221). Soon afterward, he says, "It is only to men, according to Aristotle, that the highest soul . . . is given, that is, the faculty of reasoning, corresponding to what we have called the 'psychoid' as regulating action" (p. 222). Later (p. 229) Driesch uses "our psychoid or Entelechy" interchangeably.

7. *What the life force operates in, however, is depicted as a mechanism.*

"That life is a kind of mechanism I cordially agree" (Bergson, 1911, p. 31).
"Every part of these organic systems has been placed by entelechy where it must be placed to act well in the service of the whole, but the part itself acts like a part of a machine" (Driesch, 1929, p. 248).
Freud's doctrine of psychic energy shows striking similarity to vitalism on each of these particulars. First, it is generally a dualistic doctrine, as Rubinstein (1965) has pointed out in detail and as I have just reviewed. Second, to the extent that Freud says that his model is *not* a physiological / anatomical one, he removes the possibility that psychic energy operates in space:

> Strictly speaking, there is no need for the hypothesis that the psychical systems are actually arranged in a *spatial* order. It would be sufficient if a fixed order were established by the fact that in a given psychical process the excitation passes through the systems in a particular *temporal* sequence. (Freud, 1900a, p. 537)

The result must either be a metaphysical mentalism or a nonexistential interpretation of psychic energy. (Rubinstein, 1967 a).[12] Third, the central concept of cathexis is repeatedly called an energy, analogous to but not identical with the energy of physics.
Fourth, it is directional in the same way as vitalistic forces are: It exists in sexual and aggressive forms, qualitative differences which amount to the assumption that the energy bears a certain kind of end in itself—destructive, or one of uniting and binding all things together. Moreover, each of these is further subdivisible into energies of varying degrees of neutralization, a concept which in turn hinges on the immanent direction or goal, whether the energy is directed toward some form of crude and immediate gratification, or is "*aim*-inhibited," directed toward socially acceptable and neutral ends. Libido in particular is often differentiated into specific kinds according to the object it is directed toward: the self ("narcissistic"), persons of the same sex ("homosexual"), or normal and appropriate partners of opposite

sex (when it is usually just called "object libido"). Thus, psychic energy is a teleological concept. It might appear that these are all shorthand expressions and that it is actually assumed that the energy itself does not contain its goal; Rapaport (1959) maintained as much. Yet one examines in vain the texts of Freud and also those of most of his followers for any explicit statement that the direction is given by structures or by some informational concept; the assumption clearly is that each form of energy itself is intrinsically directional, and the particular direction can be gotten out of it only with difficulty, as by neutralization.[13]

Fifth, it should hardly need demonstration that the standard procedure in psychoanalysis has been to follow Freud's habit of speaking about psychic energy anthropomorphically. It "struggles," "presses for discharge," is "ever on the alert for opportunities," and so on and on. I hope that the dangers and fallacies of this practice are self-evident. The sixth point I quoted about vitalism was that its proponents frequently tended to equate the essence of life with that of the mind, so that the living–nonliving dualism was assimilated to that of mind versus matter, and the life energy was also a psychic energy. This constitutes a bridge to psychic energy rather than a point of possible similarity.

Finally, Freud's theory is surely like the recent vitalists' in that it postulates a mechanistic structure within which the energy operates. Most of the time he called it the "psychic apparatus," but as we saw in Chapter 5, it remained a passive reflex model that required an input of a disturbing energy to make it work. Without the cybernetic features of the Project, it had to rely for its control on an ego interpreted as a homunculus. In this sense, it was at best the same kind of mixture as the combined mechanistic-vitalistic systems of such neovitalists as Reinke, Pflueger, and Driesch. "Driesch called himself, not without justice, a 'consistent mechanist' because his theory presupposes a machine model of the organism and an extreme preformationist view, in which the entelechy 'is the engineer who sets this machine in motion'"(Mainx, 1955, p. 628).

The demonstration above amounts to nothing more than circumstantial evidence for the proposition that Freud was probably influenced by the vitalistic concepts that were then widely used and defended by reputable scientists, when he came to frame his own concept of cathexis, the "excitation" that operated his psychic apparatus. He did not directly discuss the matter. I have not found any reference to vitalism nor to any well-known vitalist in anything of his I have read, nor do the authors he refers to in the volumes of the *Standard Edition* include any vitalists (if one leaves out of consideration such nature-philosophers as Lamarck, Goethe, and Fechner).[14] Doubtless he would have rejected any attempt to identify cathectic energy with *élan vital* or entelechy. It is therefore not my intention to maintain that he knowingly turned from mechanism to vitalism. I do submit, however, that psychic energy is a vitalistic concept in the sense of being similar to and influenced by vital force, and being to a large extent functionally equivalent to it. They are at the least historically and methodologically homologous—buds from the same branch.

OBJECTIONS TO VITALISM AS THEY APPLY TO PSYCHIC ENERGY

The facts that vitalism has been effectively refuted and that its adherents are a vanishing breed do not constitute an effective or sufficient argument against psychic energy. Biology and psychology are separate disciplines, and what is fallacious for one *may* not be for the other. Let us take a brief look at the major objections to vitalism and see to what extent they may be applicable to corresponding aspects of psychic energy.

First, a few telling points against vitalists are clearly specific to them. Schneirla (1949), for example, points out how the vitalists, in arguing for a monolithic explanatory life force, obscure "the fact that somewhat similar effectiveness in adaptive behavior may exist on rather different biological and psychological levels of organization" (p. 281). Also,

> Although orthodox teleologists generously endow all animals with . . . [the capacity to project themselves] into an organized sequence of specialized adjustments of representational character dominated by the expected development of a given outcome—a "goal" . . . its presence has been demonstrated adequately only in the mammals. (p. 275)

Likewise, he demonstrates the weakness of the attempt made by many vitalists to prove their theory through eliminating mechanistic alternatives; the trouble, of course, is that it is impossible to eliminate the possibility that someone will develop an adequate theory that is neither mechanistic nor vitalistic.

Another favorite, but dangerous, form of argument on which vitalists rely is analogy. As Schneirla (1949) notes, "A common feature of Vitalism . . . and other procedures featuring the use of analogy is that the organization of processes underlying behavioral systems is not subjected to very close study" (p. 250). This becomes part of a larger point that, with a few notable exceptions like Driesch in his early years, vitalists have not been led by their theory into fruitful experimentation or new types of observation; their methods of seeking truth have been sterile.

Hempel and Oppenheim (quoted by Nagel, 1953) make a similar point even more forcefully: All statements about entelechy are inaccessible to empirical test, because there is no provision for any means of testing assertions about it. For similar reasons, Frank (1955, p. 434) called the concept of vital energy "useless" since "we have no 'practical' operation to define the energy of life."

This is a serious charge, even if one adopts the generally permissive and moderate versions of operationism that philosophers of science advocate today (e.g., Kaplan, 1964, pp. 36 ff.). Not all terms—particularly theoretical terms, which get their meaning from the network of propositions in which they are embedded—need to have operational definitions; but ultimately, "it must be possible to deduce determinate consequences from the assumptions of the theory," and "at least some theoretical notions must be tied down to fairly definite and unambiguously specified observable materials" (Polanyi, 1962, p. 40). But not only does the dualism of vitalism doom its central concept to unmeasurability, "it has no explanatory import, because it does not function in a set of general laws" (Hempel & Oppenheim, quoted by Nagel, 1960).

And how is it with psychic energy—is it vulnerable to the same charges? They have surely been leveled against it. In the New York University symposium on psychoanalysis and philosophy of science, Nagel (1960, p. 41) said that he had no objection to metaphor as such, but "in Freudian theory metaphors are employed without even half-way definite rules for expanding them, and that in consequence admitted metaphors such as 'energy' or 'level of excitation' have no specific content and can be filled in to suit one's fancy." A dozen years earlier, Kubie (1947) had attacked psychic energy as an unmeasurable, metaphorical concept. Moreover, the theory lacks the tightness of structure that would give its theoretical terms what Kaplan (1964) calls "systemic meaning," for it is "formulated in such a manner that it can always be construed and manipulated so as to explain whatever the actual facts are" (Nagel, 1960, p. 40). Psychic energy has been criticized by Kardiner, Karush, and Ovesey (1959) and by Rubinstein (1967a) as tautologous: The only data by means of which it can be assessed are the very ones it is invoked to explain.

I believe that Nagel is unduly harsh in his strictures and that the picture is not so wholly black. The doctrine of psychic energy has not been quite as sterile as he implies; a number of experimenters (e.g., Silverman, 1967[15]) have obtained researchable ideas from it, and shortly before his death David Rapaport had started on a broad program of laboratory research explicitly devoted to measuring psychic energy, which has given rise to a fair amount of published research (e.g., Schwartz & Rouse, 1961). Proceeding on quite a different, more clinical tack, Ostow (1962) launched a program of drug research in which psychic energy is a central variable. So long as there is investigative mileage in a concept, it has some claim to scientific usefulness. But the same thing was once true of phlogiston, caloric, and the other "imponderables" of physics, which does not blind us to the fact that in the end they proved empty and useless.

Despite their otherwise considerable differences of approach, the attempts of both Rapaport and Ostow (and their coworkers) to measure psychic energy have in common a noteworthy indirectness. Libido or hypercathexis can only be rated or estimated from behavioral signs that are coordinated to psychic energy by fiat, and the nomological net in which the theoretical statements using such energy are woven is far too loose-meshed to permit a crucial test of basic assumptions like a conservation law. I find it difficult to believe that psychic energy and related concepts play an essential role in the generation of empirical studies in either of these programs. Rather, they appear to serve as a language in which to discuss cases and experiments, much as Lewin's topological-vector theory served him in relation to his investigative work. Although Lewin (1935) was as fertile a source of experimental ideas as any psychologist of his time, the theory lost its vogue quickly after his death because it seemed intrinsically not well suited to generating new questions to put to nature. The same fate can be predicted for the economic theory of psychoanalysis, however long it may linger in the less exacting atmosphere of the clinic.

To return to vitalism: It is generally conceded that the strongest argument for it is the adaptiveness of organisms, with its strong implication of purpose. The apparent goal of many metabolic and adaptive processes, writes Schlick (1953, p. 527), "is the preservation and development . . . both of the individual and of the species . . . reference to the teleology of organic life constituted throughout the ages the strongest argument in favor of the autonomy of organic life." The facts of purposiveness are undeniable in biology as well as in psychoanalysis; what is questionable is whether they require the assumption of some finalistic, teleological concept of purpose, or whether they can be explained by means of the causal concepts of natural science.

"Modern science . . . regards final causes to be vestal virgins which bear no fruit in the study of physical and chemical phenomena" (Nagel, 1953, p. 540). A final cause is the answer to the question *why*; it is the kind of ultimate explanation that essentialism fosters.[16] By contrast, the way of a modern scientist is to ask *how*, to describe what happens as precisely as possible, and to determine its contingency on as many conditions as he can. Newton accounted for the movement of physical objects by his interlocking, mathematical, yet operational laws of motion. Interestingly enough, he was still enough a child of his time that he did not feel satisfied by his own explanation of planetary movement, but turned to religious and metaphysical speculation about supernatural spirits, in search of the "real causes" of motion (Koryé, 1956, p. 21).

Nagel's most impressive refutation of teleology is his detailed demonstration that it is possible to construct causal, nonteleological explanations such that "the former can be replaced by the latter without loss in asserted content" (1953, p. 541). He writes, "The structure of character of so-called 'teleological' systems is . . . expressed by the . . . conditions for a directively organized system; and these conditions can be stated . . . in a manner not requiring the adoption of teleology as a fundamental or unanalyzable category" (1953, p. 549). And without the use of any energy concept, it should be added; direction is a matter of structure and information (see also Nagel, 1961).

Such analysis of goal-directed behavior into nonteleological elements has enabled engineers to build servomechanisms, using negative feedback, which are to an increasing extent self-regulating, self-maintaining, and goal-directed. A few cyberneticists have been tempted to attribute purpose to such machines, but even if one wants to do so, it is not as an explanatory concept and it has no metaphysical dualistic implications.

Thus, the last stronghold of vitalism has fallen. But note well that the death of vitalism has not been a victory of mechanism. Indeed, in the end mechanism and vitalism turn out to have had a good deal in common—a common heritage of Greek philosophy, of silent and fallacious assumptions about causality. In the realm of animal behavior, Schneirla (1949, p. 244) writes, mechanism and vitalism alike went astray, "the former by endeavoring to fit all adaptive capacities directly under physico-chemical rubrics, the latter by setting out to bring all cases under a universal supernatural causal principle." Mainx (1955) adds:

> Regarded from the empiricist standpoint, the mechanistic and vitalistic systems [of theoretical biology] show a fundamental affinity, while the contrasts between them seem to lie more in the formulation. Common to both systems, in the first place, is the view of causality in the sense of an executive causality, while in the empirical science of the present day the causal connection is usually conceived only in the sense of a consecutive causality. Both systems seek for an "explanation" of the organic event by reducing it to a "principle" or "category" which is "at work" in it, which "causes" it. (p. 628)

In psychoanalysis, this approach to explanation takes the form of the pleasure principle and reality principle, and the executive ego, superego, and id, as well as an energy that is defined as being directional.

Mainx (1955) continues,

> A further common feature of mechanistic and vitalistic system is the tautological character of their general statements. . . . In the statements in which the concept of entelechy . . . occurs these concepts are, for the most part, defined only by their connection with the processes which they are to cause. In this way such statements escape empirical testing either by experiment or by observation. It is for this reason that the formulations of mechanism and vitalism [in biology] have been discussed for many decades on the purely speculative plane, without the great progress meanwhile reached in research having permitted a decision in this controversy. (pp. 628–629)

In physics, mechanism died near the turn of the present century. Field theory, the special and general theories of relativity, quantum theory, and related developments destroyed any hope that all science could be unified around Newtonian dynamics. Today, laymen like ourselves find it difficult to grasp the nonintuitive picture of reality implied in the physics of elementary particles, which have properties both of energy and of matter in the old sense; a physics that postulates antimatter as well as matter; time that is conceived in certain laws as flowing in either direction; not one fundamental force of attraction and repulsion, but at least four and possibly five basic and apparently irreducible types of physical force. It is surely easy to long for the comfortable and intelligible world of mechanism, and the mysteriousness and disembodied quality of some physical concepts tempt some nonphysicists (e.g., Teilhard de Chardin, 1959) to revive mystical concepts such as the "life principle," which *seems* no more intangible than a field of force. [For further discussion, see Chapter 14, this volume.]

But there is a major, critical difference. However esoteric the new physical terms, they are given precise mathematical formulation; they are embedded in a tight system of laws; they generate testable consequences and lead directly to research and new empirical discoveries. There may be a Heraclitean cast to a world view in which the elemental starting points are fields and operant processes rather than substantial Democritean atoms, but the resemblance is quite superficial. From Heraclitus to Koffka, the emphasis on process and gestalt was opposed to analysis, empirical or mathematical. We have learned, however, that structure *is* analyzable, that one can be precise about the impalpable, and that mathematics does not destroy.

Some of the most scientifically sophisticated among psychoanalysts are not satisfied with the argument to this point. They are perfectly willing to abandon the mystical implications—argument by analogy, reification, and anthropomorphism—that have characterized the treatment of psychic energy in much of the psychoanalytic literature and which are so reminiscent of vitalism. All of that may have been true in the past, they argue, but none of it is a necessary aspect of psychic energy, and we have given it up long ago. What is wrong with psychic energy interpreted nondirectionally and nonexistentially as an abstract, quantitative construct with qualities and direction contributed by structures? True, it is not directly measurable, but not every concept needs to be operational in any simple sense, and even in physics energy is only indirectly measurable. Such is the concept of psychic energy as used by Rapaport (1951a, 1959) and by his students (e.g., Schwartz & Rouse, 1961).

In this version, the concept is, of course, more nearly acceptable. But let us consider first the issue of measurability. The only *directly* measurable concepts in physics are the basic dimensions of time, space and mass. A great many other concepts may be quite precisely and determinately measured by means of these three, however, because of the network of laws that define concepts and relationships among them. As Rapaport (1959) himself pointed out, psychology lacks dimensional quantification; psychological measurement is possible, but there is as yet no known way of tightly and systematically relating the resulting quantities to one another or to higher-order constructs. As a result, there is no true analogy in the situations of the two sciences; the indirectness of measurement in physics has never raised the suspicion that energy is a tautologous concept. In psychoanalysis and psychology, however, the burden of proof is on anyone who defends psychic energy to show that it can be measured in a useful way, so that it is estimated independently of the very phenomena it is to explain.

And then it is not so easy to escape the necessity of accepting a rather extreme metaphysical position in order to retain psychic energy. To be both consistent and comprehensive, one must adopt interactionism and postulate a break in the chain of physical causality, which will expose one to the constant temptation to avoid any theoretical embarrassment by escaping into the second world of metaphysical mentalism. This will make it increasingly difficult for the theory to be tested in any definitive way. Psychoanalysis is already much too invulnerable to the refutation of its theoretical statements—a purely illusory safety, since philosophers of science agree that the usefulness of a theory is a function of its capacity to generate testable consequences, which means to stick its neck out and suffer the possibility of becoming extinct. A better theory usually arises from the ashes of the one that expires, however.

What is needed in place of psychic energy is not simply a better concept, but a new set of basic assumptions about the nature of the behaving organism and how it operates. In psychoanalysis, such propositions are contained for the most part in metapsychology, on a level of theory that is considerably removed from clinical observation. What Rapaport (1959) called the clinical theory is the distillation of actual work with patients; it is known to and is used daily by every analyst and by most clinical psychologists, psychiatrists, and psychiatric social workers as well. This was Freud's most original and lasting contribution, and for the most part it will stand unaffected by changes in the general theory. As Freud recognized, "basic concepts . . . are not the foundation of science, upon which everything rests: that foundation is observation alone. They are not the bottom but the top of the whole structure, and they can be replaced and discarded without damaging it" (1914c, p. 77).

CONCLUSION

I will conclude with two points about metapsychology as a whole. To the extent that the dynamic and structural points of view involve existentially interpreted *psychic* forces and *psychic* structures, they are subject to the same criticism that has been made above with respect to psychic energy and the mind–body problem. Partly because of the necessary ambiguities and vaguenesses that therefore exist in metapsychology, it is at best (e.g., as stated by Rapaport, 1959, and Rapaport and Gill, 1959) only a sketch and a program, not a developed and elaborated model which can thoroughly explain a complete behavioral process. As we saw [Chapter 5], its basic assumptions were taken from currently accepted scientific (including neurological and physiological) doctrine during Freud's student days. Many of these assumptions have subsequently been proved erroneous and need to be replaced.

Theories are not dragons to be dispatched by a single stroke of a methodological sword; they are much more like social systems, which can be overthrown only by being replaced by another, no matter how creaking and inadequate the other may be. It would be naive to expect psychoanalysts to drop all reference to psychic energy as soon as they understand the fallacies and basic untenability of the term. With the best will in the world, the working analyst still needs a conceptual system in terms of which to organize his data and his thoughts about them.[17] Even though I believe that the clinical theory could be rewritten without reference to energy, and still not lose its recognizable character and its explanatory power, the fact is that economic considerations have been written into it quite extensively. As long as a new roadworthy model is not actually competing with it, the old one will have to serve, patched up as best it can be.

It will be a major job, requiring many hands for many years, for a new theory to become elaborated enough to compete successfully with the old. Some scientific developments of the years since Freud's death have made many of the assumptions of metapsychology anachronistic and suggest some of the features of the kind of alternative theory that seems to me most likely to develop, transcending the old alternatives of vitalism and mechanism.

To begin with, thermodynamics has been generalized to take into account not only the closed systems Helmholtz usually assumed, but open systems—systems like living organisms, characterized not by equilibria but by steady states, a dynamic balance of inputs and outputs (Bertalanffy, 1950; Miller, 1978). An organism is an energy *user*, not a closed system within which a fixed quantity of energy reverberates, is conserved, and is stored in reservoirs. Of course, Freud always maintained that there were inputs (principally from the instinctual drives) and outputs (which he called "discharge"); what he did not realize was that this state of affairs destroyed the assumption of a closed system, and that only within a closed system did his *economic* conceptions make sense. The fundamental working assumption of the economic point of view is that there is a fixed quantity of libido, and so if one object or system is cathected, there are lawful and necessary consequences: It must be withdrawn from elsewhere. This is an elegant and appealing conception, with the one major flaw that its quantitative precision is illusory because cathectic energy cannot be measured.

The thermodynamics of open systems has the great advantage that it can account for the otherwise paradoxical observation of negative entropy in living systems of which Bergson made so much: that they do often tend toward greater complexity rather than the simplicity that classical or closed-system thermodynamics would necessitate.[18] But, since we can now conceptualize negative entropy along with positive in a precise mathematical way, the facts of creativity and growth do not necessitate any Bergsonian, mystical forces or energies of a nonphysical kind.

I have already referred to another recent great development in hard science of fundamental relevance to any consideration of energies in psychoanalysis: cybernetics, the theory of self-regulating systems (living or nonliving), which control themselves by use of informational feedback. It is fascinating to go back to the Project after reading Wiener (1948), for this 1895 work is an astonishingly sophisticated, virtually cybernetic theory containing no less than five feedback loops! By contrast, at the time of Freud's death behavioristic psychology had only one such loop—as indeed any scheme based on an uncomplicated reflex arc must have, and that includes the topographic theory. Yet Freud was too many decades ahead of his time to make full use of his own insights, and so he thought that he had to supplement his self-regulating device of defense by a *deus ex machina*, the Ego—not this time an ego as the total of cathected neurones, but in the old philosophical sense contemporaneously described by William James (1890) as "the pure ego or self of selves," an ultimate prime mover and knower. Quite a voluntaristic and teleological concept for a man who also advocated exceptionless psychic determinism! Also, it is an unnecessary one.[19] If he were alive, I am sure Freud would be delighted to know that there are now servomechanisms that regulate themselves via negative feedback loops and can even respond defensively to signals of danger, without requiring any homunculus or any hypercathectic energies of attention.

Today, we can measure the quantities of energy propagated through the nervous system; we can even measure the slight variations of potential in various parts of single nerve cells. Psychoanalysts are not much interested in such measurements (no doubt properly so), for the kinds of motivational phenomena they have in mind when they talk about energies have little to do with these microvolt quantities. They observe people who have violent, importunate impulses; people who strive to attain their goals for long periods of time against tremendous odds and despite physical exhaustion; people who differ strikingly in the amount of pep, initiative, and zest they have, as against depression, lethargy, inertia, or fatigue. All of these observations seem to cry out for some kind of energy concept—not just the energy that is released by the metabolism of food, but some kind of directly experienced, *psychological* energy.[20] So, too, does the fact that thinking is hard work; if you try to make that into a quantitative statement, however, you end up with the assumption that thinking must use a great deal of psychic energy—quite the contrary of what Freud postulated.

Is his psychic energy, then, not the same thing as the energy we feel full of sometimes, drained of at others? No, it is not; it is something a good deal more abstract, a construct in a theoretical system and not *directly* detectable or measureable in any way. Where does that leave us with our conscious experience that *feels* like energy? Freud long ago decided that conscious experience is a poor and unreliable indicator of the most important events that go on in the psychic apparatus. The conscious feeling of energy is an epiphenomenon, a clinical observation that is to be regarded seriously and used for its behavioral import, but not to be taken literally.

What is loosely called the psychoanalytic theory of instinctual drives covers a great deal, from observed clinical correlations and generalizations about the unconscious goals for which people strive, to a poorly integrated set of assumptions about psychic energy and its assumed sources in excitatory processes in various bodily zones. Again, I want to emphasize that my objection is to the latter part of the theory, not the former. Psychoanalysis must have a motivational theory that will account for unconscious striving, for the importunacy of many kinds of driven behavior, and for the phenomena of indirect or symbolic substitute-gratification. The basic outlines of a revised and more tenable psychoanalytic theory of motivation may be seen in two papers by Klein (1967) and Rubinstein (1967a). The directional aspect of motivation is given by cognitive and structural concepts, like Klein's ideomotor system. The general activation and impulsion of the theory may be provided by making use of discoveries about cortical activation systems, notably the reticular formation. Pleasure and unpleasure can now be viewed as affective feedback from the consequences of behavior without commitment to a tension reduction theory.

Psychoanalysis cannot afford to ignore such major discoveries from the general area of neurophysiology as those just mentioned, yet it cannot take account of them with a theory that relies on a *psychic* apparatus operating with *psychic* energy. With Rubinstein (1965, 1967a), I believe that we must turn to a protoneurophysiological model of the operating system; that is, our concepts will be based primarily on clinical and other behavioral observations and need only be reducible in principle and ultimately to neurophysiology. To postulate a general theory that is not incompatible with the findings of the relevant biological disciplines will facilitate more fruitful dialogue across the boundaries of the sciences and will enable psychoanalysis to conceptualize psychosomatic matters without inconsistency or metaphysical embarrassment. In clinical discussions, we shall surely not be talking about commissures and dendritic potentials instead of impulse and defense; it will be enough to clarify and redefine our clinical terminology, making sure to keep it consistent with our general theory, which will be testable from several independent directions and thus may more rapidly approximate truth. Growing by contributions from both clinic and laboratory, it will take a rightful and unquestioned place among the sciences. So long as it tries to hold on to an anachronism like psychic energy, however, psychoanalysis will have great difficulty in progressing beyond Freud's monumental contribution.

PART III

Instinct Theory:
The Dynamic Point of View

CHAPTER 7

Drive or Wish?:
A Reconsideration of the
Psychoanalytic Theory of Motivation

*Characteristically, Freud nowhere gave clear, comprehensive, textbook
definitions of his metapsychological points of view. In his major statement
of 1915 (1915e, p. 180), he was pretty explicit about the topographic and
economic points of view, but seemed to consider that it was more self-
evident what he meant by "dynamic." Nevertheless, it is evident from the
context that when he proposed (speaking about "psychical acts" in general),
"to classify and correlate them . . .* according to their relation to instincts
and aims, *according to their composition and according to which of the
hierarchy of psychical systems they belong to" (1915e, p. 172), he meant the
words I have italicized to be equivalent to what, on the next page, he calls
the "dynamic view of mental processes." (The reference to psychical systems is plainly a taking "account of psychical topography" [p. 173]; the
phrase "according to their composition" is obscure and does not recur;
presumably it alludes to the* economic *point of view.)*

*In their influential reformulation of "The Points of View and Assump-
tions of Metapsychology," Rapaport and Gill (1959) proposed a much
narrower reading: that the central focus of the dynamic point of view is the
concept of psychic force. There is undoubtedly an appealing elegance to
their interpretation, but the fact remains that it is theirs and not Freud's.
Doubtless he would have agreed that propositions involving forces are
dynamic, but he probably would not have wanted to be faithful to such a
restrictive definition.*

*I take it, then, that the theory of instincts is not only part of metapsy-
chology, but that it is the dynamic part. The chapter that follows is, with the
most minor retouching, my own major effort to critique instinct theory and
to consider some alternative ideas.*

*As to the concept of psychic force, I have nothing much to add to what
I have said about it in Chapters 5 and 6. It is closely related to psychic
energy, like the latter, it is an obvious borrowing from physics—along with
the ubiquitous term "dynamics," now routinely misconstrued as a plural.
Many clinicians evidently feel a strong sense of being on the side of psychological profundity when they talk about "this dynamic" or characterize their
psychotherapeutic orientation as "dynamic." I doubt very much that the
vast majority of them have any idea how classically mechanistic this lan-*

guage is, or that it is an anachronistic hangover from Freud's unsuccessful attempts to make psychoanalysis a respectably tough-minded member of the natural sciences.

Its theory of motivation is at once the glory of psychoanalysis and its shame. What is loosely known as the theory of instincts includes both a number of Freud's most important and lasting insights and some of his most regrettable theoretical failings. It badly needs fundamental revision; but the process must be both radical and conservative—what is not good must be extirpated at the root, but what is good must be retained.

From the beginning, this part of psychoanalytic theory has been the most intensely controversial, the focus of several apostasies and of the most violent and personal attacks on Freud himself: the traducer of innocent children, the slanderer of holy men and women, the sexual monomaniac, and so on, *ad nauseam*. Analysts therefore have good reasons to view with considerable suspicion any proposals to reconsider Freudian motivational theory, especially one that proposes to do away with the concept of instinctual drive itself. It is only natural to rally round the flag when it is under unfair assault, and to feel that any doctrine so often viciously attacked for so many bad reasons must be not only heroic but true—a conclusion, unfortunately, that is not necessarily accurate. When I used the deliberately overdramatic phrase, "the shame of psychoanalysis," in reference to the theory of instinctual drives, I meant to prepare the way for a demonstration that this central part of psychoanalysis is so riddled with philosophical and factual errors and fallacies that nothing less than discarding the concept of drive or instinct will do. At the same time, just because this concept contains so much of value, we must be quite sure before we abandon it that a viable alternative is at hand which does not sacrifice any of the hard-won gains of psychoanalysis. In particular, there is a danger of repeating the error made in the course of some earlier efforts to revise the theory, which have begun by ignoring or repudiating a number of *facts*.

Let me emphasize, then, that a first necessity of any revised psychoanalytic theory of motivation is that it *save the data of observation*. We must not let any theoretical novelty cause us to deny the facts that people have blind rages, wild lusts, and parasitic infantile longings, any of which may not be present as conscious desires, or that they are also capable of mature interests, genuine altruism, and intense devotion to principle. If it seems that throwing out the dual-instinct theory, psychic energy, or the notion of drive as the cause of behavior threatens to turn psychoanalysis into a pallid game of disembodied and feeble cognitive operations, we should ponder long and hard before we make any such radical changes. For these very reasons,

I hesitated for some years to publish this chapter, not because its stance is radical, but because I wanted to be sure that it did not inadvertently undermine any part of the central observational core of psychoanalysis. And I believe that some of these same reasons may account for the fact that George Klein (1967) did not call attention to the truly radical nature of his contribution to a revised psychoanalytic theory of motivation, or explicitly call for abandonment of the prevalent theory.

I shall list briefly some empirical propositions that I believe include the most important motivational facts of psychoanalytic observation, which must be adequately conceptualized. Often, people are unaware of the goals toward which their behavior is directed and strongly resist any efforts to help them become aware of these goals. After psychoanalytic work (analysis of defenses, interpretation of dreams, etc.) or in altered states of consciousness (drug states, fever deliria, hypnosis, etc.), they frequently become aware of previously disavowed wishes (positive or negative—longings and aversions) and offer new confirmatory memories or other material. People can have somatic symptoms for which no organic cause can be found, but which can be shown (by the just-mentioned means) to be the bodily expression of wishes or fears and defenses against them. When a wished-for form of behavior is (or seems) impossible, people are capable of getting some gratification by engaging in other behavior, which at times seems to them unrelated. Almost all people are more interested in getting sexual pleasure than they will admit, often pursuing it in devious and complicated ways. Symptoms and other forms of puzzling behavior are frequently motivated by unconscious fears concerning, or wishes for, sensual (including narrowly sexual) pleasure. Several parts of the body other than the genitals—notably the mouth and anus—are capable of yielding pleasure that has a sensuous, exciting quality very similar to that provided by stimulating the genitals. (Rather than stating the facts of infantile sexuality and the perversions propositionally, let me merely allude to them in this parenthesis.) If a person is forbidden one form of sexual pleasure, he will often turn to another. Children living in the Western nuclear family (and in many more or less similar family structures found in other societies) regularly develop sexual attraction to the adults with whom they come into close, repeated contact during the first few years of life, as well as jealousies, fears, and hatreds, many of which feelings (incestuous, parricidal, etc.) are culturally taboo and are not easily avowed; but they continue to exist and to have demonstrable effects on behavior (especially on dreams, fantasies, and symptoms). Boys commonly develop fears of body mutilation after having experienced and more or less openly expressed erotic wishes toward their mothers—frequently fears that the father or some surrogate will harm their penises. Girls often develop feelings of having lost a penis and/or envious wishes to get one. There is an intrinsic connection between certain universal types of wishes (e.g., sexual and destructive), certain biochemical and other organismic states (hormones and catecholamines in the blood), and associated affects (sexual excitement and anger). When adults are severely thwarted or exposed to other kinds of intense stress, they frequently abandon goal-seeking behavior of a kind appropriate to their developmental status and re-experience wishes that were characteristic of earlier stages. Much of the time all people experience motivational conflicts; that is, they have mutually incompatible wishes, though these may or may not be wholly conscious. Finally, a great deal of human behavior is motivated by one or another form of a need to maintain a satisfactory self-evaluation.

Though I have tried to state this brief inventory of motivational observations (which does not aim to be exhaustive) in as untheoretical terms as possible, we are more familiar with most of them as cast in the form of propositions from what Rapaport (1959) called the "clinical theory" of psychoanalysis. Indeed, it is virtually the hallmark of the clinical theory that it is quite close to the factual, observational core of psychoanalysis, as opposed to metapsychology, which Rapaport called the "general theory" of psychoanalysis. I might epitomize the rest of this chapter by saying that it is an attempt to recover and rehabilitate the clinical theory of motivation by clearing away the deadwood of metapsychology, which has buried it to a great extent. Indeed, at first it is difficult to decide what aspects of the body of psychoanalytic propositions about motivation belong to the one theory and what to the other. Freud did not make any such distinction: He even tended to lose sight of the basic distinction between observations and concepts or theories. For that reason, many analysts believe (mistakenly, in my opinion) that Freud derived the notion of instinct or drive and many of his propositions about it directly from clinical experience, and that this whole segment of psychoanalysis is part of the clinical theory. On the contrary, historical studies (such as those of Amacher, 1965; Spehlmann, 1953; and Ellenberger, 1970) make it plain that the conception of *Trieb*, particularly as set forth in the *Three Essays* (Freud, 1905d) and in *Instincts and Their Vicissitudes* (Freud, 1915c), is a direct outgrowth and elaboration of a physicalistic model of the organism presented by his predecessors and teachers. In my view, then, a large part of what we know as the theory of instincts, including the concept of instinct or drive itself, is part of metapsychology and not of the clinical theory; and my own estimation is that this chapter does not make nearly as radical a proposal as anyone who is accustomed to considering instinct theory as being close to the clinical heart of psychoanalysis might think.

METHODOLOGICAL CRITIQUE

In this section, I propose first to push further the distinction between the metapsychology of motivation and clinical motivational theory. Then I shall review the respects in which Freud's metapsychology of instinctual drives contains fallacies, factual errors, inconsistencies, and other philosophical shortcomings. Little of what I will have to say is original, and because many of these criticisms are familiar or have been made by myself or others more fully elsewhere, I shall not document the points extensively. My aim, instead, is to show the cumulative impact of these criticisms.

The two psychoanalytic theories of motivation (see Klein, 1976) are not only difficult to separate; paradoxically they sharply contradict one another in many ways. In its starkest and clearest form—essentially as stated in the "Project"[1] (Freud, 1950 [1895])—the metapsychology of motivation is an explicit, coherent, but untenably mechanistic theory, which has the virtue of being testable and the misfortune of being mostly wrong. It is demonstrably the result of Freud's effort to remain true to Helmholtz and Brücke, his scientific ideal father-imagoes; about all that is original to him in his theory is his synthesis of his teachers' ideas. With nonessential changes in terminology, the same ideas persisted in his various reworkings of metapsychology (see particularly 1915c) until the end. The clinical theory, by contrast, originated in Freud's work with patients, and he never brought it together in any one place. It is partly implicit, partly scattered throughout his writings, and I cannot undertake the task of assembling the bits here. [See, however, Rubinstein, 1975.] My present concern is not with specific formulations about the kinds of goals people strive for and the regularities of conflict and defense—the kinds of topics with which the clinical theory deals—but primarily with more fundamental, underlying conceptions of an explanatory sort. In the final section, however, I shall return to the task of explicating the clinical theory of motivation and completing its extrication from metapsychological entanglements. In doing so, I hope to hold fast to what is essential and original in Freud's treatment of motivational issues, and to free it from the residues of 19th-century physiology, which threaten to conceal the true merits of what he had to teach us.

Let me concentrate now on stating the important testable propositions of the metapsychological theory.

The basic model of the organism is the hypothetical reflex arc, conceived of as stimulus → internal processing → response. That is, all behavior originates in the intrusion of physical energies either from the external world or from intrasomatic sources into the nervous system, which is conceived of as passive, without energies of its own, and functioning so as to rid itself of the noxious input via action. Since the inner processing may be very complex, involving much delay and the apparent violation of the constancy principle in the building up and maintenance of tension over some time in the service of the reality principle, the basic, pleasure-principle functioning may not be apparent though it is assumed to be there. Only adaptive, realistic behavior with biologically adequate objects can reduce tension by removing the inner organic sources of input; hence the necessity of paying attention to the real world and acting in a sensible, purposive fashion, instead of making impulsive but futile lunges after direct gratification.

This is a complex first formulation, and there are several testable propositions inherent in it.[2] Item: The nervous system is passive and functions only when stimulated from outside itself. Testable neurophysiologically, and on the whole found wanting. Item: All stimulation is inherently and originally noxious ("primal hate of objects," Freud, 1915c) and becomes of positive interest only when the child has learned that even more painful inner sources of unpleasure cannot be eliminated except by pursuing external need-satisfying objects. Testable from infant observation, and found wanting. There is a large body of contemporary behavioral observation in man and other animals attesting to the independence and elemental nature of curiosity, an exploratory motive, stimulus hunger, or the like; indeed, Freud himself, especially during the decade 1905–1914, made many statements that there are autonomous, nonvoyeuristic sources of curiosity or the drive for research. Item: Increases in intrapsychic tension are unpleasant, and pleasure may be obtained only from reducing tension. Freud explicitly tells us that his observations contradict this proposition, which is clearly demanded by the theory; there is a considerable and growing literature of contemporary observations that confute tension reduction as a basic principle of motivation; and there is neurophysiological evidence for anatomically separate pleasure and unpleasure centers. In sum, the passive reflex model must be abandoned.

Motivated behavior differs from ordinary reflex action, Freud often asserted, in that external stimuli act as simple impacts, which may be removed or escaped, whereas drive stimuli are internal, act continuously, and cannot be escaped. (At times in later papers, he sharpened this contrast by contending that there are thresholds protecting against external stimuli, but no thresholds to give shelter even momentarily against the incessant input of the instinctual drives.) Here the model of the external stimulus seems to be the neurologist's rubber hammer, which Freud had wielded for so many years in eliciting reflexes. But as any experimenter in the field of stimulus deprivation knows, it is virtually impossible to protect a person from physiologically effective, external stimuli and keep him alive. We are bathed in a continuous sea of inescapable stimulation, and in fact our normal functioning seems to be dependent on an average expectable environment of varied stimuli. By contrast, the motives that seem most clearly to fit Freud's drive model—the evacuative needs, hunger, and thirst, as well as genital sexuality—are all capable of satiation and exhibit refractory phases after full consummation.

The facts are, then, that to the extent that internal stimuli can be physiologically detected, they are relatively phasic rather than "always . . . constant" (1915c, p. 118), whereas external stimuli may be of all durations, from a microsecond flash of light to the eternal background of noise (except when extraordinary efforts are made to achieve silence). The assertion that we cannot literally run away from inner stimulation is, of course, true, but it is not a fact on which it is possible to build much useful theory.

In attempting to draw that distinction, Freud was leading up to a central proposition in his metapsychology of motivation, which is that instincts involve inputs of stimuli to the nervous system from within the body; indeed, he wrote, "instincts are wholly determined by their origin in a somatic source" (1915c, p. 123). Even though Freud said that "The study of the sources of instincts lies outside the scope of psychology" (p. 123), he made it explicit in several contexts (1905d, 1911b) that all motivation originates in bodily stimuli, which meant that complete satisfaction of whatever motive is possible only through commerce with an object (which might be part of one's own body, but which is clearly enough a physical entity) that alters the offending endosomatic inputs. This is a rather extreme formulation, and it is surprising that it has attracted so little questioning from within psychoanalysis. I do not hesitate to say that it is impossible to demonstrate any relevant somatic stimulation connected with the vast majority of human motives; surely, the burden of proof was on Freud to find it, and neither he nor any of his followers has apparently felt it necessary to do so.

It is instructive to read reviews of the contemporary literature on the so-called physiological needs or basic drives (e.g., Wayner & Carey, 1973), which generations of us have unquestioningly assumed, with Freud, intimately involve stimuli to enteroceptors of some kind—for example, stimuli arising in the stomach and buccal mucous membranes have long been thought to play a major role in hunger and thirst. While such sensations undoubtedly exist and are part of the *experience* of being hungry and thirsty, important especially in infancy, they are not necessary to food- and water-seeking behavior; numerous studies (some of which I shall cite shortly) have demonstrated that they play no crucial role in these motives (which is not to deny the clinical importance of experienced hunger and thirst). The fact that people have no sense of being hungry after they have starved themselves for a few days creates a life-threatening danger for anorectic patients. Quite aside from the nature of their specific unconscious fantasies and the role these may have in interfering with food intake, such patients lack the usual conscious urge to eat.

Please notice that if we reject the passive reflex model and the conception that internal stimuli play a decisive role in motivation, very little is left of Freud's celebrated summary statement in *Instincts and Their Vicissitudes*:

> from a *biological* point of view, an 'instinct' appears to us as a concept on the frontier between the mental and the somatic, as the psychical representative of the stimuli originating from within the organism and reaching the mind, as a measure of the demand made upon the mind for work in consequence of its connection with the body. (1915c, pp. 121–122)

Very little, that is, except one of Freud's baldest commitments to a dualistic interactionism, a solution to the mind–body problem that holds little favor among contemporary philosophers. After he left the consistent and defensible parallelism he clearly enunciated in his book on aphasia (Freud, 1891b), Freud did not squarely face up to the issue and attempt to think it through. Rather, he seems to have adopted whatever position seemed expedient in any context where it came up, disarming criticism by a wry self-depreciation—he had, he said, a constitutional incapacity for and antipathy to philosophical thinking, and a predilection to stick to the facts of clinical observation. Or, as in the passage I just quoted, Freud would paper over an issue by a literary device: He would take refuge in a metaphor— here, that of a frontier between territories—instead of committing himself to a conceptual analysis.

However inclined we may be to empathize with Freud in his dilemmas, in its effort to become a science, psychoanalysis cannot avoid the responsibility of adopting a consistent philosophical position. It should be some form of identity theory, I believe, a monistic conception of the body–mind relation in which we think of the biological and the psychosocial as different levels of conceptual analysis of a complex unity: the behaving person in his context. In this frame of reference, there is no "mysterious leap from body to mind," any more than there is either a concrete or a metaphysical chasm to be jumped between electronics and information theory. There is surely no need to assume that a process, such as a physiological need, starts out on the bodily level and then at some point suddenly becomes "psychical," in Freud's term, only to return to a physical level of existence again if a somatic symptom is involved. Rather, the same complex event must be studied from beginning to end on the physiological level, and likewise on the psychological level—that is, in terms of wishes, fantasies, and other meanings. As long as we are consistent and comprehensive on each level, the two analyses are complementary, and both contribute to our total understanding without getting in each other's way.

Part of Freud's difficulty, as others and I (Klein, 1976; Yankelovich & Barrett, 1970; Chapter 5, this volume) have argued elsewhere, stemmed from his inability to see any way to make a true science in other than physicalistic terms, although he dealt always and almost exclusively with patterns of meanings.[3] That fact poses no insuperable difficulty for the contemporary philosopher of science, nor need it do so for the psychoanalytic theorist.

The disinterested contemporary reader must be struck by another feature of Freud's discussion of motives or instincts—his treating them constantly as if they were real, concrete entities. In short, he reifies (and often, even personifies) concepts that should remain abstract. For example, Freud wrote of the sexual instincts that they are numerous and "*act* in the first instance independently of one another. . . . The aim which each of them *strives* for is the attainment of 'organ pleasure'" (1915c, pp. 125–126; emphasis supplied). Here, as he was often to do elsewhere, he spoke of an instinctual drive not only as if it were capable of acting—serving as an efficient cause—but as if it were a sentient being capable of exerting effort, of persisting in its need to attain discharge (despite internal defense and external blocking), and even of adopting wily disguises. This charge is anything but novel; psychoanalysts are justifiably weary of hearing it, for the fallacy is not truly intrinsic to the theory. The psychoanalytic theory of motivation *can* be stated and used without reification or personification. The fact is, however, that almost all of us stumble into these fallacies at least occasionally, and I venture to say that most of the time when psychoanalysts use motivational concepts—instinct, drive, libido, energy, force, cathexis— as if they were causally efficacious entities, they do so fallaciously. Schafer (1976) is so much impressed with the insidious pervasiveness of this error that he has embarked on the radical program of doing without substantive nominal concepts almost entirely. The only nouns he allows in his "action language" are words denoting persons, actions (plus classes and modes of action), situations, and to some extent dispositions. I find his proposals for such fundamental changes in our scientific language rather breathtaking, and am reluctant to conclude that radical surgery of this extent is needed. [See also Chapters 12 and 13, this volume.]

Another curious feature of Freud's various versions of his theory of instinctual drives is his strong preference for only two fundamental motives, to which all others could be reduced. True, in various places he did assert that there were numerous sexual and ego instincts, and the final conception of "life instinct" clearly contains a good many diverse motives. It was as if his conviction about the central importance of *conflict* forced him always to postulate an opposed duality of basic drives, even if it became necessary to lump together disparate motives with anatomically and physiologically quite separate bases. But all we need to do is to hold fast to the clinical facts about conflict, accounting in an alternative theory for its ubiquity and pathogenicity, and then we are freed from the artificial necessity to assume that all motives may be reduced to any two. It is clinically obvious that sex and aggression, in their many manifestations, are overridingly important; but fear, anxiety, dependence, self-esteem, curiosity, and group belonging- ness (to name only an obvious handful) cannot validly be reduced to sex and aggression, and are motivational themes the therapist cannot afford to ignore. For that matter, I do not believe that love, affection, friendship, and related themes can be satisfactorily reduced to sex either, despite the fact that Freud's authority has made us accept the reduction all too unquestion- ingly for years. Again, let me emphasize the fact that the dual-instinct theory belongs to metapsychology, not to the clinical theory.

If you have followed me so far, you may nevertheless feel that I have disposed of only the most mechanistic version of the metapsychology of motivation. What about the sophisticated version Rapaport (1960b) proposed in one of his last papers?[4] "*Motives are appetitive internal forces*," he wrote, going on to define *appetitive* in terms of "(a) peremptoriness, (b) cyclic character, (c) selectiveness, and (d) displaceability" (p. 865). Peremptoriness corresponds to Freud's pressure (*Drang*); Rubinstein (1967a) calls this concept the hypothesis of motive pressure, and it has been highlighted in Klein's (1967) paper on peremptory ideation.

If we were to ask, "What is the evidence for the existence of such internal forces as Rapaport postulates?," we would find that he adduces none. He merely invokes clinical experience generally and leans on the authority of William James (1890), who pointed out as a basic unsolved problem of psychology the distinction between behaviors we are impelled to carry out and those that are optional. Now, it is surely a fact of observation that some impulses and desires are relatively weak and easily managed by voluntary activity, while other impulses bring to mind vivid metaphors: They erupt from ego-alien sources, take over the organism, and drive it to an inexorable conclusion. But this is a kind of data to be explained, not in itself conclusive evidence for any theory.

The analogy of the sorcerer's apprentice comes to my mind at this point. Surely, when the obliging broom kept bringing water beyond the point where it was wanted, when it indeed began to be a threat to the hapless apprentice's life, its behavior appeared as inexorable and peremptory as one could imagine. Yet all that was involved was the necessary signal to halt the mechanism that had been started: the magic word that would serve as a negative feedback or switch-off. Or, closer to home, if we consider any machine that is not self-regulating, like an automobile, once it has been turned on it will go until its energy supply has been exhausted. Whether or not it seems "peremptory" is entirely a matter of control—if the car's throttle is stuck and no one is at the wheel, it is as much of a menace, and in much the same way, as a person in an epileptic furor or psychotic rage. A biological phenomenon even more analogous to the runaway car is a cat with a cauterized interpeduncular nucleus: It walks straight ahead, remorselessly and undeterred by any barriers put in its way, until it literally knocks itself out or collapses from exhaustion (Bailey & Davis, 1942). These examples suggest the possibility that the peremptoriness of some kinds of motivated behavior is at least as well explained in terms of defects in the controlling mechanism of negative feedback as by a theory of elusive psychic forces and energies pressing for discharge. Indeed, as Rubinstein (1967a) has demonstrated, the existing doctrine of psychic energy lacks any explanatory power and is merely a set of descriptive metaphors. They owe their survival not to enhancing our understanding or providing any new insights into the detailed workings of behavior, thought, and affect, but to their rich literary suggestiveness.

I do not wish to discuss the concepts of psychic energies and forces, however, since their emptiness has been extensively and adequately argued elsewhere, by a number of others (e.g., Kubie, 1947; Rubinstein, 1967a; Peterfreund, 1971) and in the preceding chapters. I want instead to attack a central remaining notion of instinct theory: that motives are a buildup of something—if not energy, perhaps tension[5]—that must be discharged, goading the person into action. Let me begin by recalling some relevant developments in the experimental psychology of motivation, a field worthy of our study despite the fact that it has mostly used nonhuman subjects.

LESSONS FROM THE EXPERIMENTAL PSYCHOLOGY OF DRIVE

For about 40 years (from approximately 1915 to 1955), research on the experimental psychology of motivation was dominated by the concept of drive. This conception arose from studies of the effects of *deprivation*: When an animal was deprived of food or water, for example, it would eat and drink more than a nondeprived animal when it got the chance, and would work, learn, dare to attempt hazards like electrified grids, and generally be more active and restless. Drive was conceived, then, as a state of unpleasant internal stimulation arising out of the physiological deficits induced by the deprivation and impelling the organism into some kind of behavior. It was assumed, further, that consummatory action with the need-satisfying object led to objective satisfaction of the tissue needs, so that the noxious drive stimuli were reduced. As Cofer and Appley (1964) point out, this conception strikingly parallels that of psychoanalysis, which preceded it by a few years. (Indeed, to the extent that Freud does talk about the bodily sources of drive, he treats them in much the same way.)

Since this concept of drive seemed so fruitful as an explanation of hunger and thirst, it was extended to all the so-called physiological needs, including sex. Initially, the experimentalists conceived of sex just as Freud had done in his paper on anxiety neurosis (1895b [1894]): Deprivation caused the accumulation of sexual products (at least in the male) and an uncomfortable state of distention rather than of deficit. Later, with the discovery of hormonal influences on sexual behavior, the position adopted by drive theorists was much like Freud's in the *Three Essays*, particularly the later editions. What accumulated with deprivation was not secretions like seminal fluid, they now thought, but blood levels of androgens or estrogens. When these hormones were abolished by castrating the animal, sexual behavior tended to stop, only to be dramatically reinstated after injections of the missing substance. But more detailed analysis of the role of sex hormones led to puzzling findings, which did not support the tension reduction notion at all. In the first place, circulating androgens and estro-gens are, if anything, only partly necessary and never sufficient conditions for sexual excitement and activity, and an impressive body of observations on many species, including man, has indicated that libido, the physiological capacity to engage in intercourse, and even orgasm (if not ejaculation) can persist for as long as 30 years after removal of the gonads, and thus without (or at best with extremely low titers of), the presumably necessary hor-mones. Moreover, it has never been found that orgasm *reduces* blood levels of hormones, nor is there any plausible means by which such swift biochem-ical change could take place.

What is even more significant is that no infrahuman species shows the expected buildup of sexuality with increasing deprivation. As long as the animal has the general health and bodily preconditions for adequate perfor-mance, and leaving aside the phenomenon of estrus in many mammalian females, once a minimal recovery time has elapsed after an orgasm, the overwhelmingly important determiner of subsequent sexual excitement and activity is the presence of a more or less suitable partner.

As the most distinguished authority on the sexual behavior of animals, Frank Beach (1956), has put it:

> To a much greater extent than is true of hunger or thirst, the sexual tendencies depend for their arousal upon external stimuli. The quasi-romantic concept of the rutting stag actively seeking a mate is quite misleading. When he encounters a receptive female, the male animal may or may not become sexually excited, but it is most unlikely that in the absence of erotic stimuli he exists in a constant state of undischarged sexual tensions. This would be equally true for the human male, were it not for the potent effects of symbolic stimuli which he tends to carry with him wherever he goes. (p. 5)

Thus, Beach is not blind to the fact that human beings do act *as if* they had such accumulations of drive tension, but he argues that these in fact amount to self-stimulation mediated by imagery, fantasy, and internal language.

The late Kurt Goldstein used to tell of a striking clinical demonstration of Beach's point. One of his severely brain-damaged patients had lost the capac-ity for imagery, and his abstract ability was so impaired that he had virtually no capacity for autonomous thought—he seemed entirely stimulus-bound. Although he was physically healthy and vigorous, he never showed any evidence of sexual desire or spontaneous erections. Even when his wife visited him in a private room and disrobed him as well as herself, he lacked sexual interest until she directly touched his genitals. At that point, he became fully potent and was able to have intercourse with her to their mutual satisfaction.

After many years of detailed study of sexual motivation in animals, Beach (1956) has concluded that sex is better conceptualized as an appetite than as a drive. There is no evidence that any physiologically measurable "tensions" build up in or near the genitals with deprivation; indeed, when the whole genital area has been denervated, male animals of several species still become excited by receptive females and successfully copulate with them, though the mechanism of ejaculation does seem to depend upon intact sensory feedback from the penis.

What seems to be critical in sexual arousal is sensory awareness of the sexual partner. If inexperienced rats are deprived of two or more senses, they do not attempt copulation when they have the opportunity. Sexually experienced rats continue with success despite the loss of any two senses, and cease only when three senses are eliminated, a fact that suggests that, even in the rat, sexual excitement may be achieved to some degree from memory of previous experience of gratification. (Compare, in this context, Fisher's [1966] case of the elderly castrate with a sexual dream.) Another dramatic demonstration of the importance of external arousal comes from repeated experimental findings that when a male has been allowed to copulate with a female to the point where he shows no further interest in her and appears "sexually exhausted," his capacity to perform sexually is immediately restored when a new mate is offered to him. This phenomenon has been found in the rat, rooster, guinea pig, monkey, and bull, and anecdotal evidence suggests that it may occur on the human level as well! It is very difficult to account for these facts by means of a conception of sex as a drive arising out of an inner buildup of tension that must be discharged.

There is a good deal of other evidence that external stimuli play an important role in sex. The frequency of mating is affected by various environmental conditions—temperature and illumination, for example. Mammalian mating takes place more frequently and successfully in familiar as compared to strange surroundings, though any inhibitory effect is chiefly experienced by the male. This fact is strikingly confirmed on the human level by the observations of Masters and Johnson (1966) that it was primarily male subjects who were initially inhibited by being called on to have sexual intercourse in their laboratory under observation.

Incidentally, in both males and females, much evidence supports Beach's (1956) suggestion that two separate mechanisms are involved in genital sexuality: one governing sexual arousal, the other governing ejaculation and orgasm. Thus, there are two separate thresholds: one for the onset of sexual excitement and tumescence, which in nonhuman animals is determined largely by an interaction of internal hormones and external stimuli, supplemented increasingly at ascending levels in the evolutionary series by subjective or symbolic self-stimulation; and a threshold of orgasm, which is determined by sensory feedback primarily from penis and clitoris. Though only orgasm reduces sexual tension, there is ample evidence that preorgastic sexual sensations are pleasurable and are eagerly sought by all species even if orgasm is denied (Kagan, 1955; Sheffield et al., 1951).

In short, recent careful observational and experimental studies of nonhuman animals, which were the classical embodiments of "animal instinct," do *not* support the notion of sex as an internally arising drive or tension that causes the organism to seek out need-satisfying objects.[6]

Let us turn to the evidence on aggression. Though rage, fighting among members of the same species, and other aggressive phenomena are widespread among animals, including many birds, fishes, and other submammalian species, and though such behavior has been meticulously studied, there is little convincing evidence that a need for aggression builds up after an animal has been deprived of it, Lorenz (1963) to the contrary notwithstanding. No animal, after being deprived of fighting, responds to the opportunity afforded by a suitable antagonist in the way it does to food after being kept hungry for a while. The bulk of the systematic experimental and observational work in man as well as in animals supports the conception that aggression is an innately determined (though extensively modifiable) reaction to certain classes of provocations, chiefly assault, frustration, and threat (including, in animals, trespass on property). In these respects, it closely resembles fear or the avoidance of pain, which seems to be equally "instinctive." It can hardly be a coincidence that the physiological and biochemical substrates of fighting and flight are extremely similar and at the least closely interrelated, so much so that it seems artificial to consider (as Freud did) aggression a drive and fear merely an affect—a point cogently made by Murray (1938) many years ago. Fear and anxiety have such an obvious outward reference that it is understandable that Freud was even more reluctant to consider them instinctual or motivational in nature; but the attempt to treat them as affects runs into serious difficulty. In *The Unconscious* (1915e), Freud wrote that it was meaningless to speak of unconscious affects, since an affect was by definition a conscious phenomenon of energic discharge; yet clinical observations forced him, as they have the rest of us, to speak constantly albeit apologetically about unconscious anxiety.

If neither sex nor aggression is considered by most experimental psychologists and ethologists to fit the drive notion, what about hunger and thirst? Hunger seems to be the original model for the drive concept,[7] in psychoanalysis as well as in experimental psychology; see the Project (1950 [1895]), as well as Freud's (1900a) hypothesis about the origins of ideation in the hallucinatory gratification of the hunger need in infants. The great physiologist Walter B. Cannon (1929) was much impressed by the role of local, unpleasant stimuli in both hunger and thirst (hunger pangs from the activity of the empty stomach, and oral sensations from dehydration of the mucous membranes); he lent his prestige to this drive conception of hunger and thirst and adduced a good deal of evidence for it. Yet it had long been known that animals might go empty for periods of weeks or months without any food-seeking behavior; and it was known that although stomach contractions might cease with the first bite or even with the sight of food, eating and hunger do continue for a while. Even so, the hungry feeling stops long before the objective tissue need has been supplied.

As I have already suggested, recent years have seen the accumulation of much more evidence undermining the applicability of the drive model to hunger. Eating is governed by strong preferences for specific substances, some of which—like saccharine—may be non-nutritive and thus incapable of providing release from "tension." In a series of experiments, the role of sensations from stomach contractions has been shown to be minimal; for example, gastrectomy or denervation of the stomach does not have any major effect on hunger. Most patients who had been vagotomized for peptic ulcer, according to a study by Grossman and Stein (1948), failed to notice any change in the character of their hunger sensations as a result of the surgery.

Both behavioral and neurological findings strongly point to the existence of at least two separate mechanisms controlling food intake: one concerns eating, the other satiety. The whole business turns out to be astonishingly complex: Hunger and eating are governed by other areas of the brain besides the lateral hypothalamus and the hypothalamic ventromedial nuclei (the satiety center, which also seems to contain glucostats); brain thermostats may be involved too, for the temperatue as well as the glucose concentration of the blood seems to affect the activity of the relevant hypothalamus and eating. Under normal circumstances, sensations from the stomach and other parts of the body do play some role, as do visual, olfactory, gustatory, and other oral sensations from chewing and swallowing. The role of learning in all this is only beginning to be investigated. Even the phenomenon of behavioral restlessness following deprivation of food no longer seems explicable in terms of accumulated tension; rather, there is good evidence that when it occurs (which is by no means all the time), it may be a mechanism for maintaining bodily temperature, which drops in starved animals if they are inactive.

The preceding summary (originally prepared for a panel discussion on drive theory at a meeting of the American Psychoanalytic Association in December 1967—see Dahl, 1968) is both out of date and too brief to give an adequate account of the complexities of the four classical drives—sex, aggression, hunger, and thirst. But the more recent literature, to the extent that I have been able to follow it, is, if anything, more open in its rejection of the drive concept, which is the main point I have been trying to make by this excursion into an unfamiliar literature.

In sum, the classical "self-preservative" or ego motive of hunger operates in much more complicated ways than was supposed a few decades ago, and does *not* fit the tension reduction model of drive, which had been originally framed to fit it. Much less can the drive concept be generalized to other types of motives, however peremptory. The metapsychological concept of *Trieb*—of instinct or drive—is thus, in all major respects indefensible: philosophically shaky, factually mistaken, and, I believe, often clinically misleading (see Klein, 1976). We must give it up.

TOWARD A NEW THEORY

As an alternative to the metapsychological concept of instinctual drive, I propose, first, that we focus attention on its counterpart in the clinical theory, Freud's concept of wish; second, that psychoanalytic theorists consider the potentialities of the theory of wishing proposed by George Klein (1967); and third, that it may ultimately be possible to build a systems conception in terms of which Klein's theory will be a microscopic look at one sector which, though important, is only part of a larger picture. In the remainder of this chapter, I shall expand on each of these proposals.

First, then, wish as a clinical concept. Let me remind you that Freud worked productively for his first fifteen years as a psychoanalyst without the concept of *Trieb*, relying primarily on wish as his motivational term. The main dynamic concept in *Studies on Hysteria* (Breuer & Freud, 1895)— affect-charged, repressed memories—has most of the major defining properties of wish: It is a cognitive–affective concept, framed in terms of meanings and potentially pleasant or unpleasant outcomes of possible courses of action. The principal motivational concept used in the case history of Dora (Freud, 1905e [1901]) and in Freud's (1900a) masterpiece of combined clinical insight and theoretical elaboration, *The Interpretation of Dreams*, is wish. With it, he was able to do almost everything that an analyst needs to be able to do with a motivational concept, and even after introducing *Trieb*, he did not cease to make frequent use of wish. Therefore, substituting wish for drive means coming back to clinical homeground, while abandoning a largely redundant part of metapsychology that has failed to work, despite its popularity among analysts who have the mistaken impression that drive has the better scientific footing.

One of the advantages of wish is that it does not easily lend itself to the reifying and personifying (anthropomorphic) fallacies with which drive is so rife. A wish implies a person doing the wishing, and we are unaccustomed to speaking of a wish as if it had a life and mind of its own, as the Freudian *Triebe* so often seem to. A wish can be conscious or unconscious; it can conflict with another one; it can be countered, blocked, or modified by defenses and controls. Wishes are plainly near-cousins to *plans* on one side (secondary process) and to fantasies on the other (primary process); they are concrete, often immediately available to introspection, not lofty or vague abstractions.

With the concept of wish, we can reassert, in answer to the behaviorists and other mechanistically inclined theorists, that behavior *is* purposive; that fears, longings, plans, fantasies, and other mental processes are not epiphenomena, but must be central to any adequate psychology of human behavior; and that the person is often not conscious of what his purposes are. Those who find it hard to shake off reductionistic habits of thought may find these ideas more acceptable if they think of wishes and plans as strictly analogous to the programs of computers.

To those who object that wishes are not biological enough, that they do not readily lend themselves to the explanation of psychosomatic problems, I would say that they can express our limited understanding just as well as the metapsychological language of instincts or drives, and have the advantage of not committing us to a great deal of pseudoexplanatory mythology that does not have satisfactory grounding in fact. Before we can begin to make any more progress in this complicated area, we have to agree to stop pretending that we have answers to insoluble philosophical problems. No matter what metaphysical position you take, there remains an impenetrable mystery in the fact that subjective experience exists in a physiochemical world. Perhaps we shall someday learn what are the sufficient conditions for a physiochemical system to take on attributes we call mental; at present, we just do not know.

I will briefy summarize Klein's proposals, but the serious student will want to study his paper on "Peremptory Ideation" (1967; see especially his Fig. 1, p. 89). Klein diagrams the sequence of events that occur in what he calls a "cognitive unit of motivation," from the initial desire to the final experience of gratification, as a closed feedback loop. It begins with what he termed a "Primary Region of Imbalance" (PRI), an unusual state of affairs in one brain region that facilitates, successively, various components of thought, affect, and action. At the end, the PRI is canceled or "switched off" by an appropriate kind of feedback from experience.

Klein's theory is basically a translation into modern terminology of Freud's account (in Chapter VII of *The Interpretation of Dreams*) of the nature of wishing: A wish begins with "the excitations produced by internal needs" (cf. the PRI), and ends when

> an 'experience of satisfaction' can be achieved which puts an end to the internal stimulus. An essential component of this experience of satisfaction is a particular perception . . . the mnemic image of which remains associated thenceforward with the memory trace of the excitation produced by the need. . . . next time this need arises a psychical impulse will at once emerge which will seek to re-cathect the mnemic image of the perception and to re-evoke the perception itself, that is to say, to re-establish the situation of the original satisfaction. An impulse of this kind is what we call a wish. (Freud, 1900a, pp. 565–566)

Klein (1967) has taken the essentials of Freud's account of wishing, has stripped it of its anthropormorphism and its energic economics, and has elaborated it in a number of interesting respects. In particular, his representations of the activity of a repressed unconscious fantasy and the various ways it can complicate ideomotor systems constitute an important contribution to the clarification and formalization of the clinical theory of psychoanalysis. Yet, to my ear, his phrase "Primary Region of Imbalance" is an unfortunately vague metaphor implying something very much like the old drive notion of need-generated "excitations" or "tensions" that must be discharged. Indeed, in an effort not to cut all ties to existing theory, Klein retains the misleading term "discharge" as well, even though he attempts to give it a new meaning. In his examples of thirst (p. 91) and sexual wish (p. 94), he tends to regress to simplistic, tension-reducing conceptions that motives originate in enteroceptive stimuli. I believe that it will strengthen his theory if all these remnants of the old drive conception are abandoned.

I propose, then, that we replace "imbalance" by "perceptual–evaluative mismatch"—hardly a gain in euphony, but, I hope, one in explicitness. "Mismatch" implies a process (which may be conscious, preconscious, or unconscious) of comparing *both* a perceptual pattern (input) and a centrally generated one (mainly from memory), *and* value judgments attached to each pattern. In more phenomenological terms, that means testing an existing and a potential state of affairs for the degree to which they coincide, as well as for any significant discrepancy in value. When what exists is less valuable than what might be, we usually call the fantasied scenario of closing the gap a wish; when what exists is more highly valued, what might be is usually considered a threat or danger, the fantasy a *fear* or an *aversion*. (I intend the term "wish" to be understood, most of the time, to include these negative forms) The (sometimes unconsciously) felt gap between actuality and potentiality can obviously be abolished by a change in reality, so that what exists is what was wanted, or what threatened has been successfully averted; then a discrepancy no longer exists, and the motivational unit goes out of existence. A sequence of the kind Klein diagrammed—a wish—is thus initiated not by some unspecified kind of imbalance, but by a cognitive–affective state something like dissatisfaction, which arouses anticipations of pleasure and/or unpleasure (I repeat, not necessarily conscious) as a consequence of various courses of action or inaction.[8] The condition of perceptual–evaluative mismatch typically originates when the person faces some opportunity or threat, or something not itself particularly desirable or undesirable but which is (directly or indirectly) associated with some such valued state.

My use of the term "value" instead of the more usual "pleasure and unpleasure" is deliberate: It is to remind us that human beings tend to conceptualize their affective responses, to crystallize them into values and ideals. Eventually, I hope that it will be possible to integrate the wise insights of Schafer's (1967) paper on "Ideals, the Ego Ideal, and the Ideal Self" with Klein's theory.

There is a strong and by no means accidental resemblance between this theory and Freud's account in the Project of what he called "judgment," in terms of a wishful cathexis (what might be) and a perceptual cathexis (what exists). Those who are familiar with the work of von Holst and Mittelstaedt

(1950) may see an interesting similarity to their conception of reafference; and the concept of mismatch has been borrowed from a contemporary Russian psychologist, Sokolov (1960). Thus, Klein's and my suggested modifications have roots in Freud's own thinking and parallels in theories proposed by some major contemporary workers in ethology and neuropsychology.

Let me turn now to a consideration of what seem to be the next steps in the building of Klein's suggestions into a complete motivational theory. At present, I cannot do more than put up a few signposts pointing in some necessary directions for further theoretical work.

One of the immediate consequences of Klein's starting point, his intention to conceptualize peremptory ideation, is the fact that his theory is limited to negative feedback systems. Here is another bit of heritage from the tradition of drive theory, which takes as the type case of motivation self-limiting sequences like that of urination. Yet it is obvious that a great deal of behavior in everyday life does not have this episodic character; most of us spend most of our time in continuing, long-term activities, many of which have no logical stopping points. We have to add the conception of *positive* feedback systems, which do not involve any "discharge" or even "switch-off." Rather, our theory must recognize that as long as a pattern of behavior yields a balance of gratification over negative affect, it will tend to be continued. In Klein's terms, the transmissions from the final stage to the primary region are not inhibitory but facilitating, and the cycle continues until it is interrupted by something external to it—for example, considerations of scheduling, or the intrusion of demands from other people. The fact that the person resumes the behavior in question when it is opportune to do so usually makes it plain enough that there had been no cancellation of an initiating perceptual–evaluative mismatch by an experience of match, but only a temporary interruption. Concrete instances of behavior undoubtedly will at times require both types of explanation (positive and negative feedback systems, or perhaps complex hybrid types).

Klein (1967) only briefly touched on a closely related issue: the relation between momentary trains of motivated thought (or wishes) and the long-run ideals, fears, defensive strategies, career plans, persistently recurring symptoms, and sustained repetitive strivings of human beings. The scheme he set forth is best adapted to explain the behavior of the moment, especially self-terminating segments of behavior. A more generally useful system will have to explain how such temporary systems come into being (Klein accounts well enough for their disappearance) and how they attain the varying degrees of specificity as well as personal consistency that observation compels us to assign them. Here again I hope for a link-up with Schafer's (1967) paper on ideals.

Another direction of needed theoretical work is one in which Klein often moved: constantly to keep in mind, and make theoretical allowance for, individual variations of all kinds on the general theoretical themes. Psychoanalysis has justly been criticized for presenting too monolithic a conception of personality, as if people were all organized in very much the same ways and developed along standard lines. Here is another locus of great discrepancy between theory and practice, for while metapsychology states the general case so insistently as to seem to allow no room for a psychology of personality, the psychoanalytic method allows the working clinician to get to know the unique individuality of each patient as few others can. It is time for theory to catch up with practice. I believe that Klein's theory can account for many types of individual differences in motives, but its potentiality needs to be actualized.

A related direction is a developmental one. Klein presupposes a mature person; but of course, we must eventually be able to conceptualize motivation at all levels of personal development, and to account for the ways in which growth takes place. The capacity to entertain simultaneously a present percept of the world and an imagined image of what it might be is a developmental cognitive achievement of no mean order. Piaget has presented in useful detail the sequential stages through which relevant cognitive operations pass, but the motivational implications of each stage have hardly begun to be worked out. The nearest approximation may be found in the work of Jane Loevinger (1976; Loevinger, Wessler, & Redmore, 1970) on ego development; she describes different kinds of goals and of goal-seeking behavior at each of the nine or so levels of development she has isolated, working largely with sentence completion test data from girls and women. I can mention only a couple of ways in which her work suggests fruitful reconceptualization of motivational issues. Much of what has been treated in the psychoanalytic literature as degrees of ego autonomy can be viewed as parts of specifiable stages of development. Freud, being a highly autonomous and mature person himself, tended at times to write as if other people were much like himself; he may not have realized how much less freedom to choose among alternative courses of action was possessed by the great majority of otherwise normal persons.

I have found it interesting to extract from the case of Dora (Freud, 1905e [1901]) the implicit, common-sense theory of motivation Freud used when dealing with ordinary, nonpathological behavior (see Chapter 8, this volume). [Rubinstein (1975) has incorporated these implicit aspects of the clinical theory in his explicit reformulation and systematization.] Freud never thought to make this theory explicit or take it seriously, since his emphasis was always on going beyond it to explain puzzling behavior; but intelligible behavior is motivated too, and a comprehensive theory must account for it. Freud's implicit view was that healthy, normal people typically act in rational ways; that is, they foresee the consequences of available courses of action and choose the one realistically likely to result in the most gratification and the least unpleasantness. Elsewhere, to be sure, he did describe the secondary process as characterized by delay and the experimental action of thought rather than by an impulsive grab for immediate gratification; but it was not always obvious that these discussions are relevant to motivation as well as to thought. And though Freud clearly stated that a developmental sequence is involved, he did not extend the phasic conceptualization of psychosexual development beyond the first few years of life. We can and should do so; I am convinced that the facts of motivation will lend themselves to a sequence of phase changes such as Kohlberg (1969) has described in the area of moral judgment. The structure of wishing as Klein has diagrammed it undoubtedly grows more complex stage by stage, and his scheme will lend itself, I believe, to the conceptual clarification of wishing at each developmental level. His developmental hypotheses about types of pleasure (Klein, 1972) can fruitfully be drawn on in this effort.

Another way in which Klein's theory needs to be evolved is to take into account self and self-evaluation, the importance of which I believe analysts are increasingly appreciating. One of the most painful kinds of mismatch is that between a person's sense of his present self and his desired self. As we know clinically, self-loathing can reach the point where suicide seems necessary to put a stop to intolerable pain. Yet this entire, highly important realm of motivation is at present only crudely conceptualized under the cloudy heading of narcissism. We know something about how the negative self-feelings of shame and guilt develop, but I believe that the whole area of self-evaluation and feelings concerning the self stands in great need of developmental reconsideration. If it is to be as useful as I believe it potentially to be, Klein's theory must find an explicit place for an explanation of self-esteem, self-hatred, narcissistic self-love, mature self-respect, and all the other varieties of self-evaluations. This requirement is much more than a specification of content; it will entail a substantial extension of the theory.

Finally, it should be evident that Klein's paper, like most antecedent psychoanalytic theories, is concerned almost entirely with psychological, intrapersonal matters. To use one of his favorite metaphors, it is a glimpse through a reduction screen, which artificially—but usefully—restricts our vision to a sector small enough to conceptualize. Klein would surely not have maintained that it was a sufficient account of motivation, or that motivation could for long be considered without reference to most of the rest of psychology. For years, Klein understood and taught the complex and many-layered nature of human concerns, and he steadily urged that we look on behavior as a seamless unity. We might for our convenience abstract emotion from thought, or perception from motivation, but we should do so at a risk of forgetting their ultimate integrity. From this standpoint, we should not proceed to develop one theory for motivation, one to explain memory, and another for each of the traditional divisions of the old elementary texts, in the vain expectation that the unity of observed human functioning will somehow emerge from the joint, even "interactive," operation of these several attempts. Nature may be orderly, but it is not the creation of an obsessive-compulsive God who created thought one day and motivation another, and saw to it that there were proper boundaries between all such categories. As an explanation of motivation grows more adequate, it begins to look like a complete theory of personality. If we ask of this ultimate theory, "How does the person get to know his surroundings?" the answer will be in a set of perceptual propositions; if we ask, "How can we understand the directional, goal-seeking nature of the person's behavior?" the answer will be put in a set of motivational propositions; but the general conception of the behaving person remains the same.

Perhaps at this point it might be useful to restate the obvious: Behavior is a complex function of internal determinants—genic, biochemical, hormonal, and other biological determinants, the residues of past learning and maturation; and external determinants—the social structure and culture within which the person lives, tonic supports [Chapter 9, this volume], and the immediately present press (potential harms, benefits, and opportunities). If this full range of behavioral determinants is to be taken into account, nothing less than the most comprehensive theoretical framework available today will do—a systems conception. This framework can satisfactorily coordinate the resources of the other human sciences that are plainly needed for a complete and generally useful psychoanalytic theory of motivation.

Among the most relevant neighboring disciplines are many of the branches of biology. We cannot content ourselves with having disposed of the notion that the body makes its contribution merely by bombarding the brain with enteroceptive stimulations; there are many important somatic aspects of sex and aggression (as well as the so-called physiological drives). Let us begin with the difficult problem of aggression.

Behavior genetics is as yet a new science, and though it is well established that we are not blank slates on which experience can write whatever she likes, the detailed structures and processes through which behavioral predispositions are inherited are far from being well understood. Nevertheless, as Moyer (1973) puts it, "the brain contains inborn neural systems that, when active *in the presence of particular stimuli*, result in aggressive behavior toward these stimuli" (p. 35). The only change I would make in that formulation would be to substitute "press" for "stimuli" (see below). Electrical inputs to certain areas in the amygdala can set off aggressive behavior, which demonstrates the point. The thresholds for the production of anger and hostility can be lowered biochemically, or by the pressure of tumors in or near the amygdala.

In terms of our theory, people have an inborn readiness to value positively *either* escape from or inflicting harm to persons, animals, or objects that harm them, threaten to do so, or block the attainment of important goals, and a readiness to act in these same ways. (What seem to be separate cases may in a way reduce to one, since injuring an enemy is a way of putting a stop to his inflicting harm on you, just as running away is. It all comes down to the negative valuing of being injured or frustrated—which has obvious survival value—and the consequent need to have a variety of response patterns to prevent being injured or blocked from attaining gratifications—a capability that is also obviously adaptive. I can see no need to postulate any direct pleasure in causing or perceiving injury to another unless that other is perceived as threatening or thwarting.)[9]

Whether a given person will tend to choose aggression or flight as a means of coping with threat or frustration seems to be in considerable part a matter of intrauterine hormonal setting of the nervous system. A great deal of fascinating work is currently going on concerning the effects of hormones and other biochemical agents on both sexual and aggressive behavior (and, more generally, on sex-linked "masculine" and "feminine" behavior). The impression with which I come away from reading accounts of this research is that the effects seem to be of two kinds: First, parts of the central nervous system may become programmed during fetal development with a readiness to produce certain patterns of behavior—most strikingly, greater aggressiveness, general activity, interest in rough games and sports, and possibly career-oriented achievement motivation—in boys and in girls who were virilized *in utero* because their mothers had had injections of progestins or had suffered from the adrenogenital syndrome (Money & Ehrhardt, 1972). (Boys are virilized by their own fetal testosterone.) Second, granted that the capacity for producing a form of behavior is present in the brain, the threshold for its production may be raised or lowered by the biochemical *milieu intern*—notably, by the amount of circulating testosterone. (Other biochemical influences, like the degree of hypoglycemia or the responsiveness of the adrenals, are also important, but the details are less important for present purposes than the basic principles.) Past learning also plays an enormously important role. If in early life a person is consistently and severely punished for any display of aggressiveness, later provocations will obviously tend to evoke fear and avoidance. If his aggressiveness has been ignored or encouraged, he will later probably fight rather than take flight.

Notice, however, that the role of a biologically adequate external releaser is still crucial. When, for example, 6-hydroxydopa was injected into the ventricles of rats' brains, fighting as a response to being electrically shocked was greatly increased and the rats also tried to bite the experimenter when handled, but there was "little or no intraspecific aggression when the animals were in their home cages"—that is, there was no aggression without provocation (Thoa, Eichelman, Richardson, & Jacobowitz, 1972, p. 76).

At a first approximation, then, the modified Klein theory links up with the biological in this way: Any particular situation is more or less likely to arouse a perceptual–evaluative mismatch and thus a wish, depending on the hormonal (and, more generally, the biochemical) history and contemporary state of the person's body, which also influence the availability of various behavior sequences as elements in the completed wish cycle or ideomotor system.

As I argue in Chapter 9, the phenomena that psychoanalysts have long conceptualized in purely intrapsychic (or intraorganismic) terms must be accounted for in a way that takes serious account of the person's environment, especially the threats and opportunities it presents. Once we replace imbalance by valued mismatch between a perceived and an imagined world, it becomes evident that the single feedback loop Klein diagrammed and discussed is only part of a larger, more complex system comprising the person and his environment. One of the incidental by-products of the current ecological movement is the rise of environmental psychology, a slogan that may help redirect the attention of psychologists to behaviorally relevant aspects of man's surroundings other than obvious positive and negative reinforcers. Again, Murray (1938) is proved to have been unusually foresighted: after a couple of generations, his concept of "press"—the motivationally relevant aspects of a person's environment—and his pioneering classification of its major types remain virtually without competition.

Since I am surely not ignorant of the notorious emphasis of behaviorists, social learning theorists, and in fact most American psychologists on "stimulus control of behavior," the just-preceding statement must sound like a willful perversity. If so, which of these colleagues has produced a psychologically useful or systematic classification of "stimuli"? If any such exists, it has remained obscure. The trouble is our old heritage of physicalism: Stimuli are almost never *clearly* defined by psychologists in any but physical terms. Outside of psychophysics, where it is appropriate and necessary to define sounds (for example) as pressure waves measured in hertz and dynes/cm^2, it is misleading to talk about situations, people, and other interesting features of a person's environment in terms of *stimuli*. Even when you attempt to define the word in psychological terms, it still carries a physicalistic, submeaningful connotation.

It was part of Murray's genius to grasp this point, to reject the misleading term "stimulus," and to substitute for it a new term clearly defined in terms of meaning, to serve as a unit for the analysis of the psychological environment. If you imagine that press are nothing more than a classification of stimuli in terms of response, let me commend to you Murray's wise exposition (1938, pp. 116 ff.). Press are not defined by reference to the subject's response to them, but in terms of consensually established meanings—essentially the same approach as that of sociologists and anthropologists. Indeed, these disciplines may be said to be the principal ones concerned with press, though they do not use the term, and psychologists have left systematic treatment of the environment almost entirely to them, to architects, geographers, climatologists, and other social scientists.

By way of summary, let me give very briefly the present status of the theory of wish as I see it. It is protoneurophysiological (Rubinstein, 1967a), in that the operative concepts are stated in generalized terms suitable for eventual translation into anatomical and physiological language, on the one hand, and into terms that are meanings, on the other. The relation between the two sets of terms is one of encoding: It is assumed that all subjective, phenomenological events are coded assemblages of information being transmitted and processed in the nervous system in biochemical and biophysical form. Some degree of isomorphism is thus assumed (if a phenomenal unity appears, there is in some sense a corresponding unity of process in the biological substrate). Units are defined predominantly in terms of meanings,[10] but care is taken constantly not to postulate anything that conflicts with the contemporary state of knowledge in the neurosciences.

All behavior is caused, but not necessarily (and not in all its details) determined, by wishes.[11] Much of it is determined simply by the detailed structure of a person's body, by the adequacy of his physiological functioning, and by genetic programs. The activity of the gastrointestinal system, for example, can be accounted for in the terms of the preceding sentence, and no doubt for such reasons is not usually considered "behavior." But consider a boy playing baseball: His native strength, coordination, and state of bodily vigor at the moment obviously have a lot to do with the style and adequacy of his playing, and even with whether he plays at all or not. Ordinarily, when we say that all behavior is motivated, we imply a definition of behavior as the part of the person's total activity that is caused by identifiable motives. I see no need to get into that kind of game here. Let us simply note that some aspects of the most obviously wish-determined behavior are caused nonpsychologically, and also that activities ordinarily considered to be "purely physiological" may be affected in some respects by wishes. Psychosomatic medicine teaches us, for example, that unconscious wishes to be filled up or emptied out can greatly interfere with the normal functioning of the gastrointestinal tract.

As part of the normal functioning of the sensory organs and the central nervous system, healthy people continually construct a phenomenal world while awake. Part of that activity is a continuous matching of inputs against stored memories of past perceptual experience. Satisfactory matching results in the sense of recognition, and it appears that a general silent precondition for normal behavior is a steady background of such implicitly reassuring matches: The person is oriented; he finds most aspects of his experience at least generally familiar. Let us assume, following Piaget (1936) and a good many other contemporary theorists, that moderate degrees of mismatch arouse mild degrees of pleasure and interest, which we call curiosity, and which initiate and sustain exploratory behavior. Let us assume, also, that when mismatch is sudden and considerable in extent passively suffered), the person experiences startle and some innately programmed unpleasure.

In the foregoing, I am assuming that there are brain centers the activity of which is accompanied by positive and negative affective experiences, and which are genetically "wired into" various innate programs (e.g., the pleasures associated with stimulation of the various erogenous zones). When infants or children happen to experience something that is in this way innately gratifying, they use whatever sensorimotor schemes they have at their disposal to prolong the pleasure—a positive feedback system (or, in Piaget's terminology, a circular reaction).

Such positive feedback systems are the main supplementation required by Klein's model, which deals only with negative feedback loops. With these two types of systems, we can explain most of the kinds of motives with which psychoanalysts are concerned. When we get more ambitious and hope to cover all aspects of behavior and inner life, what began as a systematization of clinical theory starts to look like an attempted replacement for metapsychology. Indeed, the program for theoretical development already sketched out here is ambitious enough to betray the fact that I share yearnings that Freud recognized as speculative and philosophical. Like him, however, I shall at least for the moment suppress them and break off.

In conclusion: Drive is dead; long live wish! Freud's concept of *Trieb* served a useful function in his own theoretical development, but for us it is an anachronism beyond hope of rehabilitation. With relatively few terminological changes, however, his earlier but never abandoned concept of wish can be made a clinically usable substitute. And as it has been sharply restated by Klein, the theory of wish promises to become the nucleus for a fully developed, recognizably psychoanalytic, and generally useful theory of human motivation.

PART IV

Ego Psychology and
the Theory of Thinking:
The Structural Point of View

CHAPTER 8

The Past and Future of Ego Psychology

If I were to be consistent with the outlook of the introduction to Chapter 7, this new section would contain chapters dealing primarily with the topographic point of view and Freud's theories about consciousness and unconsciousness. Instead, it deals primarily with ego psychology, with a special emphasis on two topics: autonomy and the theory of thinking. Why such an imbalance?

The first reason is that I have found not much to say about the topographic theory itself, after Gill (1963) finished with it (see also Arlow & Brenner, 1964). Of course, a lot could be said about the problems of consciousness and unconsciousness, but I do not feel ready to do so, and it would not be part of a critique of metapsychology.

Second, although Chapter 8 is primarily about ego psychology, it does contain most of what I have to say about other aspects of the structural point of view that replaced the topographic. The id has very little meaning aside from the theory of instincts, just treated in the last chapter; and after reading Schafer's two excellent papers on the superego (1960, 1967), I felt that I had nothing much to add to them.

The present chapter was first written as part of a panel discussion at a meeting of the American Psychoanalytic Association, celebrating the 50th anniversary of the publication of The Ego and the Id *(Freud, 1923b). The centerpiece of that panel was a paper by Jacob Arlow (1975), and my invitation was to comment on his presentation. Some traces of that original orientation still remain in the present chapter, though I have tried to make unnecessary for a reader first to become familiar with Dr. Arlow's paper.*

Ego psychology is one of several disciplines of which it may be said that it has a short history but a long past. Its history, which has been adequately covered elsewhere (e.g., Rapaport, 1958b), is often thought to begin in 1923 with *The Ego and the Id*, but its past extends back beyond human history.

THE PAST

The past of ego psychology may be said to extend so far back because the conception of the ego manifestly grows out of a number of observational roots: ways of noticing certain kinds of phenomena which today occur in the early life of almost every human being and which are the inevitable consequences of the person's structure and organization.

"The ego is first and foremost a bodily ego" (Freud, 1923b, p. 26). In these words, Freud asserts that the first observational root of the ego concept is the fact that the bodily part of an organism is persistently perceptible. A baby spends much of his time looking at, feeling, and otherwise getting perceptually familiar with all parts of his body, and the continuity and relative sameness of these percepts is often cited as a core for the "sense of self." We know nothing of any sense of self in nonverbal animals, but plainly many species can and do become aware of their own bodies and treat them as something special in their perceptual worlds. This quality of specialness, as Freud points out, is attributable to the unique dual perceptibility of the body. For instance, I can see my hand and feel it with my other hand, while at the same time enjoying proprioceptive information about it from within. Following Schilder (1935), psychoanalysts have come to refer to the lasting precipitate of many such perceptions as the "body image," and to accept Freud's declaration that it is an important constituent of the ego.[1]

A second historical root extends as far back as the first observation of the fact of death—another perceptual event that is older than mankind itself. We know from studies of chimpanzees that they not only can discriminate the difference between a living and dead organism, but that they react to a dead member of their own species in a way that suggests they feel something close to the human experience of uncanniness—an irrational fear and ambivalent loathing (Hebb & Thompson, 1954). I suspect that by the time Homo sapiens was a clear-cut species, this reaction was elaborated into superstitious awe and, quite possibly, into the beginning of a concept that there is a distinction between the body and a "something else"—something that has to do with breathing, with initiating movement, and with conscious awareness—all of which constituted life. Even today, each of us struggles with the profound philosophical problems of life and death in early childhood, when the dying of a family member makes death very real. Grandfather is there, cold and still, and at the same time, as we say, "gone." Even a nonreligious family finds it hard to explain this paradox to the bewildered grandchild without recourse to some version of the soul theory.

From anthropology, we know that something very much like the soul of Judeo-Christian theology is part of almost every culture's religion. As elaborated by the early church fathers, the animistic conception of the soul had already many recognizable aspects of what we today call "ego psychology." Despite his personal irreligiousness, Freud was a participant in a culture in which these religious ideas were thoroughly ingrained—quite aside from the influence of his Catholic nanny with her terrifying stories of souls burning in hell. [See also Vitz, 1988.]

On a slightly higher developmental level, many of the elements of the animistic soul theory reappear as the vitalism of *Naturphilosophie*, to which Freud seems to have been exposed during his adolescence. These were some of the philosophical inclinations, he told Jones, to which he had found it so tempting to yield, and which he had deliberately suppressed by immersing himself in the reductionistic scientism of physicalistic physiology. In Chapter 6, I have said that the influence of vitalistic concepts may be plainly seen in the concept of psychic energy, and that the speculative works of Freud's later years, from *Totem and Taboo* through *Moses and Monotheism*, embody many returns of the exiled *Naturphilosophie*.

This second, relatively unrecognized source of ego psychology is important, I believe, and not a mere intellectual curiosity, because the primitive animism of the soul theory is the intellectual equivalent of a fixation: Not just Freud, but all of us are exposed to the constant temptation and danger of regressing to it. We must not neglect to apply to ourselves this lasting contribution of psychoanalysis not only to psychology but to the understanding of all intellectual work: That most of autonomy is relative and that the capacity to think maturely—according to the secondary process—is a fragile, never securely won achievement, with developmentally earlier (primary-process) ways of thinking always operating in the background and always ready to influence conscious thought when the going gets difficult.

In this sense, therefore, the soul theory is not only a historical antecedent of ego psychology, but an omnipresent mode of thought (or, in Piaget's term, "scheme") that any of us is in danger of falling back on at times. That observation is cast in the form of a warning because animism involves a number of serious philosophical fallacies, which may be found cropping up in ego psychology quite pervasively if one is attuned to them—dualism,[2] anthropomorphism, reification, essentialism, and the like. More specifically, the soul is a reification of the sense of self and of the abstract concepts of life and consciousness; it is the essence of a personality or individuality. These closely related, rather primitive ways of trying to grapple with basic observations about people are dualistic in that they assume that the body is one kind of reality, temporarily inhabited by a spirit or essence which in some ghostly way epitomizes the psychological facts about a person and is conceived to be somehow ontologically different from its "tenement of clay." And while it may seem strange to think that anthropomorphism could be inappropriate in a discussion of *anthropos*, the criticism is valid, for the whole is not identical with any of its parts.

Anthropomorphism points to the redundant and confusing custom of postulating an additional entity beyond the observable organism and then giving this abstraction many of the properties of an entire person. Freud's (1900a) concept of consciousness as "*a sense organ for the perception of psychical qualities*" (p. 615) is an excellent example of this kind of tautologous and concretistic confusion as it shows itself in ego psychology. The eye is a sense organ; there is no need to postulate any little man crouching behind it to perceive its pictures—or if there were, there would be no escape from the infinite regress of homunculi each taking in the perceptual laundry of his predecessor in line. The very concept of ego exposes us to all these temptations, and surely in its everyday use by most of us it becomes a prime mover, a kind of insubstantial *shabbas goy* who is called upon to do everything for the indolent, unemployed, and (by psychoanalysts) almost totally ignored *person*. [See, however, Rubinstein, 1981.]

A third observational root of the ego concept is linguistic, and therefore distinctively human. The process of individuation, or what Schafer (1973b) calls "representational differentiation," makes an important advance as the infant gradually becomes aware that the adults who tend him consistently use one word to refer to him, a personal name. It has long been noticed (e.g., Preyer, 1882) that the child learns and uses his own name well before any personal pronoun, the correct use of which marks another conceptual advance (see Gesell & Ilg, 1943; Moore, 1986).

For present purposes, these and many related facts may be lumped together into the statement that human beings universally learn to employ their own personal names, and later first-person pronouns and other words to refer to themselves. This fact is often cited as another nucleus of self, as a point around which the self-concept crystallizes, and the like. A less obvious point, which I wish to emphasize, is that language is both freeing and confining. On the one hand, the ability to name oneself gives the infant the power not only to observe himself but to think about himself, which is the beginning of a kind of autonomy. It is Descartes inverted: If *I* exist, I can think; therefore, I am a third force—something beyond other people and objects that make demands on me, and something beyond the aches and urges that trouble my sense of well-being (or, if you prefer, the exigencies of such wishes as hunger and pain avoidance). On the other hand, we are all vulnerable to the danger of assuming that when a word exists, a thing must exist to which it refers. This is the familiar fallacy of reification, which arises from such paleological pseudosyllogisms as this: All things have names (concrete nouns); therefore, any name or noun must refer to a thing. The necessity of first-person pronouns and names is attested to by the fact that all known languages contain them and no tribe or similar group of people has ever been found who did not use them. But the legitimacy of "I" does not necessarily imply that there is an entity, "*the* I," widespread though such a concept was long before Freud. This feature of language is another reason for the treacherousness of the ego concept and its liability to fallacious misuse.

A fourth observational root of ego psychology seems to be another uniquely human capacity: self-observation beyond mere bodily perception. As soon as a child notices not only the world but also the fact that he *notices* the world, this reflexive awareness introduces a new paradox, a new set of philosophical dilemmas that are intrinsically difficult enough to have provided intellectual fodder for generations of our best philosophers. Small wonder that the most gifted of us, as children, necessarily solve these problems in ways that do not stand up well to adult scrutiny. If I find that I can observe myself, even in the reflexive act itself, it is difficult to resist the conclusion that two entities must be present, signified by the two different words "I" and "myself." The "I" is what does the observing, and it seems subjectively identical with the internal possessor of sensations and memories, and with the wisher who conceives of goals and plans, or strategies to get them, and originates actions of all kinds. This "I" does not seem identical to or completely coterminous with the body image, or with the total person or organism, though it is inextricably and bafflingly interwoven with them. This set of observations lies behind the familiar Freudian concept of the "observing ego," with whom the therapeutic alliance is made. (For a highly sophisticated modern treatment of these issues, see Chein, 1972.)

I am following the British tradition of substituting the Latin "ego" for Freud's straightforward "*Ich*" when I refer to his terminology, but it is not unimportant to recall that he himself did not particularly like and very seldom used the word "ego." From the beginning, he adopted the prevalent practice of speaking about "the I" (*das Ich*) to mean that hypothetical entity, the part of the person that does the self-observing and seems generally in charge. As Strachey points out (Strachey, 1961), "the term had of course been in familiar use before the days of Freud" (p. 7), though he does not remind us that it was used as a technical term by such teachers of Freud's as Meynert, whose theory of primary and secondary *Ich* anticipates Freud's distinctions between id and ego, primary and secondary processes.

But Meynert was himself the inheritor of a considerable psychiatric tradition, a major figure in which was Wilhelm Griesinger. In 1867, two years before his death, Griesinger published an enlarged and widely read edition of his 1845 textbook on psychiatry. There, in the words of the distinguished historian of psychiatry, Ellenberger (1970), he "developed an entire ego-psychology. Distortions of the ego can result from nonassimilated clusters of representations, which then may face the ego as though they were a stranger and come in conflict with it" (p. 241). These ideas were hardly original even with Griesinger but were in general currency; his French contemporary Durand, for example,

> claimed that the human organism consisted of anatomical segments, each of which had a psychic ego of its own, and all of them subjected to a general ego,

the Ego-in-Chief, which was our usual consciousness. . . . The sum total of these subegos constituted our unconscious life. (Ellenberger, 1970, p. 146)

Notice how similar these propositions are to the following from Freud's 1892 paper in which he made his first published use of *"das Ich."* He was dealing with the problem of how it is that what he called "antithetic" ideas (which seem to be the same ones called "pathogenic" in *Studies on Hysteria*) "gain the upper hand" in cases of exhaustion. The exhaustion is only partial, he says. "What are exhausted are those elements of the nervous system which form the material foundation of the ideas associated with the primary consciousness . . . the chain of associations of *the normal ego*" (emphasis added). The ideas excluded from it, "the inhibited and suppressed ideas, are *not* exhausted . . . [but] . . . emerge like bad spirits and take control of the body, which is as a rule under the orders of the predominant ego-consciousness" (Freud, 1892–1893, pp. 126, 127).

These usages point to a fifth root of ego psychology, another ancient piece of self-observation—the fact that we have two kinds of impulses or desires, which Freud called "ego-syntonic" and "ego-alien." Before him, they were better known as voluntary and involuntary actions. The notion of a division of the self into higher and lower natures, the former—the source of voluntary actions—controlling the latter—the source of involuntary actions—is virtually as old as philosophy. By Freud's time, the discussion of that and a great many other problems, which we subsume under the heading "ego psychology," had become a substantial part of academic psychology. Fortunately, for anyone interested in looking into the then-contemporary status of these discussions, there is a readily available and deliciously readable source: William James's masterpiece of 1890, *Principles of Psychology*, especially Chapter X, "The Consciousness of Self." As Rapaport (1960b) reminds us, James spoke of the distinction between actions that were voluntary, a matter of conscious will, and those that were peremptory or involuntary as "one of the basic unsolved problems of psychology" (p. 869). Some other topics covered in James's Chapter X are the empirical self or "me"; the material self; the social self; the spiritual self; emotions of self; what self we love in self-love; the pure ego; the verifiable ground of the sense of personal identity; theories of self-consciousness; the mutations of the self; insane delusions; alternating selves.

Later, James became an admirer of Freud and read a fair amount of his work, but there is no record that Freud read James. I do not mean to imply that Freud should have read James or that he would have learned much from him: the mature Freud did not learn by reading philosophical books, no matter how profound or brilliant. Indeed, he frequently complained of a disinclination to read philosophy, aided by what he called a "constitutional incapacity" (Freud, 1925d, p. 59). Freud's way of learning was primarily observational; his main teachers after 1890 were his patients.[3] And when he came to write about what he had seen and heard, though he seldom shrank back from the desirability of conceptualizing his findings and even spinning theories about them, his theorizing was almost always focused on the matter at hand—the puzzling behavior that confronted him and which he needed to understand. Only in the Project (Freud, 1950 [1895]) did he set out to write a virtually complete psychology for neurologists, probably modeled on Exner's (1894) similar attempt to synthesize the ideas of their common teachers, Brücke and Meynert. The Project contains not only an ego, a subset of cortical neurones with striking resemblances to Meynert's secondary ego, but an extensive discussion of topics we now think of as being within the province of ego psychology, particularly in Part III, "Attempt to Represent Normal ψ Processes." Thereafter, however, just because he was not an academic professor deliberately trying to construct a comprehensive system of psychology, but a psychotherapist whose patients brought him baffling symptoms, his attention was constantly engaged by the pathological, rarely by the normal.

Freud first defined his theoretical attempts, the construction of a metapsychology, as a "psychology that leads behind consciousness." The fact that the traditional definition of *Ich* or ego had virtually equated it with consciousness is a plausible explanation for the relatively late emergence of ego psychology as an explicit focus of psychoanalytic theorizing—it was what psychoanalysis was to transcend, not incorporate. Implicitly, however, much of it was there all along. The contemporary academic psychology dealt with such topics as conscious perception, thought, will (voluntary action)—in short, with adaptive ego-syntonic functions; it was a psychology not only of consciousness but of normal, conflict-free, everyday behavior. Much of it was little more than the formalization (or translation into jargon) of common sense. Freud saw no need to traverse this well-trodden ground. He wanted to make original discoveries, and he had a method superbly adapted for doing so but not well suited for helping him contribute to normal psychology. Even after Hartmann (1939) sounded the call for psychoanalysis to become a general or total psychology, not just a theory of neurosis or psychopathology, this limitation of method held back his efforts as well as those of other classical psychoanalysts whose experience was confined primarily to treating patients in private practice. Freud's own feeling was that he was limited in what he could learn about ego psychology because the psychoanalytic method did not seem suitable for treating schizophrenics and others who suffered from major interferences with ego functions.[4]

Recently, I made a special scrutiny of the Dora case (Freud, 1905e [1901]) and attempted to identify every theoretical proposition, explicit or implicit. Implicitly, there are a large number of concepts and assumed propositions that make up the common-sense psychology of the time, which Freud took for granted and which, closely examined, turns out to be what today we call ego psychology. One might call this psychology the explanation of nonpuzzling behavior—the very kind of phenomena Freud found of little interest because they were so perspicuous and the prevalent theory so self-evident. For instance, let us consider the following explanations of why people act as they do.

1. Some experiences (e.g., sex, eating) are directly pleasant and we act to attain them for that reason, while others (notably pain) are unpleasant and we act to avoid them. It is perfectly evident that Freud believed this proposition, which is in fact a way of formulating the pleasure–unpleasure principle, even though by 1905 he had not yet stated it in so many words. (It is put in metapsychological terms in *The Interpretation of Dreams*.) Similarly, his occasional references to an instinct of self-preservation indicated his implicit subscription to the next proposition.

2. Some activities (breathing, eating, drinking, evacuating, avoiding pain) are obviously necessary for survival, and others are indirectly necessary for survival (working for a living, fighting off threats), which is, at least in part, why we do them.

3. There are a number of states that do not seem obviously necessary to life yet are almost universally wanted and sought (the good opinion of others and oneself; love; security; power and competence generally), and there are complementary or opposite states which we feel it is perfectly natural to dislike and to act so as to avoid experiencing them (shame; inferiority; guilt; anxiety; contempt; etc.). Similarly, if the reaction is proportional to the grievance, people will feel hurt and angry, become irritated, or develop rages and hatreds when they are thwarted by others in getting what they need or want, or when they are insulted or assaulted.

When we limit our purview to such forms of behavior (as academic psychologists tend to do), it is easy to believe that people are mostly rational; that is, they choose to do what is obviously good or leads efficiently to rewarding experiences and to shun what is bad, self-defeating, or hurtful. Moreover, people seem to act as they do because of conscious intentions and values. As every science must at some point include the precise formulation of the obvious, let us examine more closely the common-sense ego psychology contained between the lines of the "Fragment of an Analysis of a Case of Hysteria."

In the Dora case, Freud frequently uses such terms as "wish," "desire," and "longing," which imply much of what I have already spelled out, in particular the proposition that everyday behavior is motivated by subjective representations to yourself of what you want or do not want. But Freud also uses another set of similar terms, "intention," "will," and "conscious effort," which imply that at some point a wish ceases being just a state of desire and passes into the status of what Klein (1970) has called an "executive intention"—a process of choice or decision made to carry out a line of action in order to satisfy the wish. Further, terms like "will" imply that it is possible for a person to make a difficult decision and to stick by it. When something wanted is not easy to obtain or when there are obstacles, a process we call "effort" is possible. By summoning up a certain conscious state of mind, sometimes called "will," a person can redouble his level of activity and striving for a goal. When, during his early therapeutic work, Freud presented his patients with "the solution" to an understanding of their neurotic symptoms, he expected them to be able to face unpleasant facts, which implied his faith that they could summon up the effort to do what they naturally and normally would not want to do. "Where id was, there shall ego be" makes no sense if we do not include under it the recognition that mature, non-neurotic people usually have the capacity to make free choices [see Chapter 9, this volume].

To summarize, ego psychology has a long past because it is founded on five virtually universal kinds of observations: the body image, the fact of death, the use of self-words, reflexive self-awareness, and the feeling that we are in control of some impulses but not of others. Moreover, ego psychology is often briefly defined as "relations to reality," reality being construed as what appears real to ordinary observation. But the very fact of its prescientific beginnings means that ego psychology began with an unrecognized heritage of conceptual problems. All of these observations give rise to a number of extraordinarily subtle, complicated, and controversial issues when one tries to conceptualize them in a systematic and consistent way, issues that are central to a great deal of philosophy.

Unfortunately, ego psychology has been developed by persons—predominantly by Freud, of course, but also by other psychoanalysts—who were not well read in philosophy and who therefore tended to take relatively naive positions on complicated issues as if they were self-evident. This is one major source for some of the fallacies built into ego psychology. My contention is that ego psychology has a short history because Freud was mainly concerned with conceptualizing his clinical observations, and because he felt, I believe erroneously, that his commitment to strict determinism limited the degree of ego autonomy he could postulate. The fact that his method required him and his patients to focus on precisely those areas of their lives in which their freedom was limited also must have tended to delay his emphasis on "the primacy of the intelligence" (Freud, 1927c). Nevertheless, if we define ego psychology in terms of its propositional content, then we must admit that there is quite a bit of ego psychology in Freud's writings from the beginning.

THE EGO AND THE ID RECONSIDERED

The Ego and the Id (Freud, 1923b), marks the formal beginning of ego psychology. Arlow (1975) believes that this was so fundamental a theoretical change that it can be called a "paradigm shift," in Kuhn's (1970) phrase. I do not agree; to me it is not a revolution, but is one of several periods of slightly accelerated evolutionary change in Freud's thinking.

Freud used the term *das Ich* almost from the beginning. Except for a few passages dealing with the egotistical nature of dreams (Freud, 1900a, pp. 267, 322, ff.) he abandoned it temporarily for a decade when he began to work on *The Interpretation of Dreams*, in which he introduced the topographic theory. In the works written during this ten-year period, the term occurs rarely and unsystematically. But starting in 1909 with his revisions of the dream book and with the lectures delivered at Clark, he began to use the term regularly, particularly in connection with the idea of defense and other oppositions to the libido, the opponent of which for a while became the *Ichtriebe* (ego instincts). By the time of the metapsychological papers, Freud was using it frequently and in an increasingly technical and systematic way.

By contrast, a remarkable fact about the topographic theory is how rarely Freud used it after setting it forth in 1900. The *Five Lectures on Psycho-Analysis* (Freud, 1910a [1909]) given at Clark contain no mention of it, though this was Freud's first major public summary of his ideas. *The Psychopathology of Everyday Life* (Freud, 1901b) contains but a couple of passing references to preconscious and unconscious *systems*. (Of course, throughout his career Freud wrote about unconscious wishes, ideas, memories, etc., and often referred to them collectively as "the unconscious," but that is different from using the topographic system *Ucs.*) The book on jokes (Freud, 1905c) contains a fairly extensive passage in the discussion of the joke work that uses the topographic terminology, but most of the volumes of the *Standard Edition* between that and the one containing the metapsychological paper (Freud, 1917d [1915]) where the topographic theory is explicitly reconsidered have not even a single index entry for "preconscious."

I can see two major reasons for Freud's neglect of his set of topographic concepts during this period. First, it was not intended to be a theoretical basis for his clinical work or for any of the other tasks for which he needed conceptual tools, except the understanding of dreams. And second, it was not a systematically constructed theory, nor one oriented to data, but more of an expository device. As such, it served him well in helping to organize the presentation of his ideas on how a dream came about, but we should not forget that the title of Chapter VII is "The Psychology of the Dream-Processes"; that was Freud's deliberately limited intent. As if daunted by the failure of his ambitious Project to create a total neuropsychology, he probably intended a strategic retreat into modesty; and he was undoubtedly right in his feeling that it had been a mistake to try to create a grand, all-purpose, abstract model of the nervous system that would account for normal and abnormal behavior, thought, affect, and other human functioning. Even today, it may be premature.

Freud was clearly ambivalent about the topographic theory even as a rhetorical device: No sooner had he expounded it than he began to find difficulties with it and, to his evident satisfaction, managed "to replace a topographical way of representing things by a dynamic one," which, as Gill (1963, p. 8 n.) notes, would today be called economic—"the existence of two kinds of *processes of excitation* or *modes of its discharge*" (Freud, 1900a, p. 610). Yet on the next page, Freud argues that it is "expedient and justifiable to continue to make use of the figurative image of the two systems." His phrase "figurative image" indicates that he conceived of it in more nearly rhetorical than theoretical terms, as does his immediately following attempt to justify it by analogy to the vital image of a telescope, in which connection he remarked again that the systems "are not in any way psychical entities themselves and can never be accessible to our psychical perception" (1900a, p. 611). Elsewhere in the same work, he had introduced yet a third way of conceptualizing the difference between preconscious and unconscious ideas: The former alone were connected with verbal memories. He left these three conceptualizations standing side by side without any attempt at synthesis.

The concept of *das Ich*, by contrast, with its many observational roots, seemed more nearly "accessible to our psychical perception" and was already established in nontechnical usage. Hence it was undoubtedly more palatable to his followers and perhaps to Freud himself than a confusingly abstract *system Pcs.*, or *Cs.*, or *Pcs-Cs.*, for Freud could not make up his mind which to invoke as the antithesis of the *system Ucs.* As Schafer (1973a, 1976) has argued, the person—the obvious originator of action—has no conceptual status in the theory, and the ego is more nearly suitable as a stand-in for it than any of the topographic systems. The later clinical utility claimed for the ego–id model (Arlow, 1975) may very well lie in its susceptibility to anthropomorphic reification, a back-door entry for the concealed idea of the person.

The clinical observation that was apparently most salient for Freud was the ubiquity of conflict in his patients. There are doubtless other reasons for his pervasive interest in binary concepts, but that seems to be the main clinical basis for his feeling that there must be two types of drives or instincts, constantly clashing. And when he did postulate systems or structures in triads, in practice he almost always reduced them to an antagonistic pair: *Pcs.* versus *Ucs.*, ego versus *Ucs.*, ego versus id. Unfortunately, these ways of conceptualizing conflict are not only unnecessary but strongly facilitate the anthropomorphic fallacy; they lend themselves all too easily to vivid figurative writing depicting struggles between homunculi. Surely *The Ego and the Id* is pervaded by just such personification.

To return to the topographic theory, in their respective monographs, Gill (1963) and Arlow and Brenner (1964) have well summarized the difficulties Freud found with it in the metapsychological papers. In those papers

Freud (1915e, pp. 186, 190–193, 195; 1917d [1915], p. 232) not only anticipated the principal objection to the old notions in his 1923 critique but went
beyond it, bringing out two other difficulties. As Gill (1963) notes, the
solution to the main problem, the necessity to classify not only the repressed
but also the repressing forces as unconscious, did not resolve these other
problems, and in his subsequent works, Freud did not specifically address
these problems. They derive from the fact that he had set up two criteria by
which mental contents were to be assigned to the various systems—relation
to consciousness and mode of organization (primary process versus secondary process)—but these criteria were not perfectly correlated. There were
conscious contents (e.g., dreams, jokes) that were organized in a primary-
process way, and there were unconscious contents (certain fantasies) that
seemed to be organized in a secondary-process way. Defining the ego as in
large part unconscious did nothing to account for either of these problematic observations.

Even in terms of his own critique of his topographic theory then,
Freud's new substitute was no great advance, nor did it contain conceptual
novelties. The term "superego" was new, but the "agency" referred to had
been introduced under the name "ego ideal" (Freud, 1914c), and the new
theory did not clarify the relationships among the three systems or structures.

The topographic theory had numerous grave deficiencies which made
it methodologically untenable and practically unworkable. Unfortunately,
almost all of them were carried over into the structural replacement, never
having been explicitly noted by Freud. A good many theorists have enumer-
ated these flaws (e.g., Apfelbaum, 1966; Klein, 1976; Rubinstein, 1967a;
Schafer, 1973a, 1973b, 1973c). What I wish to emphasize here is that Freud's
theoretical models are an intrinsic part of his metapsychology, being the
embodiment of first the topographic and later the structural point of view.

I am unable to follow or agree with Arlow's (1975) contention that the
conception of the ego and the id is part of the clinical theory (as opposed to
metapsychology) or that it is more intimately connected to clinical observation than the topographic notions. The concept of ego is no more observable
than that of the *system Pcs.*, and the inferential chain between clinical
observation and either set of concepts is of equal length. Concepts like
projection and isolation, unconscious guilt, and regressive impulses are close
to direct observation and are undoubtedly integral parts of the clinical
theory. When we try to assign them to different parts of a hypothetical
psychic apparatus, however, we are doing precisely what Freud urged as
one of the three tasks of metapsychology. Likewise, I do not find convincing the argument that various theoretical and technical developments of the
past 50 years demonstrate the value of the structural theory. An equally
plausible case may be that since it was quickly adopted as the official

language of psychoanalysis, any new formulations had to be couched in its terms. Could it not be argued just as well that the change from German to English as the dominant tongue of psychoanalytic authors has made possible and "cleared the way for" the principal contributions to ego psychology of the subsequent 30 years? As to therapeutic technique, I find more persuasive Schafer's (1973c) argument that it has been hampered than Arlow's (1975) that it was significantly advanced.

My critical position, therefore, is not that "the paradigm of psychoanalysis advanced in *The Ego and the Id* . . . no longer fits the data of observation (Arlow, 1975, p. 513). I see no real change in the degree to which the theory fits psychoanalytic data; in my estimation, neither one ever fit them in a usable way. As I have already said, it is extremely difficult to use it without reification or personification; instead, the very concepts themselves as well as Freud's own habit of slipping into these philosophical fallacies have encouraged clinicians to lose sight of the fact that it is the patient who talks, dreams, and acts in the real world, not his ego, superego, or id, or some coalition of these soul-like entities.

As I see it, the crisis of psychoanalytic theory generally is not that new facts have been piling up that embarrass the old theory, but that its fundamental methodological—that is, basically philosophical and conceptual—weaknesses and fallacies have been exposed. Similarly, psychoanalysis needs new biological foundations because the old, hidden but immanent ones are outdated biology. When Klein (1976) wrote: "physiological terms cannot substitute for psychoanalytic terms descriptive of the meanings of object relations; for it is these purely psychological considerations, not the physiological ones, which make behavior coherent to the analyst" (p. 49—a passage quoted approvingly by Arlow), he misunderstood what Rubinstein (1967a) and I intended in our calls for a new protoneurophysiological model: We have no intent to attack or replace clinical concepts or observations, nor to reduce meanings to physiological measurements. The issue is very simple, as I see it. Is psychoanalysis to try to become a pure psychology by turning its back upon the body, or is it to remain faithful to its psychosomatic heritage? Surely the mind is not disembodied; sex, for example, is ineluctably a biochemical, anatomical, physiological, even genic matter, as well as one of conscious and unconscious meanings—longings, passions, fantasies, and interpersonal transactions. And, I would add, it also has important legal, institutional, cultural, economic, and even political aspects. It is true that a good deal of the time, psychoanalysts can manage most patients' sexual problems by paying attention only to intrapsychic conflicts and meanings; but to try to build up a systematic and comprehensive understanding of sexual behavior with this restriction seems to me false to Freud's example and his ambition for psychoanalysis. [See also Chapter 12, this volume.]

TWO EGO PSYCHOLOGIES: NARROW AND BROAD

As Arlow (1975) notes, there were a great many important contributions to ego psychology in the first decades following its formal promulgation. Yet, ego psychology, as I have known it and identified myself with it, and as it was expounded by Rapaport (e.g., 1951a, 1960a), is missing. It would seem that Arlow, and Joseph (1975), propose the implicit definition of ego psychology as the adoption of the ego–superego–id framework; for them, and a good many other psychoanalysts, its definition centers on the replacement of the topographic by the structural point of view, and structures mean what Freud called (so confusingly to English-speaking readers unfamiliar with German jurisprudence) the three great "psychic instances."

It is curious that the 1923 book should have introduced an era of ego psychology in this narrow sense, for the term has come to mean, for many of us within the psychoanalytic movement, a great broadening of what had been a deep but narrow inquiry into intrapsychic conflicts. *The Ego and the Id* merely renames and slightly reorganizes the terms and field of such conflicts, yet I believe that Arlow may be right in contending that it was a liberating moment for psychoanalysis—not because it was a paradigm shift in Kuhn's (1970) sense, but perhaps because it *seemed* to be a fundamental shakeup in the theory. Freud's willingness to bring the ego to center stage and see it in a new relation to consciousness, his renaming the ego ideal, and his adoption of Groddeck's term (*das Es*) for a slightly revised *Ucs.*, coming as they did just after the revised dual-instinct theory, may have signaled his coworkers that it was time to re-examine old data and old assumptions and to strike out in new directions.

Though I do not see that many of the clinical innovations cited by Arlow and Joseph are logical or necessary consequences of *The Ego and the Id*, they probably are psychological consequences. In particular, I do not see that the new–old signal theory of anxiety (Freud, 1926d) had to await the structural theory before Freud could abandon his economic notion of anxiety as transformed libido and could revive an adaptive conception which he had sketched in its main outlines in the Project (Freud, 1950 [1895], pp. 324, 357 ff.) and had occasionally invoked on a number of seldom-noticed occasions thereafter (1895b [1894], p. 112; 1900a, pp. 601 ff.; 1905c, p. 178; 1915e, pp. 182 ff.; 1916–1917, pp. 394 ff., 405). The 1923 work did, however, foreshadow two important changes to which ego psychology in its second and broader sense may perhaps be traced: the revived and extended conception of defenses (repression again being construed as one among several kinds of defense), and the increased role of reality as a determinant of behavior. The first of these opened the door for Anna Freud's (1937) important work on defenses, and the second paved the way for Hartmann's (1939) introduction of the adaptive point of view and Erikson's (1950) psychosocial and (1958) psychohistorical outlook.

There are, then, two somewhat different meanings of ego psychology. The first, the one emphasized in the papers by Arlow (1975) and Joseph (1975), implies by the term only the addition to psychoanalysis of the ego–superego–id triad plus a restricted group of clinical contributions seen as having been directly stimulated by it: the signal theory of anxiety; a systematic consideration of a full spectrum of defenses and their implications for the understanding of perversions and borderline states and of therapeutic techniques in a widening scope of applicability for psychoanalysis; and "many other contributions regarding superego function, identification, and object relations" (Arlow, 1975, p. 513).

The second meaning of ego psychology, the one to which I was introduced by Rapaport, stems in large measure from Hartmann and Erikson, though also from Anna Freud (1937) and Reich (1933). To someone trained in academic experimental psychology and the social sciences, it presented psychoanalysis as a reasonable, intelligible discipline, by no means exclusively focused on intrapsychic conflict and unconscious infantile wishes, but with much concern for a person's real setting—especially his social, cultural, and historical milieu; the groups and traditions that shaped his identity; and the *mise-en-scene* of interpersonal relations in which his life was played out. In other words, psychoanalysis offered not a physicalistic but a differentiated and structured view of reality as a habitat containing ecological niches and a social structure of role opportunities and societal modalities into which a person's own modes of behaving can fit.

In their revision of metapsychology, Rapaport and Gill (1959) also proposed that the topographic point of view be reinterpreted as structural. But in so doing, they meant much more than exchanging systems *Ucs.*, *Pcs.*, and *Cs.* for id, superego, and ego. Rapaport taught that individual behavior was far-reachingly determined by relatively stable, slowly changing internal configurations that set limits on what behavioral options were open to a person and gave an individual a distinctive, persistent, and thus recognizable style. This closely interrelated pattern of defenses and abilities Rapaport called a person's "ego structure." He taught the diagnostic use of psychological tests through conceptualizing a typology of ego structures corresponding to recurrent diagnostic entities (see Rapaport et al., 1945-1946). His students learned to recognize obsessive–compulsive, paranoid, or schizoid types of ego structure, for example, from the patterns of abilities—achievements of people functioning as best they could with neutral materials in a testing situation made as conflict-free as possible.

To a young psychologist learning his diagnostic trade in this way, there was no question that psychoanalysis was a broad enough theory to accommodate the contributions of academic psychology: They were simply the fruits of systematically studying behavior in the "conflict-free sphere." Hartmann's program of expanding psychoanalysis into a general and comprehensive psychology by building conceptual bridges to existing academic disciplines (including sociology and anthropology as well as psychology) seemed to us the most natural, indeed inevitable of developments. *Psychological Issues*, founded at Rapaport's urging by George S. Klein, was a means for bringing about this extension of psychoanalysis. In the experimental work that issued from his laboratories at the Menninger Foundation, Harvard, and New York University's Research Center for Mental Health, Klein (1970) showed the fertility of Rapaport's ego-structural conceptions: Cognitive style is a major conceptual and empirical embodiment of ego psychology in the second sense. With his students and coworkers, Klein developed a series of practical means of assessing a person's characteristic and stable ways of taking in and processing information about his world—structural characteristics (in Rapaport's sense), which helped to make sense out of previously chaotic data. An unselected sample of subjects would often contain people who responded in diametrically opposed ways to an experimental intervention (Klein, 1970, Chapter 6), so that until they were separated by tests of cognitive controls (Gardner et al., 1959), such powerful but antithetical effects could misleadingly look like no effect at all.

Because of my own immersion in diagnostic and research work, the usefulness of Rapaport's ego psychology for these two fields of endeavor was most salient. I leave it to others to evaluate its therapeutic implications. Erikson's well-known work (e.g., 1964, 1968, 1969) is ample testimony to the fruitfulness for psychohistorical studies of this second type of ego psychology.

THE FUTURE

Yet in the end, Rapaport's students have become disenchanted with ego psychology. In a word, its fatal flaw proved to be its foundation on metapsychology. We all agree that metapsychology is moribund if not actually dead, and I find it hard to imagine that the concept of ego will survive the general collapse.

Thus, I foresee a future for ego psychology similar in one main respect to its prehistory: The problems it is addressed to will remain, the observations collected under its umbrella will stand, and even some of its conceptual components (e.g., the defenses) will doubtless survive, but I doubt that ego psychology will be the applicable rubric for many more years. In the long run, I am not even sure that psychoanalysis will have a general theory of its own, nor that there will be any valid scientific need for a recognizable psychoanalytic theory to replace metapsychology. As sciences mature, schools wither. We are not yet at a high enough level of scientific maturity that it is evident to all that there can and should be one general, all-purpose theory of the human person. *A necessary and absolutely indispensable prerequisite to any such theory is that it incorporate all of the clinical discoveries of psychoanalysis*; and I believe that, as a second prerequisite, general psychology will have to give up its unfortunate enchantment with behavioristic reductionism. Neither of these prerequisites is met in any adequate theory I know of, but I do not doubt that the time will come. For the foreseeable future, psychoanalysis is in the awkward position of having to abandon metapsychology without having any equally comprehensive and more tenable substitute ready at hand.

AFTERWORD

In retrospect, it seems to me that one important issue was not discussed in this chapter, nor in any of my published papers. This is the ontological status of the concept of structure: In what sense can psychic structures be said to exist? I devoted a good deal of attention to talking about issues of this kind in relation to energy, but so far have bypassed such philosophical considerations in the present section. Let me take them up here, therefore, albeit briefly. (For a definition and further discussion of the concept, see Chapter 10, note 4.)

In the book Force and Matter, *which had such an impact upon the adolescent Freud (Holt, 1988), the old materialist Büchner (1855) did not distinguish clearly between force (Kraft) and energy, but saw both as necessarily linked to matter (Stoff). Earlier generations had called the former two imponderable, the latter ponderable. To a mechanistically minded era, matter comprised the world engine, while energy (e.g., from steam) made it run. In the everyday world, unlimited supplies of energy are useless to do work unless one has material structures through which forces may be applied and energy degraded (used up).*

As a young physician, Freud dealt constantly with the body, the neuroanatomical structure of which he studied in a good deal of his research. Perhaps because it was so obvious, right before one's eyes, the structural side of things did not call for as much theoretical attention as the more inferential energic concepts he felt the necessity of postulating in order to account for the analogue of work that seemed to be done in the psychological realm. Perhaps his critics have been similarly diverted from asking about the structural concepts he did use, "What is their nature? How are we to understand them?"

As I have already pointed out, Freud only reluctantly gave up the "real world" of anatomy and physiology and started building psychological theory. When he came to write the theoretical chapter of his dream book (1900a), his constant temptation was to speak as if he was still dealing with the brain, its pathways and their innervations, for both such terms crop up repeatedly even after he explicitly stated that he was going to build a purely psychological theory. He proceeded to describe a psychic apparatus— oddly ambivalent term!—which is transparently modeled on his conception of the brain as outlined in the Project (1950 [1895])

If one takes Freud at his word, that he had (provisionally at least) given up the attempt to work with anatomical structures, replacing the brain with the psychic apparatus, it is fair to ask what kind of existence he postulated for the latter. Psychic energy presumably is transmitted through pathways in psychic structures; examples of the latter are the systems, Ucs., Pcs., and Cs., and later, the ego, superego, and id. Even as late as 1923, Freud would occasionally write of the ego as if it were (at least in one of its guises) to be identified with parts of the brain such as the cortical homunculus, the projection areas where the sensory nerves from the different parts of the body terminate (1923b, pp. 25–26). And yet in the same work he defined it in several other quite different ways, which are difficult to reconcile with one another: "a coherent organization of mental processes" (p. 17); "that part of the id which has been modified by the direct influence of the external world" (p. 25); "first and foremost a bodily ego . . . the projection of a surface" (p. 26); "a precipitate of abandoned object-cathexes" (p. 29); and so on. He attributes to it both strength and weakness, and many remarkable powers or functions: "it gives mental processes an order in time and submits them to 'reality-testing.' . . . it secures a postponement of motor discharges and controls the access to motility. . . . It withdraws libido from the id and transforms the object-cathexes of the id into ego-structures" (1923b, p. 55). All this and more, in a single work, not to mention later elaborations!

Some of the time, then (e.g., when it is a body ego or a set of identifications), he seems to treat the ego as a psychological structure in the same sense that one's mastery of a foreign language may be thought of as a psychological structure: structural, in that it is an enduring pattern, but one whose elements are subjective meanings, hence psychological. Some of the time, it is a part of the psychic apparatus, itself a term of uncertain ontological status. In this guise, it perceives, plots against, submits to, or seduces other "psychic instances"; deploys defenses; and in general acts like an active little homunculus. By and large, the superego has a parallel set of attributes, whereas the id usually appears as one of the agonists of interstructural conflict and/or as either the instincts themselves or a kind of cage within which they are kept.

What are we to make of this confusion in philosophical terms? One possibility, at which Freud hinted at times without ever explicitly committing himself to it, is that the psychic structures have their being in a realm fundamentally separate from that of ordinary physical reality. In this world, "the psychic," exist such entities as psychic energy and psychic structure, of which we have no subjective knowledge, and also all the contents of consciousness, notably including words, plastic images, feelings and emotions, and abstract meanings. In this interactional dualism, just as physical energies at times may be transmuted into the psychic and vice versa, Freud apparently assumed hypothetical points of contact between anatomical and psychic structures.

Although I feel that this is the most nearly comprehensive solution, and although it seems to me clearly implied by countless of Freud's statements, it still leaves much to be desired even if one is comfortable with interaction-ism, as some reputable philosophers are. It does no better job than any other philosophical system of accounting for the mystery of consciousness, for the realm of the psychic explicitly includes a great deal more than the phenome-nal, which is not conscious; hence there is no saving in the number of arbitrary assumptions required to account for it. Everything about the psychic realm has to be postulated ad hoc; there is no way to make any observations about psychic structures other than those that are supposedly to be explained by reference to them. And it is not all obvious how uncon-scious meanings are supposed to function as the equivalent of anatomical pathways or barriers.

The only alternative I can see, however, is to admit frankly that Freud did not attempt to solve the ontological question, but simply ignored it and other philosophical embarrassments. That would be to admit defeat from the outset, renouncing any attempt to rationalize or invent philosophical ingenuities to shore up his theoretical lapses. It is the simplest way, but an opponent of metapsychology must be reluctant to take it without at least making a valiant attempt to make sure that no philosophically tenable alternative is being overlooked. When I became aware of this embarrass-ment of psychoanalytic theory, I was strongly enough identified with it to be highly motivated to make the necessary effort. As the years have gone on, however, and no solution appeared either out of my own struggles or from the pens of others, I have concluded that none is likely to emerge—not, for certain, before the publication of this book.

In any event, at the time the chapters in the present section were written, I had not reached any conclusion. I began with the hope that "structure" (not further specified) was a safe term to use, not being saddled with the vitalistic implications of psychic energy, and took the recourse of rather abstract definitions that simply bypassed the ontological issue. Prop-ositions that took no stand on whether the structures involved were psycho-logical or physical would be useful, I hoped, so long as they did not contradict existing physiological knowledge if they were anatomically inter-preted. That is the "protoneurophysiological" strategy of Rubinstein (1967a), which is explained somewhat more fully in some of the chapters that follow.

CHAPTER 9

Ego Autonomy and the Problem of Human Freedom

In the fall of 1961, I was invited to be a discussant of a paper by Stuart C. Miller, M.D., in a meeting at the Austen Riggs Center when he was to receive a prize for it. Later, I turned the discussion into a paper, which was published in 1965 in the International Journal of Psycho-Analysis. *The paper created a minor stir: I was invited to present it to the New York Psychoanalytic Association, with prepared discussions by several distinguished psychoanalysts beginning with Heinz Hartmann and including Benjamin Rubinstein and Kurt Eissler; it was then reprinted in the* International Journal of Psychiatry *with critiques by Stuart C. Miller, Alfredo Namnum, Benjamin Rubinstein, Joseph Sandler and W. G. Joffe, Roy Schafer, and Herbert Weiner. I was also given an opportunity to write a rejoinder, which I prefaced by some further reflections on the problem of freedom.*

Since then, I have returned to the problem of free will a couple of times, most extensively in a recent paper (Holt, 1984b) that I considered including here but decided not to, since it contains no further critique of metapsychology. I have tried to make one chapter out of these published sources, plus various notes and new thoughts that have come to me in the course of trying to bring my ideas reasonably up to date. It has been an unusually difficult task, for the 1965 paper was anything but single-pointed and my views on a number of the issues discussed in it have changed considerably. I have taken advantage of the various critiques of the paper, also, probably without adequately acknowledging all the sources of the corrections I was able to make.

There remain problems with the chapter, which is still poorly integrated. I have tried to concentrate on deepening the critique of metapsychology, but the topics insistently lead off into a series of extremely fundamental questions: What is the role of reality (the environment, sensory–perceptual inputs, all the larger systems in which the person participates) in the instigation, support, control, and organization of behavior? What is the nature and the role of determinants originating within the person—notably motives, but also all forms of inner control and organization? What were Freud's views on these matters, and what problems are there not just with his answers to the questions but with those of various subsequent theorists? In addition to these psychological issues, there is a group of metaphysical conundrums: What is reality? How are we to solve the mind–body problem? How can personal freedom be reconciled with

218

the deterministic universe seemingly required by science? Then, it is difficult to leave such important topics without stating one's own ideas about appropriate solutions in light of contemporary knowledge, although to do so adequately means having solved most of the basic theoretical problems of psychology! Therefore, I have had to leave matters in some disarray, in varying degrees of partial solution.

In a presidential address to the Society for the Psychological Study of Social Issues, Chein (1962) declared that psychology "must choose between two images" of man[1]—two basic conceptions of human nature, which he finds implicit in all of the general theories of behavior.

> The first is that of Man as an *active, responsible agent* . . . a being who actively does something with regard to some of the things that happen to him . . . who insists on injecting himself into the causal process of the world around him. . . . The contrasting and, among psychologists whose careers are devoted to the advancement of the science, the prevailing image of Man is that of an impotent reactor, with its responses completely determined by two distinct and separate, albeit interacting, sets of factors: (1) the forces impinging on it and (2) its constitution (including . . . momentary physiological states). (pp. 2–3)

To the reader who is conversant with the recent literature on psychoanalytic ego psychology, it sounds as if Professor Chein is pointedly posing the question of ego autonomy. Change his term "Man" to "ego" and one alternative sounds like the autonomous ego of Rapaport and Hartmann, which actively intervenes as a "third force" in the operation of causal pressures from the environmental "forces impinging on it" and from the id (cf. "physiological states") and does not merely submit to them, being pitted against the familiar conception of the passive "ego as a poor creature owing service to three masters and consequently menaced by three dangers: from the external world, from the libido of the id, and from the severity of the superego" (Freud, 1923b, p. 56). This is the question of ego autonomy, clearly; and Chein's paper shows that the issues entailed pervade all of modern psychology, far beyond the realm of psychoanalytic theory.

Indeed, it is possible to see that Chein and the ego psychologists are dealing with a modern form of one of the great pendular swings in the history of ideas: the conception of the nature of man as a free agent, the rational master of nature, as against the antithetical and more pessimistic view that he is the servant of powerful and inscrutable forces—a machine operated by his environment, or the plaything of his own instincts. It is the classic, Apollonian view (in Nietzsche's phrase) against the romantic, Dionysian one. Throughout history these conceptions, or as Chein has it, images, have alternated in the writings of philosophers, poets, and other belletristic writers as well as psychologists. The theological and ethical antitheses, such as free will versus necessity, and individual responsibility versus sociological or psychological determinism, are derivatives of this polarity.

The sense of freedom, of the ability to choose and master one's own life, is a real and clinically important phenomenon. Knight (1946) observes that

> this kind of "freedom" is experienced only by emotionally mature, well-integrated persons; it is the goal sought for one's patients in psychotherapy; and this freedom has nothing whatever to do with free will as a principle governing human behavior, but is a subjective experience which is itself causally determined. (p. 256)

[I shall return, below, to his contention that felt freedom and "free will" have nothing to do with each other.] There is no tenable alternative to determinism for science, Knight continues, but the scientific method does not require us to deny that some people are gripped by compulsions, addictions, and other ego-alien, unconscious types of acting out, or are sedulous conformists whose every choice is dictated by external models and norms—while others are free to perceive reality in nonstereotyped ways, to choose personally congenial paths to personally gratifying goals, and thus to be socially responsible. The behavior of the free person can be predicted from a knowledge of his past, of his structure and needs, and of the presenting situation, because it follows lawful regularities just like any other behavior. [We must therefore figure out a way to reconcile these two, seemingly contradictory ideas.]

I shall approach these issues by a brief historical survey of the way autonomy emerged as a concept in the development of ego psychology.[2]

HISTORICAL SURVEY

The 19th century began with the classical ideal of the Enlightenment still uppermost. This was the heyday of classical economics, when economic man was thought by Smith, Bentham, Ricardo, and others to be motivated by prudent self-interest and to be very much in control of his own affairs. The age of reason had pictured the human being as a logical, potentially (if not actually always) rational creature who was almost infinitely educable and needed only to be informed in order to choose order and justice over the opposites. In the philosophical psychology of the time, it was taken for granted that we have the freedom to make moral choices or to decide the direction of our own behavior. In a series of irregular waves, however, opposing romantic currents made all these calm waters turbulent and muddy: Schopenhauer, Kierkegaard, and Nietzsche were heard instead of Kant, the Encyclopedists, and Hegel; Byron and Shelley sang the dangerous life of the passions, which composers like Beethoven and Wagner expressed in tempestuous music; even economics turned toward voluntarism with Marshall and Pareto. Was man "noble in reason, infinite in faculty," as Shakespeare has Hamlet exclaim? No, said the followers of Darwin, man is an animal; no, said the Marxists, he is a pawn in a historical process; no, said many who were impressed by the growth of physical science, man is an ingenious machine.

Freud grew up under the influence of these contending classical and romantic ideas, absorbing and later using both, with varying degrees of synthesis. In *Studies on Hysteria*, for example, Breuer and Freud (1895) followed the common custom of speaking about an *Ich*—"I," "me"—conceived of as the conscious, willing self. They attributed to it considerable power to master its fate: It strives for consistency and unity (Freud, 1894a, pp. 45, 47); it *chooses* its defenses (Freud, 1894a, p. 54), which it has *at its disposal* (Breuer & Freud, 1895, p. 123); it maintains contact with reality and exercises censorship. At the same time, however, it is clear from many contemporary passages that Freud longed to replace such "philosophical" concepts as the *Ich* (so impersonally translated in English as "ego") by a strictly mechanistic terminology. In the flush of his youth, he longed to be as scientific as possible, and in those days mechanics was the very model of a modern science. His greatest effort to produce a strictly mechanistic neuropsychology, the "Project," failed even as he was writing it; he noted as he was going along that he was unable to make the apparatus completely "automatic" and thus to do without a willing ego as psychic prime mover [see Chapter 6, this volume].

In the second phase of psychoanalytic theory, which was inaugurated by *The Interpretation of Dreams* and lasted for approximately 20 years, the concept of instinctual drive came into its own and the dominance of the dynamic point of view largely obstructed the development of ego psychology. The impressive discoveries of the defenses, the dream work, the devious and powerful workings of unconscious motives, plus Freud's developing the theory of the primary process so that the unconscious language of the id could be read—all of these fundamental discoveries dominated the psychoanalytic scene, and the very term "ego" appeared rarely. Yet the theory of the secondary process and of defense that were developed in Freud's metapsychological writings of this period contained a good many implications and occasional explicit statements of ego autonomy, mostly in the explication of ways in which the system *Pcs.* and the secondary process make possible realistic gratification through the *delay* of immediate discharge. And in a couple of places in Chapter VII, Freud (1900a) clearly hints that the structure that is responsible for the secondary process is present, at least in germ, from the beginning of life and gradually develops. This is one of the first precursors of what Hartmann was to call "primary autonomy." Beginning with the paper on narcissism (1914c), the term "ego" began to appear with increasing frequency; it was now given its own source of energy, the ego instincts, which provided it with power to oppose the drives and the automatic, "almost omnipotent pleasure principle."

With *The Ego and the Id* (Freud, 1923b), we begin to find side by side statements attributing to the ego both far-reaching autonomy and abject subservience to the id. The introduction of the concepts of identification and narcissism had opened a way to conceptualize the ego's energies as being ultimately derived from the id. Nevertheless, some autonomy is implicit in the idea that this libidinal energy was neutralized and became freely available to the ego for such work as "the activity of thinking" (1923b, p. 45). From the standpoint of structure, *The Ego and the Id* contains many of the clearest statements of the antiautonomy point of view: The ego is the part of the id modified by the influence of the external world (p. 25), and the two never become fully and sharply differentiated (p. 28). Yet in the same breath, Freud says that the ego starts from its nucleus, the *Pcpt.* or perceptual apparatuses, which clearly implies a differentiated and structured part of the personality present from birth and capable of mediating contact with reality. Here the idea of ego rudiments alluded to in 1900 is made more explicit, and a basis is laid down for a conception of primary roots of autonomy. Freud's approving quotation from Groddeck, that "we are 'lived' by unknown and uncontrollable forces," (p. 23), is the "lowest depths" of the nonautonomy standpoint, as Rapaport put it in a seminar. Not much further on, impressive strengths of the ego are listed: It organizes the thoughts, tests reality, controls motility, and delays motor discharge by interposing thought (p. 55). What Rapaport called the "proudest sentence" then follows: "The ego develops from perceiving instincts to controlling them, from obeying instincts to inhibiting them." On the very next page, however, Freud is again impressed by the power of the drives: The ego placates the id by such devices as rationalization (p. 56). Identification plays a large role in this work, with two antithetical implications for autonomy. Identification entails the ego's subservience to the id, but also its control of the id, since by a seductive self-offering the ego causes the id to give up its other objects, and captures and desexualizes some id energy.

In his subsequent writings, Freud did not add a great deal to these points, though depending on the context he emphasized either the ego's strength or its weakness, and in a famous passage in *Analysis Terminable and Interminable* (1937c, pp. 240 ff.), he was even more explicit than he had been before about there being innate rudiments of the ego with respect to which persons differed—one of his relatively rare statements about individual differences. This is the principal passage cited by Hartmann as the basis for his concept of primary autonomy.

We owe to Hartmann (1939) the very term "autonomy of the ego" and most of the propositions in the doctrine. The ego's autonomy is heralded in his basic formulation about development: that the ego and the id differentiate from a common matrix, the undifferentiated phase, in which the ego's precursors are inborn *apparatuses of primary autonomy*: "perception, intention, object comprehension, thinking, language, recall-phenomena, productivity . . . motor development . . . and . . . the maturation and learning processes implicit in all these" (p. 8). These functions, which develop outside of conflict and from innate structures, refer to aspects of behavior that show no obvious dependence on drives and their vicissitudes. Therefore they are the primary basis of the ego's autonomy from the id. But the ego's conflict-free sphere can be enlarged and further functions can be sequestered from drive domination, so that a *secondary autonomy* also exists. For example, Hartmann (1939) writes,

An attitude which arose originally in the service of defense against an instinctual drive may, in the course of time, become an independent structure, in which case the instinctual drive merely triggers this automatized apparatus . . . but . . . does not determine the details of its action. Such an apparatus may . . . come to serve other functions (adaptation, synthesis, etc.); it may also . . . through a change of function turn from a means into a goal in its own right. (p. 26)

Hartmann's theory of the ego's autonomy from the id has an economic aspect, too: He has been the principal proponent of the view that some of the ego's energies may derive from nondrive sources, and his concept of neutralization has been one of his best-known contributions to ego psychology. This is a generalization to both major drives of Freud's concept of sublimation or desexualization; neutralization provides the ego with energies, and since it is carried out by the ego, the extent to which instinctual energy seems to be neutralized (indicated by breadth of interests and affects) is a measure of ego strength.

Hartmann makes it clear that all autonomy is relative: The ego may lose its autonomy if there is too great an increase in drive; or if synthetic functioning is weakened by illness, drugs, or organic injury; or if there is a decompensation of defending and controlling structures. Then secondary autonomy may be undercut, and even apparatuses of primary autonomy may be drawn into conflict (e.g., hysterical blindness). Thus, his presentation comprehends all of Freud's versions of the ego, both strong and weak, and accounts for them by elucidating the conditions under which the ego has more or less autonomy.

Rapaport (1951b) brought together all of Hartmann's scattered remarks about autonomy, amplified and explicated them, and focused interest on the concept. In his second paper on this topic (1958a), he added a whole new dimension by highlighting an issue that Hartmann had only adumbrated by occasional remarks: the autonomy of the ego from the environment.

> Man can interpose delay and thought not only between instinctual promptings and action, modifying and even indefinitely postponing drive discharge, [he wrote, referring to autonomy from the id;] he can likewise modify and postpone his reaction to external stimulation. This independence of behavior from external stimulation we will refer to as *the autonomy of the ego from external reality*. Since the ego is never completely independent from external reality, we always speak about *relative* autonomy. (Rapaport, 1958a, p. 723)

One way that man is protected from slavery to stimuli is through the fact that he has endogenous drives. Likewise, the insistence of the real world helps to protect man against the demands of these inner instinctual pressures.

> Thus, while the *ultimate guarantees of the ego's autonomy from the id* are man's constitutionally given apparatuses of reality relatedness, the *ultimate guarantees of the ego's autonomy from the environment* are man's constitutionally given drives. [Both autonomies, be it noted, have] *proximal* (secondary) *guarantees*: namely, higher-order superego and ego structures. (Rapaport, 1958a, p. 727)

In large part, Rapaport came to these new formulations through his interest in the related topics of hypnosis and sensory deprivation or perceptual isolation—both of them environmental manipulations reputed to have extraordinary regressive effects. His treatment is the first psychoanalytic attempt to conceptualize metapsychologically a series of phenomena in which autonomy from external reality seems to be lost. Moving naturally enough from the complementarity suggested by his formulation about ultimate guarantees, Rapaport said that the two types of autonomy were reciprocally related:

> Since reality relations guarantee autonomy from the id, excessive autonomy from the environment must impair the autonomy from the id; and since drives are the ultimate guarantees of autonomy from the environment, an excessive autonomy from the id must impair the autonomy from the environment. (1958b, p. 733)

The next point in Rapaport's theory has been well summarized by Miller (1962):

> Maintenance of autonomy in relation to the id or to the environment depends on input from the environment or from within the psychic apparatus. This input is called *stimulus-nutriment*, a term adapted from the *aliment* of Piaget. Stimulus-nutriment from the environment includes all that is perceived in the ex-

ternal world, while nutriment from within is provided by ego- and superego-structures and ultimately by drives. (p. 8)

The mediating concept here is *structure*, for it is structure that nutriment replenishes: Controlling and defending "structures depend upon stimulation for their stability. . . . When such stimulus-nutriment is not available, the effectiveness of these structures in controlling id impulses may be impaired" (p. 19). As examples, Rapaport instanced sensory deprivation and hypnosis. (He also related autonomy to his analysis of the closely related concepts of activity and passivity, but for the moment I shall bypass that aspect of his paper.)

In the context of a valuable review of the experimental and anecdotal literature on the effects of deprivation and isolation, Miller (1962) also summarizes the theoretical contributions of Gill and Brenman (1959), especially in their chapter on the metapsychology of the hypnotic induction, which was written with Rapaport's general supervision and approval. In considering how modifications of external inputs may affect behavior, they distinguish between *press* and *information*. The latter is a purely cognitive and neural matter; the former is Murray's term for pressures, incitements, arousals, and other dynamic aspects of stimulation. There are similar inputs to the psychic apparatus from inside the organism, Gill and Brenman continue. In place of press there are urges (impelling drive derivatives); their concept of information from within includes memory but a good deal more, and (as Miller points out) is roughly equivalent to Rapaport's nutriment from within. Beyond these distinctions, which help them clarify the difference between the degree of input from a source and autonomy from it, they essentially cover much the same ground as Rapaport did (1958a); but with added perspective they were able to clarify issues on which his paper was inconsistent. Thus, reviewing many of the same facts and arguments, they come to the conclusion that autonomy from id and environment are positively rather than negatively correlated.[3]

In his own theoretical discussion, Miller makes essentially four points:

1. Diminution of external stimulation, as in sensory deprivation, does not heighten ego autonomy from the environment, but tests it.
2. The relation between the autonomies, far from being reciprocal, is so symmetrical that it makes more sense to conceive of it as only a single ego autonomy.
3. Drive-dominated behavior is not autonomous with respect to the environment; though (as Gill and Brenman demonstrated) it may be *oblivious* to reality, behavior in states of extreme need tension is often enslaved with respect to drive objects in the environment.
4. Miller rejects Rapaport's definition of autonomy in terms of the ability to modify or postpone response, and Gill and Brenman's in

terms of the capacity to pit forces against drives or stimuli, showing gains in clarity and consistency that result from his definition: Ego autonomy is "a capacity for self-government in relation to both the demanding and nondemanding (informational) aspects of id and environment" (p. 15).

[A comment on this history: The reader who is not familiar with psychoanalytic theoretical writings may find this summary confusing, not to say dull. It seems to deal with abstractions, not human beings; yet these theoretical entities are constantly treated as if they actively cause things to happen or give guarantees to other abstractions. Plainly, Freud's pervasive habit of reifying and personifying his theoretical concepts has infected his followers, even so careful a writer as Rapaport.

There is a further reason why this kind of theorizing numbs the brain. At one approximation, we might call it complexity, the fact that there are so many layers of concepts with such intricate relationships among them—or at least there seem to be, but it is never made explicit. Anyone who is not an insider to these debates easily feels left out because the participants take it for granted that the definitions of terms are known and mutually agreed upon. In fact, however, that is not the case. The habit of not defining well-known terms that are "established in the literature" easily makes us overlook the fact that typically such definitions do not exist, and those that do frequently lean on or incorporate concepts that have been severely discredited. Anyone who as accepted the position argued in Chapter 7 may well wonder why I dutifully repeat, as if they made good sense, statements about drive and instinct that have been unmasked as anachronistic at best and animistic at worst.

Despite the validity of these objections, there is some value in such a review. Under all the jargon are buried serious attempts to come to grips with genuine issues. Let us begin the attempt to see what they are] by stepping back a few paces and asking, as it were, naively, "What is autonomy? What kind of concept is this?"

When one reviews the passages in which Miller discusses Hartmann's and Rapaport's usages, it becomes apparent that autonomy can be defined in either of two contrasting ways—either positively or negatively.[4] May I remind readers of the Four Freedoms in the Roosevelt–Churchill Atlantic Charter: two of them were stated negatively, two positively. Indeed, a joke current at the time highlighted the distinction between the two types of freedom by deliberately neglecting it: The Four Freedoms, it ran, are the freedom from want, freedom from fear, freedom from speech, and freedom from religion.

In the passage from a paper in which the two autonomies are most succinctly defined, Rapaport (1958a) got into trouble by relying on a negative definition. Autonomy from the id was "independence *from*" determination by drive forces, and its counterpart was "independence of behavior *from* external stimulation" (my italics). From these definitions, it follows logically enough that independence of this kind *can* be maximized by eliminating the source of determinative input in question. This kind of negative freedom is not autonomy, however—it might better be called "autarchy," if I may revive another World War II reference. Economic autarchy was the Nazi ideal of an ersatz economy that did without any imports. Similarly, the obsessive–compulsive ideal with respect to drives [or, let us now say, wishes] is not an autonomous relation of being able to accept and enjoy their gratification or to defer it, if necessary, indefinitely, but an autarchic, complete freedom *from* unwanted [sexual and aggressive impulses]. One can enforce autarchy on a person by artificially robbing him of inputs as in a deprivation experiment, but autonomy in the sense that seems most appealing to us, the positively defined "freedom *to,*" can be won only by the person himself; it can no more be thrust on him than a person can passively be made active. Compare the explanation of why he is not free to go out given by the son in the play, *Oh Dad, Poor Dad, Momma's Hung You in the Closet and I'm Feeling So Sad* (Kopit, 1960):

> Mother says I'm going to be great . . . Of course, she doesn't know exactly what I'm going to be great *in*, so she sits every afternoon for two hours and thinks about it. Naturally I've got to be here when she's thinking in case she thinks of the answer. Otherwise she might forget and I'd never know what I'm going to be great in. (p. 40)

This passage would not have its mixture of pathos and humor if the activity implied by greatness could be attained passively.

The distinction between two types of freedom seems obvious enough in the abstract, but in a concrete instance it is not so easily made. Consider the problem of distraction, an issue in autonomy from the environment. I can get freedom from distracting sights and sounds by either of two strategies: by avoiding the distractions (e.g., going into an experimental room for sensory deprivation) or by concentrating enough on something I am interested in. The difference is crucial: In the autarchic freedom from distraction, the actor remains passive; in the autonomous suppression of external inputs, the person actively attains this freedom through effort.

The trouble with this kind of positive definition of autonomy is that it gets us right into the complex and subtle issues of activity and passivity, about which Rapaport wrote a major paper in 1953, [though it was published only posthumously (1967)]. Not *any* opposition of the drives by the ego can be considered autonomy from the id, said Rapaport, for his first model of passivity is the automatic opposition of any drive impulse by a defense. Here, even though the anticathectic force is [supposedly] wielded by the ego, the latter is primarily determined by the drive itself or by the superego, not acting because of realistic considerations. It gets very tricky, therefore, to decide in the case of any particular piece of behavior whether the ego is active (autonomous) or not. Even with Miller's definition, we have to ask what are the operational criteria that enable us to know whether a person's ego is self-governing. [And if we accept the forceful case made by Schafer (1976) and Rubinstein (1981), we recognize that it makes little sense to attribute self-governance to such a hypothetical entity as an ego instead of to a *person*.]

Rapaport (1951b, p. 359) defined autonomy as "the nature and degree of this constancy and reliability"—meaning, that of "the new organization, the ego, which is pitted against" the id forces. This is a highly conceptual definition, a long way from operations, [as well as one that is committed to concepts (ego and id) that we have abandoned as more mischievous than useful. Moreover,] the definition equates autonomy with characteristics of the ego organization as a counterforce—specifically, its constancy and reliability.

Getting somewhat more clinical, Rapaport (1951b, p. 362) gives a [hypothetical] example of primary autonomy maintained despite stress: "A patient on the verge of psychosis, totally helpless to deal with his problems, and torn in every respect, may nevertheless display . . . an amazingly accurate memory, or sensitive perception, or perfection of motility." Here we get closer to observables (operations): Autonomy now equals the veridicality of memory and perception, their sensitive accuracy in creating representations of reality. As Klein (1959) has pointed out, it is by no means a simple matter to establish the accuracy of perception, however, [much less of memory; first, we must take a carefully thought-through position on difficult philosophical issues. Before attempting to do so, we can see that] Rapaport's criterion entails an even more explicit *evaluation* of perceptual and mnemic functioning, an evaluation by a presumably objective observer against a set of (assumedly) objective standards which, nevertheless, implicate a value system.[5]

Similarly, the phrase, "perfection of motility," suggests an analogous evaluation of motor functioning as being efficient or as correctly attaining the intended goal. In either event, there is an implicit subjective ideal against which actual performance is measured.[6] Later, in his second paper on ego autonomy, Rapaport (1958a) speaks as if autonomy was a more absolute and objective kind of concept, when he attempts to equate it with any opposition by the ego against the drives. Miller (1962) correctly points out the internal inconsistency of Rapaport's position when the latter speaks of the severely obsessive–compulsive patient as exemplifying maximized autonomy from the id. [Clearly, here and when Rapaport spoke in the passages quoted above about "excessive autonomy," he seems to have been thinking about a break in communication or inputs to the ego from either the organismic sources of motives or from the environment.] When Miller argues that there cannot be too much autonomy, he himself makes it fully clear that autonomy is an evaluative concept, an ideal.

[That does not mean that is is not measurable.] Like the similarly normative, value-laden concepts of health and intelligence, autonomy can be roughly quantified and objectified, and can thus prove of considerable value in research (see Kafka, 1963). It is only when we move away from the assessment of individual patients or subjects into the rarer atmosphere of metapsychology and the building of theory that evaluative concepts take a back seat.

In *Childhood and Society*, Erikson (1950, p. 87) writes: "A system must have its utopia. For psycho-analysis [that is, for id-psychology] the utopia is 'genitality.'" Similarly, I believe that autonomy is the utopian ideal of ego psychology,[7] a slogan emblazoned on the banner of the ego psychologists in their struggle against the excesses of traditional id-oriented psychoanalytic thinking. Indeed, I believe that the main reason we have a concept of autonomy is the unbalanced development of psychoanalytic theory, the fact that motivational considerations and the vagaries of defense absorbed the attention of analysts to the relative neglect of structure and the environment as determinants of behavior. Hartmann and Rapaport were writing polemics as well as theoretical contributions. If we ignore such ideological warfare and simply try to imagine what psychoanalytic theory would look like if rewritten on a clean slate, I think we may find that the concept of autonomy would not occupy an important place. One would instead be mainly concerned to describe the relative roles of drive [or wish], external stimuli and press, and various inner structures—all as determinants of behavior, along with their complex interactions.

[Or so I concluded two decades ago (Holt, 1967a). Since thinking through the problems of instinct theory (Chapter 7, this volume) and beginning to absorb the systems point of view (Ackoff, 1974; Laszlo, 1972; Weiss, 1969), I believe that Rapaport's intuition was correct when he held back from publishing his paper on activity and passivity. It did not in fact solve the problems he tackled, for in it he nowhere faced four major issues: the need for a fundamental reconsideration of metapsychology; the need for a systems view of our relationship to our environment; the need to take an explicit and carefully considered stand on the nature of reality (the ontological aspects of metaphysics); and the need to reconsider the old philosophical conundrum of freedom versus determinism. This book as a whole is an effort to supply the first of these needs; the remainder of this chapter will attempt to address the others.]

SOME SPECIFIC ASPECTS OF RELATIONS TO REALITY

[In 1965, I was groping for a new way to conceptualize reality for psychoanalytic theory, and proposed several ways in which it should be expanded. The relevant passages may serve as an introduction to the formulation I have reached today.]

The experimental studies of isolation and stress, which Miller (1962) has competently reviewed, have contributed to psychoanalytic theory in opening up for detailed consideration the question of just what kinds of roles aspects of the environment do play *vis-à-vis* behavior. I agree with Miller that there is considerable merit in the beginning made by Gill and Brenman (1959) along these lines in distinguishing between press and information.

We owe the concept of press to H. A. Murray (Murray, 1938), who divided them into two classes: Harms and Benefits. Press Harm of any kind, he pointed out, leads to the need for Harmavoidance (some type of escape) or active coping. Press Benefit leads to some appetitive, approaching need. Murray recognized that press was partly a function of the nature of the object, partly a function of need; so that, by this theory, harms and benefits do not come into being without the involvement of some kind of need— [that is, wish]. Thus, press operate through their interaction with needs, functioning in terms of a learned set of meanings and relationships—in short, with the intimate involvement of psychic structures.

Miller might have pushed his own analysis a step further, if he had not adopted the position that psychoanalysis need not concern itself with physiological explanations. In this instance, disinclination to take seriously the EEG evidence and the theories of isolation's effects that involve the function of the reticular formation leaves us with an incomplete picture. The work that has followed the basic discovery of Moruzzi and Magoun has given us ample evidence that inputs from the environment ("reality") have a third function, which might be called *tonic support*. In this phrase, I am deliberately harking back to Breuer's physiological terminology (in *Studies on Hysteria*, 1895). Breuer adopted the prevailing concept of a tonic excitation of the neurone [see Chapter 4, this volume]; it anticipated something much like the modern conception.

In the waking as opposed to the sleeping brain, Breuer said, the nerve cells are in a state of moderate, nontransmitted excitation which facilitates the propagated impulses—compare the concept of cortical activation by volleys from the reticular formations, giving rise to wakefulness and alertness. During sleep and other states of low vigilance, there may be a transmission of information from the sensory receptors to the cortex, but as long as the cortex lacks the tonic activation of these reticular volleys, it cannot make use of the potentially informational inputs. The reticular formation, in turn, issues tonic volleys because of its diffuse connections with incoming sensory fibers. They mediate a nonspecific, noninformational input of variegated stimulation, which actuates the reticular formation. If there is a steady, monotonous input from the receptors, the reticular activating system rapidly becomes habituated and no longer stimulates the cortex, so that vigilance tends to be lost.

A complicating fact, but one that may correspond in part to what Miller calls nutriment of one part of the ego by another, is the discovery that the cortex itself may stimulate the activity of the reticular formation, so that the dependence on sensory inputs is not absolute. We know from our experimental data (e.g., Goldberger & Holt, 1958) that most people are in fact not completely dependent on external stimuli to maintain cortical activation. Tonic support, then, results from the kind of varied patterns of stimulation that an average expectable environment delivers to the sense organs, plus some self-stimulation (external or internal). Psychoanalytic theory cannot afford to neglect this well-established explanation. How can it be fitted into the theory?

[At this point, I argued briefly that the solution was to abandon Freud's metapsychology and to build a new theory using "explicitly anatomical/physiological" concepts. The passage is omitted here, since I have since come to other conclusions; see Chapter 12. I then proceeded to discuss the interactions of environmental inputs and *structures*, at that time my favorite metapsychological concept.]

The interaction of reality with structures appears as an issue in psychoanalytic theory primarily in Rapaport's (1958a) discussion of *nutriment*, which was his translation and adaptation of Piaget's concept *aliment*. Rapaport's conception was, briefly, that structures require nutriment in order to be maintained, and that they get it primarily from environmental stimuli: "When such stimulus-nutriment is not available, the effectiveness of these structures in controlling id impulses may be impaired, and some of the ego's autonomy from the id may be surrendered" (1958a, p. 728). In this conception, he did not distinguish clearly between two separate issues: first, structure building—undeniably, infants and children need contact with the rich world of stimuli for the growth of adequate structures; this seems to me to have been Piaget's meaning of *aliment*. Second, structure maintenance—that is, structures allegedly need constant nutriment lest they wither away; here I think Rapaport's formulation applies to some but not all structures.

Perhaps because of his prejudice against physiological theorizing, Rapaport made no provision for any such concept as the one of tonic support that I have proposed above. Yet this conception is much better able to account for the rapid onset of the effects of isolation (sometimes after only a few minutes of homogeneous sensory stimulation) and rapid recovery as soon as a normally variegated environment is restored. If we had to assume that structures decompensated as soon as they were robbed of their usual nutriment from reality, we would be hard put to explain why it is that so many people are able to get up in the morning after eight hours deprived of such nutriment and fairly quickly get about their day's work. If the alleged hallucinations that occur after a few hours of isolation are due to the breakdown of structures, then the problem would be to explain why hypnopompic hallucinations—the vivid images that occasionally accompany the moment of awakening—are the rare exception rather than the rule.

Further, there is good evidence that certain classes of structure can be disused for periods of time up to decades, and then be found to be intact. I am referring particularly to organizations of memories.[8] By means of hypnotic age regression, brain stimulation, or psychoanalytic treatment, it has been possible to recover with great vividness detailed and verifiable memories of childhood about which the subject had not thought for years, and which had thus been completely without nutriment.

Even more damaging to the conception of nutriment is the fact that there seems to be no relation between the type of nutriment that is taken away and the effects of [brief] deprivation on structures. Thus, it is difficult to see how the kinds of stimuli of which the subject is deprived in a typical experiment have any direct relation to the ability to pursue protracted logical chains of thought. Is there any obvious relation between variegated perceptual input and orderly, purposive reasoning? On the contrary, one would think that the proper nutriment for such logical thinking would be a supply of problems plus interest in them, and that the perceptual world otherwise would be of importance primarily as a source of distraction. Moreover, the inability to think connectedly in this way during an isolation experiment does *not* occur, as one might think, because of any usurpation of the secondary process by wishful fantasies, imagery, or other manifestations of the primary process [a point independently confirmed by Zuckerman, Persky, Link, and Basu (1968)].

This discussion of nutriment does point up a further function of external inputs besides that of supplying tonic support: One might call it simply "opportunity." If I am faced by a rowboat on a lake, I have an opportunity to use my ability to row. Because I am wholly unable to row a boat without oars, should we assume that they provide the stimulus nutriment that revivifies some rowing structures, which atrophy in between the rare occasions when I find myself on the water? No, we need only assume that in the lack of appropriate opportunity, many structures simply cannot be used. To the extent that they subserve adaptation, deprivation of opportunity will cause a loss of these kinds of adaptive functioning.

It is true that a Mozart could and did write whole sonatas in his head, and some poets can complete at least brief works purely internally; but there are few enough activities involved in the work and recreation of most people that can be carried on very long without environmental opportunities. Fantasies *can*, however; they are the one human activity ideally designed for a lull of uninterrupted and undistracted time, requiring no equipment, no fellow player, no external grist. Even if a person is in a state of [gratification, all major motives temporarily fulfilled,] fantasies or idle imagining tend to take over when nothing else is possible.

[It should follow, from Rapaport's hypothesis that the lack of nutriment in an isolation experiment induces structural regression, that the controls over sexual and aggressive wishes should deteriorate likewise. Indeed, just such a hypothesis led Miller (1962) to predict that the subject would] restructure a restitutive external world in terms of his drives. This formulation is appealing, but the thing that bothers me about it is that the evidence seems so scanty. Miller suspects that there are few reports of sexual fantasies from isolation experiments because of censorship; I am not sure that that is the whole story. From my personal experience as well as contact with other subjects, I do not think that most people do in fact experience much lust or anger in the totally bland environment of isolation. To be sure, the situation is complicated by the fact that, as long as the subject is not psychotic, he knows very well that it is only going to frustrate him to get all worked up; such knowledge might give rise to a general restraint of wishes.

Consider, however, the fact that one wishful outlet is definitely possible in the experiments: gratification of oral motives. The regressive pressures of the experiment should lead to an awakened need for passive oral gratification. Yet subjects typically lose interest in food; even when on demand feedings, with plenty of food (which they themselves have selected) freely available to them, they frequently lose weight. Moreover, few of them miss smoking, even habitually heavy smokers. Is the passivity, then, itself a substitute for directly oral gratification? This hypothesis does not seem convincing; if it were true, one would expect that the passive gratification of sleep would satisfy the oral longings of ulcer patients and prevent the dreams of eating that so typically accompany and exacerbate this disorder. More likely, the appetitive aspects of the oral gratifiers are missing in perceptual deprivation. Few people like to smoke in the dark, and finicky appetites are notoriously pepped up by visually attractive presentation of food.

As I read them, the facts lend themselves to the following conceptualization: The cognitive processes of a subject in an isolation experiment undergo relatively little "takeover by drives" because the deprivation of external input directly interferes with the usual motivational processes themselves. Quite the opposite of being given free rein, wishes seem to act for the most part as if they too have been impoverished.

I suggest, accordingly, that the apparent deneutralization that takes place in isolation does *not* indicate a decompensation, through a lack of nutriment, of the structures that have been laboriously built up in sublimative pursuits. By definition, most neutralized activities get a person away from introspection about his own body and crude motivational concerns, and direct his attention toward aspects of external reality, with which he interacts in some active way. Force him into passivity, take away his brush and paints, or the followers whom he delights to organize, or his books to study, and you put out of commission those structures that make possible neutralization by taking away the particular set of external opportunities they need in order to be used. Disused, they do not automatically start to rust; as soon as the pond freezes over, the skater finds his muscles interacting with shoe, runner, and ice in their old harmony and coordination. Every year, the structures involved in such seasonal activities perforce undergo months of deprivation or lack of nutriment, without showing any signs of decomposition or destructuralization. Indeed, William James (1890) was enough struck by the way that such skilled performances often show actual improvement after a prolonged layoff to make up a special theory about this phenomenon.[9] This is half of the nutriment story, as I see it.

The other half is more interesting and complicated, and it amounts to a limited set of conditions under which the concept may be preserved much as Rapaport left it. Some of the most interesting phenomena resulting from perceptual isolation are involved: the changes in *perception* that are so obvious to the subject when he returns to the familiar world after days of deprivation. Mild forms of them can be picked up by careful testing after a matter of only a few hours of homogeneous stimulation, or even a few minutes of focusing on intensively disarranged stimulus fields. The experiments involved are, on the one hand, those of Richard Held (Held & White, 1959) and Sanford Freedman (Freedman & Greenblatt, 1959); and on the other hand, those of Ivo Kohler (1964). Both the phenomena they report and their theoretical explanations are worthy of the closest study by psychoanalysts interested in the ego psychology of reality. Briefly, the most striking finding is that the perceptual constancies are easily disturbed or broken down by an interruption of regular input of variegated stimuli, and especially by randomized or systematically disrupted inputs.

As a concrete example, I should like to quote from some notes I put down shortly after spending 36 hours in a silent isolation chamber, lying on a bed with my eyes covered by eye-cups (halved ping-pong balls):

> Immediately on coming out, and as soon as I stood up with the eye-cups off, I felt a little dizzy; this experience lasted for quite a few hours. It was not exactly like dizziness or grogginess; but rather, a kind of uncertainty in my relation to the gravitational field and the environment generally. I had a feeling as if my head was slightly large, and as if I was separated from the world by some kind of indefinable something. Walking home, I had the strange feeling that objects were a little blurred, particularly when I moved my eyes rapidly. If I made the effort to concentrate on an object, I could see it clearly enough; but if I didn't make the effort, things were slightly blurred or imprecise. It seemed to be harder to focus at a distance than nearby. In general, I had a feeling that I had my glasses off; or more exactly, the whole experience was rather like having a new pair of glasses. Motions seemed somewhat exaggerated, particularly the rapid motion of cars.

A few hours later, when I tried to read, "I had a strange experience of something like tunnel-vision: I could actually see outside of the fovea, and yet it was as if I had trouble paying attention to anything else" but the very center of my visual field. After a few more hours, however, the perceptual world was back to normal. As I recall this whole experience, it was extremely difficult to put into words the kind of change in the visual world that had been brought about by my 36 hours of exposure to diffuse, unpatterned light.

Heron, Doane, and Scott (1956) were the first to report perceptual effects of this kind; their findings have been followed up and quantified by Freedman and his coworkers (Freedman & Greenblatt, 1959; all of these studies have been summarized in Freedman, 1961). The loss of perceptual constancies was most pronounced and prolonged in the earlier work of the McGill investigators, who kept one another in perceptual deprivation for six days each, but even Freedman's eight-hour procedure produced several minutes of noticeable "shimmering, instability, undulation, and fluctuation of contours in the visual field with apparent changes in the size and shape of simple forms" (Freedman, 1961, p. 18).

Consider next some data from one of Kohler's (1964) experiments. Subjects are induced to wear lenses that invert the visual field—to wear them uninterruptedly for weeks at a time. At first, the subject is confused and disoriented; none of his visual–motor coordinations works. He reaches up into the air to pick up something down on the table, because it looks as if it is up there. But learning proceeds fairly rapidly if he keeps trying to move about, to handle things, and to keep up the usual kind of commerce with an otherwise ordinary world—he learns to get around, to reach accurately, and ultimately, to *see* the world as right-side up again. The stimulus information coming in has obviously been processed in a different way than the usual one, but in order to achieve the usual kind of adaptation. Now, take away the inverting lenses and give the subject back his usual kind of stimulation— and the world looks upside down to him! He is processing visual stimulation by the newly learned set of rules, which no longer correct for the disarrangement; so that once again he has to learn, to rebuild the structures corresponding to the transformation rules so that the result is once again adaptive, visual–motor coordination is again smooth, and the world is back in its proper orientation.

Held's (1961) explanation of phenomena like these, following that of von Holst (see von Holst & Mittelstaedt, 1950) involves a conception of the perceptual apparatus too complex and subtle to be described here, but the essence of it can be stated in terms that are assimilable to a psychoanalytic theory.

When you stop to think about it, the fact that we are in sensory contact with a stable, reliable external world, constructed and projected from fragmentary, constantly varying information, is an extraordinary achievement. The mere fact that the world holds still when we move our heads or eyes, despite the swirl of retinal information, is one of the remarkable commonplaces that are extremely easy to overlook and yet in need of explanation. To be sure, it is highly adaptive, and the simplest solution to the confusing mass of data we get from our eyes is to construct a steady world that will stand still and let us scan it by turning head or eyes; perhaps the problems involved can be shrugged off by appealing to learning. Yet the years of overlearning can be quickly undone, as happened to me after a few hours' exposure to diffuse, unpatterned visual stimulation—the world wouldn't hold still. The same thing can be observed in a much more everyday situation: Upon any marked change in prescription for his refractive error, the wearer of new glasses may be annoyed for a while by the jumpiness of the visual field, despite its new sharpness and clarity. In both of these situations, however, the world very quickly learns to stay put.

The German ethologist Erich von Holst turned his attention to this phenomenon a number of years ago and managed to encompass it under a broad theory, which he calls the "reafference principle" (von Holst & Mittlestaedt, 1950). It may be illustrated by the example of eye movements. von Holst assumes that there are at least two controlling centers for eye movement, a higher and a lower one. When an intentional eye movement is to take place, an efferent impulse goes out from the higher control center to the lower one where it gives rise to a pair of results. One is the actual command to the eye muscles; the other is what von Holst calls the "efference copy," which remains in the control center and might be looked on as the neurological equivalent of the *intention* to turn the eye. When the eye muscle acts, there results a movement of the pattern of stimulation on the retina, a report of which is fed back into the peripheral control center; this is the reafference. It now makes contact with the efference copy, and if all is well, the two cancel each other out, and no resultant message goes to the higher centers. If, however, the degree of movement on the retina does not accord with the expectation or efference copy, there is a resulting message giving rise to an experience of external movement.

Let me translate this theory into somewhat more intelligible (albeit teleological) terms. From experience, we learn that, if we move our eyes a certain amount, there will result a certain degree of jump in the external world, which needs to be prevented. Accordingly, we learn to cancel out the reported jump by exactly the amount of the intention. If the retinal pattern is moved without there being any intention—an effect one can easily produce by pressing against the eyeball with one finger—there is no efference copy or intention to cancel out the effect of the resulting retinal movement, and so there is a resulting perception that the world has moved. A corresponding and opposite illusory movement can be obtained by paralyzing the eye muscle, as with curare; then, if the person tries to move his eyes, he experiences an actual jump of the visual field despite the fact that the eye remains immobile—or rather, *because of* the fact that the immobility of the eye does not produce the necessary reafference to cancel out the efference copy from his intention.

Now what does all this have to do with nutriment? What I have been describing can be conceptualized in terms of ego psychology as a specific perceptual structure. If you like computer analogies, you might look on it as a program for processing a combination of internal and environmental information to yield a perceptual result. The great difference between the human being and the computer, however, is that the [brain] is capable of rewriting its programs continuously and automatically to take account of changes in the information fed to it. Introduce any kind of *systematic* distortion, and, sooner or later, a new program is written that makes the old sense out of the new information.

Here, then, is an example of a structure that does depend very directly on being fed its accustomed diet of stimulation from its average expectable environment, and this kind of structure does undergo precisely demonstrable change when there is a change in this input. With such a good fit to Rapaport's concept, I see no reason why we should not regard these changeably programmed structures involving reafferentation as structures in need of nutriment, just as Rapaport described.

The fact that we have such structures requiring nutriment is one reason why organisms become so profoundly incapacitated when they are brought up during the critical early stages of development in impoverished environments: The [set of structures] that develops may get a built-in rigidity and inability to cope with stimuli as chaotic as the average expectable environment if it is fed highly simplified information for a long enough time (Bruner, 1961). This marvelous self-regulating, self-constructing apparatus can, however, gradually develop a capacity to process extraordinarily subtle data and extrapolate to a real structure from tiny samples, under normal circumstances. When it does so, it typically remains quite flexible—as it must, almost by definition, if it is to remain finite in size and still be able to cope with a bewildering diversity of possible inputs. In order for organisms to adapt themselves to the kind of variegated world they encounter, the structures involved must remain flexible and adapt themselves to any marked and systematic changes in input. In the typical deprivation experiments, however, instead of systematically changing the pattern of the input, one simply robs it of pattern. Now the apparatus searches and searches for the logic that isn't there, tries in vain to make sense out of something random, and fouls up its old programs without producing anything workable.[10] Restore contact with the usual perceptual input, and you get oddly distorted results, the results of processing external inputs by means of a program that has been randomly disrupted, more so the longer the disarrangement of the input. Just because these effects are essentially random, they are hard to verbalize, and to a nonintrospective subject they may not be reportable, perhaps not even noticeable.

In general, the range of structures that seem to have this kind of dependence on nutriment seems to be roughly equivalent to the phenomena that Head and Holmes conceptualized in terms of their concept of schema, notably including positional, orientational, and coordinative sensations and responses involving the body. Incidentally, we ought to learn a good deal more about the dependence of these structures on nutriment from studying the effects of prolonged weightlessness, which is a systematic interference with the usual somatic inputs.

I believe, however, that many—perhaps most—psychic structures are not of this kind, do not depend upon reafferentation, and are not constantly reprogrammed. Even for the ones to which the concept of nutriment applies, I think it is an unfortunate metaphor, for it seems to say that a psychic structure is like a muscle, which needs both exercise and an input of substances to replace the destructive effects of metabolism. A disused muscle atrophies, and a starved man's muscles waste away likewise, being unable to keep reconstructing themselves on their standard program. Any psychic structure, on the other hand, if neglected—deprived of input entirely—seems to lie quietly in storage and remain relatively unchanged. If fed the wrong diet of stimuli, or an insufficient diet, it begins to rebuild itself on a new plan, unlike the muscle.

[Though I believe there is enough value in the passage above to reprint it, I must add that it is considerably weakened by extensive reliance on the concept of "structure." The psychoanalytic concept of psychic structure, as I learned it from Rapaport, has the attractive simplicity of a waste bin in which all kinds of stuff can be stored. As the analogy suggests, one trouble is that a gather-all lacks internal organization, and so quite different kinds of entities get filed under one heading. See note 7 above; the generalization with which the just preceding paragraph ends evidently does not hold for every type of structure. The subtypes of structure seem different enough to warrant the use of separate terms. In this chapter, it is used to refer to at least the following referents, and it surely has been applied to others as well: something that is responsible for "the" secondary process; the ego, id, and superego; the perceptual "apparatuses" and other "apparatuses of primary autonomy" (which turn out to be very generalized terms for such functions as thinking, language, memory, even "productivity"); attitudes; defenses and controls of "drive" or "instinct"; organizations of memory traces; whatever makes possible "protracted logical trains of thought," rowing a boat or ice skating, "sublimative pursuits," and neutralization; whatever corresponds to perceptual transformational rules; a program for processing information to yield a percept; the entire "psychic apparatus"! In Chapter 10 (and the afterword to Chapter 8), there is further discussion of structure and some attempt at a definition, but I have not begun to tackle the taxonomic task that would face anyone who wants to develop the theory further.]

A SYSTEMS VIEW OF REALITY—AND FREUD'S

[Freud, and other psychoanalytic theorists following him, unwittingly and unquestioning adopted the assumption that the organism or person could easily be separated from its environment, and that it was conceptually necessary to do so. From an ecological perspective, however, we are intimate parts of an ecosystem, which in turn is made up very largely of other creatures, the vast majority of which are invisible microorganisms. Millions of those pass into and through our bodies daily, while billions of others reside within us with mostly benign or helpful but occasionally lethal effects. Knowing those facts, and coming to realize the beautiful intricacy of the symbiotic relationships that make up an ecosystem, we may be tempted to reject entirely the separation of organism and environment as conceptually artificial and empirically impossible.

Not so fast. According to a fundamental tenet of the systems viewpoint (Laszlo, 1972), reality consists of many hierarchies of nested and partly overlapping systems, all equally real. That means that a person may be considered a complete system, but also as a part of larger systems and as made up of many smaller systems. The larger systems include not only the environment or ecosystem, but the family, other social systems (from a neighborhood chess club or labor union to the United Nations), and physical systems (such as the earth, solar system, galaxy, and supergalactic cluster). It may be hard to *feel*, looking up at the Milky Way, that one is an integral part of this grandiose entity, but each of us is, just as much as Sirius or Halley's comet is. (We say that systems are "nested" when we recognize such successive inclusions as that the organ is part of the person, the cell is a constituent of the organ, itself made up of organelles, which are composed of molecules, etc. They may also be interpenetrating, separately defined but overlapping in space.)

True to his predominantly analytic and reductionistic orientation, Freud naturally looked to component systems within the person when in search of explanations. He would probably have found it incomprehensible that the person's behavior can best be explained at times as a result of events in *larger* systems of which he or she is a part. Since the advent of family therapy and family systems theory (see, e.g., Bowen, 1978; Haley, 1963; Selvini Palazzoli, 1988; Watzlawick, Beavin, & Jackson, 1967), contemporary clinicians are beginning to understand the necessity of thinking this way, though the full implications of the step are far from evident. For example, a mammal's need to maintain thermal equilibrium with its environment while keeping a steady internal temperature accounts for a good deal of food seeking and water drinking (see Chapter 7, this volume), types of behavior Freud unquestioningly considered "discharges" of ego instincts or the life drive. Regardless of the particular term he chose at different times, he never wavered in his belief that the explanation had to be sought exclusively in a force or energy discharge from *within* the organism.

An attentive reader of Chapter 7 must have caught the implication that when motivated behavior is studied carefully, the inside–outside distinction becomes increasingly difficult to maintain. The clarity that seems to be given by the conception of an internal id or set of drives, and an external reality or environment, has proved illusory. Nothing like the upwelling instinctual force that Freud imagined has been discovered; even hunger, which seems to arise from purely organismic sources (at least in infants), varies greatly with a number of aspects of the environment besides the sheer availability of "need-satisfying objects." And when we look at the motives that we postulate to explain most of what people do all day, it takes an act of disciplined faith to believe that it fits the model of infantile hunger, or of Freud's speculations about male sexuality as a kind of micturition.

Instead, we find people to be parts of larger systems in which wants are stimulated or seemingly created; in which people are cajoled, seduced, and manipulated into believing that they are playing the roles assigned to them in society out of a need for self-fulfillment. If we try to detach ourselves from our own culture, and look over the shoulder of an ethnologist observing an entirely unrelated one, it becomes evident how much the needs of the society and culture are reflected in the motivated behavior of individuals.

I have, of course, covered some of this ground in Chapter 7. Here I am trying to demonstrate that it is necessary to go considerably beyond the mere substitution of "wish" for "drive," for that does not get us away from an exclusively intrapsychic orientation. Pursued relentlessly, the latter amounts to reductionism. If psychoanalysts do not simply ignore social, political, economic, and cultural systems, they mostly assume—with the Freud of *Totem and Taboo* (1912–1913) and *Group Psychology and the Analysis of the Ego* (1921c)—that the "real" explanation of all "mass" phenomena is to be sought in the depth-psychological study of the individual. So ingrained is this way of thinking, so natural does it seem to most of us, that I will not be surprised if few psychoanalysts are able to give more than lip service to the systems outlook.

Let us pause and try to summarize Freud's implicit concept of reality. Inevitably, that takes us into the metaphysical realm of ontology. As an adolescent, Freud (1900a, p. 211) tells us, he took part in "a discussion in a *German* students' club on the relation of philosophy to the natural sciences. I was a green youngster, full of materialistic theories, and thrust myself forward to give expression to an extremely one-sided point of view." Elsewhere (Holt, 1988), I have made a case that the main source of these one-sided materalistic theories was probably Büchner's (1855) *Force and Matter*, which young Sigismund and his boyhood companions read and discussed during one of their last years in the Spoerl Gymnasium. Despite his notoriety as an extreme materialist, Büchner must strike a contemporary reader as primarily a defiant atheist, and only inconsistently and waveringly a proponent of what Whitehead (1925) was later to call the *scientific materialism* of the 19th century:

> the fixed scientific cosmology which presupposes the ultimate fact of an irreducible brute matter, or material, spread throughout space in a flux of configurations.

> In itself such a material is senseless, valueless, purposeless. It just does what it does do, following a fixed routine imposed by external relations which do not spring from the nature of its being. (p. 18)

Instead, the matter of which Büchner's universe is made has a host of Platonic and idealistic connotations. It is clear that Büchner was not emotionally ready to give up the humanistic outlook of his classical Gymnasium education, but smuggled a great deal of it back in after having loudly proclaimed a no-nonsense, hard-headed belief in the ultimate reality only of the *Kraft und Stoff* of his title.

Hence, it was easy for Freud to be both a materialist and a dualist, even though the former doctrine implies a monistic skepticism that the realm of the spirit, of consciousness and ideas, is anything more than epiphenomenal froth. That is, he could echo Büchner (in the Project; 1950 [1895], p. 308) by declaring that "in the external world . . . according to the view of our natural science, to which psychology too must be subjected here, there are only masses in motion and nothing else." And yet at virtually the same time, he was concerning himself quite seriously with neurotic symptoms of an ideational kind, such as obsessions and phobias, and with the subjective phenomenon of affect. Moreover, his hypotheses about the etiology of neuroses laid great emphasis on ideas and affects (e.g., Freud, 1894a, 1895b [1894]). True, he felt uneasy about the ephemeral nature of his subject matter; in a letter of June 30, 1896 to Fliess, he wrote, "perhaps with your help I shall find the solid ground on which I can cease to give psychological explanations and begin to find a physiological foundation!" Freud, 1985 [1887–1904], p. 193).

When he spoke about "a piece of reality," it referred to the social fact that a young man had other reasons for visiting a female patient's father than a supposed romantic interest in her (1895b [1894], pp. 58–59). Where are the masses in motion here? Entirely subordinate to the cultural and interpersonal *meanings* they mediated, which Freud called "psychic reality."[11]

It might seem, therefore, that his materialism was only a passing, youthful phase, which Freud abandoned for a more conventional sort of common-sense dualism or an implicit ontological pluralism. At various times, the realm of the real was to encompass conscious ideas and affects, unconscious ideas and impulses, the more impersonal world of culture and ideas (which is Popper's [1972] "World 3"), what I called above "social facts" (the realities of everyday social interaction and relationships), and even the netherworld of the occult (Freud, 1922a, 1925i, 1941d [1921]). He nowhere directly addressed the ontological implications of this casual stretching of the concept of reality.

His dualism was much like that of Descartes, being a combination of an everyday realm of physical, material, mechanistic reality, and another (for Freud, "the psychic," for Descartes, the spiritual) interacting with it in a way that was never satisfactorily explained. Though he occasionally declared himself a psychophysical parallelist, often enough for Jones (1953) to assert flatly that this was his stand on the mind–body problem, Freud turned so decisively against philosophy after his early flirtation with it that he simply directed his attention away from metaphysical issues and did not let himself become aware of the contradictions implied by various pairs of his statements.

Not surprisingly, then, there remain some lingering aspects of material-ism in his thought. One was what Bergson (1911) posited as a general characteristic of Western thought: "Our concepts have been formed on the model of solids." Even when Freud wrote about the filmy and evanescent world of fantasies and dreams, his treatment is in sharp contrast to that of William James (1890). Nowhere is there anything comparable to the stream of consciousness. Freud was steadily under the sway of what Holton (1973) calls "the thema of atomism" (as against the continuum). It seemed to him perfectly natural to equate thoughts and words (1915e): Just as language was for him a string of separate units, so was thinking or dreaming. Even the theory of the primary process holds consistently to a punctate conception of what we often think of as a hazy, vague, plastically transforming flow. Instead of James's coursing image, a better metaphor for Freud's concep-tion would be a kaleidoscope, in which the designs shift and change but the elements remain constant. (See Chapter 11.)

In another way, Freud's pervasively analytic approach caused him to conceive of reality atomistically. "Exogenous excitation operates with a single impact," he wrote (1895b [1894], p. 112), "the endogenous excitation operates as a constant force." This tachistoscopic conception of reality crops up again and again in later works (e.g., 1900a, p. 565; 1915c, p. 118), in a way that seems curiously perverse to anyone who has ever tried to interfere with a person's contact with reality. Motives wax and wane in a truly cyclic fashion, but "exogenous excitations" keep stubbornly and steadily coming in, hard as we try to exclude them by soundproof and perfectly dark rooms. The body itself is noisy, obtrusively so when other sources of sound are excluded; and though total darkness is not hard to achieve, the lack of the usual visual attention grabbers opens the door to focal awareness of the endemic pulls of gravity on muscles and joints and to all the skin senses' busy and ceaseless inputs. To be sure, the experimental work of recent decades on sensory deprivation had not been dreamed of until well after Freud's death.

Another subtle manifestation of Freud's early materialism may be seen in one of his favoite analogies: comparing psychoanalytic work with the excavations of archeologists. It crops up in his works from the beginning to the end—from *Studies on Hysteria* (Breuer & Freud, 1895, p. 139) and the early papers (e.g., 1896c, p. 192) to the last ones. For example,

> just as the archaeologist builds up the walls of the building from the foundations that have remained standing, . . . and reconstructs the mural decorations and paintings from the remains found in the debris, so does the analyst proceed when he draws his inferences from the *fragments* of memories, from the

associations and from the behavior of the subject of the analysis. . . . the excavator is dealing with destroyed *objects* of which large and important portions have quite certainly been lost. . . . But it is different with the *psychical object* whose early history the analyst is seeking to recover. . . . it may . . . be doubted whether any *psychical structure* can really be the victim of total destruction. (1937d, pp. 259–260; emphasis supplied)

The hidden truths of archeology, for Freud, were the meaningful artifacts themselves that he so loved to collect and possess, not the abstract ancient culture to which they pointed. Likewise, he thought of his own discoveries in thing-like terms, as objects.

Archeology may be a principal basis for another aspect of Freud's conception of reality: its *stratification*. The theme of *hidden layers*, a generally accessible surface concealing unsuspected mysteries superimposed on one another in a dimension of depth (compare "depth psychology" as a synonym for psychoanalysis), seems to have had a profound appeal to him.

Yet he was far from being the originator of this conception of reality. As Bahm (1977) has shown, it is one of the characteristic features of Western (European/American) ontology. More recently, Bahm (1988, pp. 44–45) has put the Western concept of reality thus:

What lies behind the appearances of objects . . . is more real than the objects as they appear. Although the implication is not a necessary one, the search for reality behind the appearances of objects tends to signify that what is being searched for is more real than the searcher, or the self doing the searching.

He connects this "faith that reality lies behind the appearances of objects" (1988, p. 44) to the Western obsession with analysis, and to reductionism—both prominent aspects of Freud's cognitive style.

This section began with a discussion of Freud's assumption that the subject (his primary interest) could easily be separated from the environment, which was of concern only to the extent that it impinged on the individual. This "inside-out" orientation is strikingly evident in Freud's way of conceptualizing the most important part of reality, human beings. His very phrase "external reality" implies that the natural starting point is with a single person, the *subject*, from whose vantage everything else is *objects*, "outside me." Further, that outer world is made up mainly of "need-satisfying objects"—which are primarily other people, seen not as they would appear to a person (as sources of love, support, danger, instruction, etc.), but as cathectable entities suited for the gratification of a need, drive, or instinct. Here is physicalistic reductionism with a vengeance!—the great world of humankind shrunk to things with which commerce of specifiable kinds permits the discharge of psychic energy and thus the pleasurable lowering of hypothetical tension or excitation.

We should recognize, as well, that the intrapsychic focus fits extraordinarily well with our political and social culture's historically extreme and anthropologically extraordinary overemphasis on individualism (Bellah, 1985; Riesman, 1950; Triandis, 1985; Yankelovich, 1981). In this light, autonomy is strongly congruent with freedom (liberty) as a political goal and supreme value (cf. New Hampshire's state motto, "Live free or die").

The very ideal of autonomy, which is widespread in our culture far beyond the modest confines of ego psychology, is transparently a convenience to—if not a deliberate product of—a capitalist culture of hyperindividualism. It is doubtful that any secret committee of greedy millionaires ever met to perpetuate their kind of world by promoting the dream that every American can get rich by looking out for Number One. Nevertheless, this fantasy seems to have been a highly effective means of preventing the development of European-style labor movements, in which workers band together out of a sense of identification, empathically recognizing a common predicament and the need for allies against a common adversary. Even for one who is not a Marxist, but who recognizes the desperate need of our world to develop more of a sense of shared fate, it is evident that it is indeed possible to have too much autonomy, that it must be tempered always by an equal development of another potentiality. Angyal (1941) saw the counterpart to the trend toward greater autonomy in the trend toward homonomy; Bakan (1966) expresses essentially the same insight in pitting *communion* against *agency*.

Both the psychoanalytic emphasis (autonomy) and the political value (liberty) express Bakan's agency. He amasses an impressive body of evidence to support his contention that human nature has a fundamental duality: the egocentric, autonomous centrifugality of agency being balanced by an allocentric (Heath, 1965), homonomous centripetality of communion. As Bowlby (1969, 1973) and Lewis (1981, 1986) have demonstrated in great detail, we human beings are profoundly social animals, innately motivated to attach and bond ourselves to one another. If anything, the biological evidence for the innateness of communion is more impressive than that for agency, though both themes are evident in most mammalian life.

To return to the issue of the two autonomies, how does the question of "autonomy from the id (or the drives)" look, once we have freed ourselves from the necessity to cling to these outmoded motivational concepts? Clinically, there can be no doubt about the phenomenon of attaining freedom from compulsive acting out and other neurotic symptoms, in the pathogenesis of which unconscious wishes and conflicts play a central role. If anyone wants to call that the enlargement of ego autonomy, it would be hard to object as long as "ego" continued to be used adjectivally and not as a substantive. Yet I believe that emphasis should be put on the overcoming of unconscious compulsion, without the old implication that motives or wishes themselves are in some way intrinsically dangerous (as in the notion of "instinctual anxiety"). True to his strong and irrational leanings toward no more than two motive systems, Freud put both the egocentric striving for personal pleasure and sensory/sensual gratification, and all the altruistic, other-centered aspects of love, under one heading—that of Eros (life instinct, libido); he then proceeded to conceptualize it in a strictly agentic way. Thus, the same erotic needs that motivate people to break up families and those that bind them together are confusingly put into the same drawer, only partly distinguished by the notion of aim inhibition. That is, tender, loving, allocentric expressions of communion were to Freud developmentally late and highly controlled derivatives of what were originally impulses of libido, that disruptive "force that introduces disturbances into the process of life" (1923b, pp. 46–47).

Contemporary observations show that manifestations of powerful attachment motives appear so universally as to indicate their innateness; moreover, they appear as early in life as hunger. Moreover, they are so strongly present in both members of the mother–child dyad that they seem more a phenomenon of that system than of the individuals concerned. It is difficult to look at the intense love of a mother for her infant as an instance of "drive domination of the ego," and to recommend to her that she be more autonomous of her id. Yet laboratory studies (Cofer & Appley, 1964) show that in several mammalian species no other motivation is stronger than mother love; and surely not only among rats and monkeys but among human beings, mothers often behave in extraordinarily self-sacrificing ways to save their offspring. When egoistic concerns are thrust aside in that way, it may fit the definition of diminished ego autonomy, but the example surely confutes the ideal conception of autonomy as good of which one cannot have too much.

And what about autonomy from the environment, from this new perspective? It is surely evident that an individual has at most a limited or relative autonomy from the systems of which he or she is a part. One form of such participation in the family system is called by clinicians "dependence," and is generally viewed as more immature than independence. We can, of course, point out the fact that no one can ever become wholly independent of a variety of larger systems; even when an adolescent male renounces financial aid and advice from the parents, he remains subtly dependent upon the family in a number of ways (e.g., what the anthropologists call the adolescent's "attributive status" derives in considerable part from his membership in a family of higher or lower prestige). Nevertheless, attaining a kind of autonomy is undoubtedly a developmental achievement—so much so that Loevinger (1976) names the stage in her developmental scheme that is next to the top "Autonomous." Even at that stage, however, her description of the mature women on whom she based the conception emphasizes a number of aspects of communion: a wide empathic range, a high value on close interpersonal relationships, and a broad concern for social issues. Such values are even more prominent at her highest state, which she calls "Integrated."

The seeming paradox can be resolved if we make use of Piaget's concept of *decentering*. Human beings have the capacity to become aware of their involvement in larger systems and to develop strategies of partial detachment from those. A wise and mature person knows that such separation is indeed only partial, and that much is to be gained from participation in the originating groups that define one's identity. A typical pattern in young adults is a "clean break" with the parental family in a protest of independence, followed some years later by a return—not to dependence or subservience, but to a sense of membership in the family and warm relatedness to its members. Often the ex-child is not ready to accept this renewed closeness to the parental family until he or she has married and begun a new family unit. Likewise, a person can learn to give up naive, chest-beating patriotism; develop a sense of being a citizen of the world; and return to a deepened love of country, region, and locality.

It is a misunderstanding of systems theory to assume that the individual has no freedom of action because of belonging to superordinate systems (family, clan, party, nation, etc.). True, individual behavior is often silently determined to a much greater extent than one supposes by having grown up in a culture and by being part of larger institutions. But the great variation in the behavior of people who are parts of the same systems indicates that there is no rigid determinism from above, any more than there is the "microprecise determinism" from below of which Weiss (1969) speaks.]

FREE WILL: ILLUSION OR REALITY?[12]

[These considerations bring us directly to the ancient metaphysical antinomy or conflict between free will and determinism. The solution to many a paradox lies in examining closely the terms within which it is framed. Here, it is evident that many writers unquestioningly accept the traditional formulation. The very title of Immergluck's (1964) paper—"Determinism–Freedom in Contemporary Psychology: An Ancient Problem Revisited"—shows that he has not questioned it.] Even the much more substantial discussion by E. Hartmann (1966) also suffers from accepting this framework.

I wish to argue that freedom is not incompatible with strict determinism, and that it is not an illusion but a valuable indicator of true or adult autonomy. Immergluck (1964) reviews the old controversy in its original terms, coming out firmly on the side of determinism and dismissing freedom as an illusion—a real psychological phenomenon and one worth studying, just as perceptual illusions are, but not worth taking more seriously than any other curious cognitive error. As one of Immergluck's critics pointed out, it is rather remarkable to see how a man can go to such trouble to try to persuade others to choose his point of view, which is that choice is purely illusory!

No, we should all of us shut up shop, we who try to teach, do therapy, or otherwise alter behavior by the use of words, if we really believed that human beings were in fact incapable of making choices and in fact doing so on rational grounds. We *act* as if we believed Freud when he said, "The voice of the intellect is a soft one, but it does not rest till it has gained a hearing. Finally . . . it succeeds . . . a point of no small importance" (1927c, p. 53).

A good many years earlier, he pointed out the fact that we have

> . . . a special feeling of conviction that there is a free will . . . it does not give way before a belief in determinism. Like every normal feeling it must have something to warrant it. But so far as I can observe, it does not manifest itself in the great and important decisions of the will: on these occasions the feeling that we have is rather one of psychical compulsion, and we are glad to invoke it on our behalf. ('Here I stand: I can do no other.') On the other hand, it is precisely with regard to the unimportant, indifferent decisions that we would like to claim that we could just as well have acted otherwise: that we have acted of our free—and unmotivated—will. According to our analyses it is not necessary to dispute the right to the feeling of conviction of having a free will. If the distinction between conscious and unconscious motivation is taken into account, our feeling of conviction informs us that conscious motivation does not extend to all our motor decisions. *De minimis non curat lex.* But what is thus left free by the one side receives its motivation from the other side, from the unconscious; and in this way determination in the psychical sphere is still carried out without any gap. (1901b, pp. 253–254)

Note that Freud, too, saw the issue as exceptionless determinism versus "free—and unmotivated—will." Or, as Ernest Hartmann puts it, "By 'absolute free will' I mean an exception to the laws of nature implying that certain actions are initiated *ex nihilo* by an act of volition rather than forming part of a continuing chain of causes and affects" (1966, p. 521).

Freud's ingenious demonstrations of the motivational determinism of many seemingly "spontaneous" acts in the 1901 book remains the best answer to anyone who would infer from the conscious feeling that certain acts are unmotivated. But today, this is surely a pseudoissue, at least among scientists. We do not accept introspective evidence quite so naively, and we believe in the pervasive influence of unconscious motives. Yet Freud did not completely solve the problem, partly because he too accepted it in the traditional formulation. For the majority of modern scientists, supernaturalism is dead. Nevertheless, we feel—correctly, I am convinced—that there is an important difference between a person who is able to listen to the soft voice of the rational intellect and to choose adaptive, personally satisfying behavior, and someone who acts in accordance with either external pressures or internal, ego-alien necessities. As of 1901, Freud had no way of accounting for the difference.

If I introspect in the traditional way about my behavior, I feel that I can choose what I want to do. I can, for example, either continue to write or go and get a drink of water. At the moment, I want to write, and it seems subjectively obvious that this choice is in no way unmotivated—on the contrary, I write precisely because I feel strongly motivated to do so, by a wish that is more powerful than my thirst. Freud's example of Luther is another illustration of the fact that the critical characteristic of choice is not that it feels free in the sense of unmotivated; rather, the point is that the person feels that *he* has made the choice *himself*, and therefore can feel responsible for it. Knowing how many people are in poor contact with their own motives, I am not impressed by the arguments of those who claim to act out of absolute caprice: The more arbitrary and seemingly uncaused such an action, the more certainly it is caused by unconscious motives.[13]

Before we consider how best to reformulate the question of free will, it may help clear the air to take note of the philosophical tradition out of which grew the unfortunate straw-man conception of absolute freedom, so easily knocked down by modern determinism. It was, of course, heavily influenced by Judaism and Christianity. In both of these religions, ethics is formulated as a matter of individual choice of good or evil behavior: The individual is responsible for his acts because he is considered free to choose one course or another. Man fell from grace and had to leave his original earthly paradise because he acquired the knowledge of good and evil—that is, became able to foresee the consequences of his acts, to plan and guide his behavior by the affect signals deriving from a value system, and thus to choose. With the loss of his original passive innocence, man became like God in being an active force and thus himself a potential creator and initiator. With this freedom came responsibility; and our legal codification of ethics still maintains a confused recognition that when a person does not "know right from wrong" and cannot actively choose what course of action to follow, he should not be held responsible for his acts.

Ontology as well as ethics is involved: For the religious supernaturalist, ever since Descartes, the experience of free will is a proof of the existence of an immaterial soul. The human spirit, which is thought to intervene in the chains of causality that obtain in the material world, exists in a wholly different realm of being from that occupied by the body; hence the baffling paradoxes of the mind–body relation for such thinkers.

Determinism, too, tends to be conceived of in anachronistic terms. In the 19th century, it connoted mechanistic reductionism—Laplace's grand fallacy that a complete formula for the universe could be written encompassing the positions and velocities of all particles in existence, from which (by Newton's laws) all future states of the system would be predictable. As

Goodwin (1955) points out, this ignores the fact that many material aggregates are structured into feedback systems, the behavior of which cannot be so simply predicted and the precise operation of which cannot be foretold at all very far into the future, because they are self-modifying and will be guided by unforeseeable future events.

I agree with Creager (1967) that Goodwin (1965) made too simple a suggestion in his hope that the concept of feedback would be enough to put the whole controversy on a new level.

> Those concerned with responsibility surely do not use "freedom" to mean unpredictability, or chaos, but rather "self-control." . . . No one is his own prime mover. Yet the notion of self-control is not meaningless. Nor is it irrelevant to the concrete question of responsibility. What, then, is "self-control"? Clearly it is another, more subtle and complex form of determinism. Call it by some other name if you prefer. It involves organic and symbolic transactions with the environment. We deal with systems and situations with finite, but variable degrees of freedom. (Creager, 1967, p. 235)

We now have enough suggestions to be able to formulate the problem more usefully. [Freedom not only is not the antithesis of determinism, but is in fact meaningless without a belief in the strict and lawful determination of behavior. The hypothetical freedom postulated by some philosophers as the reverse of determinism is complete spontaneity, acting in a totally unpredictable fashion. It takes only a moment's thought experiment to bring the realization that such freedom would actually be a kind of slavery. If I were free in that sense, I would not be able to act in a self-consistent way, according to my own desires and values, for that would mean that my behavior was determined by something; nor could I consistently approach potential benefits nor to avoid ominous threats in my environment, for again my behavior would be determined by external press in just the way that this supposed freedom rules out.

Meaningful freedom of will or choice presupposes a stable and lawful world. That is no problem for some philosophers, since they assert that determinism holds throughout the universe *except* in the behavior of human beings. What they overlook is the fact that the significant reality for us is other persons. If everyone else were free and completely unpredictable, I could have no usable freedom; communication among persons, for example, would be impossible. The universe of the philosopher of free will in this sense must therefore be completely solipsistic: Only I have freedom; everyone else's behavior is lawfully determined. Amusingly enough, that is precisely the position of those who, like B. F. Skinner (1971), propound the opposite explicit theory, rejecting all freedom of will (except, implicitly, for themselves).

When the issue is conventionally formulated, virtually every scientist opts for determinism, even though it seems to mean that we must give up as an illusion the very freedom of choice that we manifestly do have—not all of the time, and not all of us, but the best-off persons among us at our best moments. For on the assumption of determinism, a genuine and meaningful kind of freedom becomes possible. It is the freedom that distinguishes a wise and mature woman from her willful child, trapped in a tantrum. It distinguishes a successfully analyzed person from a neurotic caught in a compulsion to repeat an unsatisfactory pattern of self-defeating behavior, or from a psychotic whose echolalia and echopraxia exhibit the most extreme form of stimulus slavery or loss of autonomy from the environment. Indeed, a patient with no remaining vestige of free will is not analyzable, for he cannot decide to cooperate, to keep his appointments, and to keep working at his problems despite the pull of resistance.

Like most other scientists of his day (and of ours too, I am afraid), Freud unquestioningly accepted the false antithesis of freedom and determinism, and had to live with the implicit contradiction between his rejection of the idea that patients could make rational (i.e., free) choices and the fact that his therapeutic method insistently required that his patients do so.]

A Suggestion Toward a Way Out

It would be possible to solve the problem of freedom if we could build a *model* of a self-governing organism—an inanimate but working model, containing no vitalistic forces or psychic energies, and no equally untestable ultimate *deus in machina* (if I may alter the phrase) like a soul. It is surely beyond anyone's means today to construct such a thing, but the attempt to imagine its specifications will be helpful.

1. First, it must be like the human organism in being sensitive to the outer world (and thus potentially open to "stimulus slavery"), and in having internally generated motives (and thus being potentially "driven" or enslaved by desire). It must have the capacity to take in external supplies of energy, like food, and to expend this ordinary physical energy in actions of various sorts; thus it will of necessity have a good deal of internal structure, processing both materials and information.

2. The model must have a control center, in which the various determinants of its behavior are arrayed, implicit conflicts among them are ironed out, and choices are made among various possible courses of action. In this control center would be assembled wishes, perceptions of the outer world (both information and press), and feedback from its own action in terms of which it would be programmed to modify itself. Such a center would have to contain devices (defenses) for slowing or delaying the effects of some peremptory inputs from either within or without, a memory system including a means of access to stored records, and a set of programs for making decisions between alternatives.

So far, the model would have an elementary degree of autonomy from both drive and environment. It would be able to recognize a given set of external inputs as offering opportunities—benefits or harms of various kinds; its action would be delayed while memory was searched for records of the consequences of accepting various opportunities. Clearly, I am skipping lightly over many matters of the greatest importance and complexity, such as how learning (self-modification) would be possible, how affect signals would work, and so on.

3. For present purposes, it is more important to inquire into the necessary devices or programs for making choices, now that their possibility has been provided for. Presumably at least two decision rules might be embodied in programs: (a) "Of the available options, choose the one that promises the most *immediate* gratification"; (b) "Of the available options, choose the one that promises the most *eventual* gratification in the long run." These rules embody the pleasure principle (id) and reality principle (ego). Still missing, however, is a decision rule of the superego type: (c) "Of the available options, choose the one that minimizes guilt and maximizes the feeling of having lived up to moral standards." Some superordinate provision of the model would have to govern which of these types of rules should predominate if they should lead to different decisions. That could be, for example, a set of weights to be attached to each choice and a means of summating the weights for each alternative and choosing the optimal one, or choosing randomly if weights are equal.

4. It is clear, however, that at least the superego rule raises the important issue of values and of self-evaluation. The model must have a *self*—an awareness of itself as a separate being (sense of identity); it must have a built-in necessity to evaluate itself continuously, and at least one set of values in terms of which to evaluate itself. Perhaps, as Sandler and Joffe (1967) suggest, it will operate well only when it has an inner climate of favorable evaluation of self and world—a modicum of self-esteem and a sense of safety. Following Schafer (1967), we should provide for various systems of values or ideals, some of which could be classified as ego, some as id, some as superego [I am using these terms as adjectives, not as nouns]. Potential courses of action become subject to a further set of weights, for each will have consequences for self-evaluation against the several value systems. By now, it is difficult to imagine how the model could function without consciousness.

Let us for the moment assume that all the above is possible, just as it seems to be for human beings. What are the consequences?

A. The model will be an automaton of the cybernetic sort, a vastly sophisticated descendant of Grey Walter's (1953) "turtles." But it will not be passive, in either Chein's (1962) or Rapaport's (1967) sense. Its behavior will *not* be predictable solely from knowledge of its current inputs from outside and inside, even supplemented by its wiring diagram and a complete history of past inputs. It will have built up an idiosyncratic history, will have modified its own programs in terms of what it encountered and the ways inner conflicts were resolved, to too great an extent. (That much is true of vastly simpler, actually realized cybernetic machines with learning programs.) It will choose at times to delay impulses, at other times to gratify them realistically; sometimes it will accept external opportunities, but at others it will reject them and seek situations more to its liking. It is hard to think of operational criteria of activity it could not meet.

B. It will make choices—in a deterministic way to be sure, but according to a complex set of criteria, so that these choices will not be easily predictable except in a statistical sense. It will therefore appear "free" or "spontaneous," even though it does not embody the absolute or ontological freedom of which E. Hartmann (1966) speaks.

C. More important, if at least part of the above-described process of consulting memory, weighing alternatives, and choosing a course of action is conscious, *and* if the model's sense of identity is closely connected with the values that govern its decisions, then it will feel that its choices are *its own*. In a real sense, since the crucial switches are thrown in a control center experienced as a self, and according to ideals that also comprise part of the self, it will be self-controlling and self-governing. If the model is taught to label the accompanying feeling one of "free will," it will be convinced that it has free will.

Clearly, consciousness is an important property of this model. Otherwise, it could make no distinction between Time 1, when the critical choices were made in accordance with the "self" value system, and Time 2, when they were made in accordance with the "id" value system. Without any internal way of detecting such a difference, the model could not successfully simulate human behavior and report itself as feeling free or not free at appropriate times in relation to its behavior. Also, if it were not possible that a certain amount of the processing went on without consciousness while the rest was taking place in consciousness, the model could not successfully simulate the behavior Freud described, when the principal determinant of a choice was an unconscious motive and the verbal report was that the decision was "free" in the sense of being "arbitrary."

This has not been merely an intellectual game. It is one way—a potentially fruitful one, I believe—of trying to construct a general theory for psychoanalysis. It is challenging indeed to try to imagine how something of the kind could construct itself, given only the various capacities of the newborn infant [placed in an "average expectable environment"]. It will be apparent that the "control center" of which I have spoken repeatedly has many of the properties usually attributed to the ego [or self. Nevertheless, to avoid misunderstanding, it will probably be safer] *not* to identify the control center of this as yet embryonic theoretical model with the familiar, but confused, concept of ego.

CHAPTER 10

The Development of the Primary Process: A Structural View

During the winter of David Rapaport's death, I was in an unusually good position to rethink some aspects of the theory of the primary process, on which I had been working for almost a decade with his encouragement and help. Though now deprived of this counsel, I had the leisure to study and the stimulating surroundings of the Center for Advanced Study in the Behavioral Sciences to do it in, with access to Merton Gill just across the bay in Berkeley. We had many valuable discussions of theoretical issues in connection with the monograph he was writing (Gill, 1963), one upshot of which was that he forced me to face a number of issues I might otherwise have blinked.

In December 1961, I wrote and presented to a couple of audiences a draft entitled "Some Reflections on the Development of the Primary and Secondary Processes." When I sent copies to a few friends, two of them— Merton Gill and Charles Fisher—sent me copies of unpublished papers on the primary process in which they had made a number of strikingly similar and congruent points. For a while, we hoped to consolidate these into a single joint paper, but the task proved beyond our collective integrative capacities. One of these turned into Chapter 6 and one into Chapter 8 [of Motives and Thought (Holt, 1967d)]; I hoped that Dr. Fisher would be able to convert his into a companion piece, but he was too heavily committed to be able to do so. I wish anyway to acknowledge the stimulation and support I received from studying his original and thoughtful paper (Fisher, 1956), which has probably influenced my subsequent revisions of the following in more ways than I am aware of. And Dr. Gill and I have discussed both of our papers so many times that it is impossible for me to do an adequate job of acknowledging my intellectual debt to him.

One of the main tenets of the psychoanalytic theory of primary and secondary processes is the proposition that when the more or less rational, realistic thinking of normal adults is replaced by cruder, more fantastic and fluid forms of ideation, this change from the relative dominance of the secondary process to that of the primary process is the regressive undoing of a developmental progression. In this chapter, I am following Freud's example of attempting to throw some light on early development by theoretical reconstruction rather than by direct observation; but I shall draw heavily on the observational work of others, notably Jean Piaget. I hope to show, first, that, as Freud described it, the primary process cannot be understood primarily in economic terms but is better regarded as the functioning of certain types of structures. Then I shall reconsider cognitive development in the light of this reorientation, arguing that the primary process itself is the product of a considerable development.

THE STRUCTURAL BASIS OF THE PRIMARY PROCESS

Being scientifically a child of the mid-19th century, Freud found explanations unsatisfactory unless they were stated in terms of forces and energies (see Holt, 1963). He had been trained by his admired teacher, Brücke, to regard dynamic and economic concepts as the ultimate explanatory resources of science; accordingly, he developed a steady bias away from structural concepts in favor of energy (Bernfeld, 1944; Gill, 1959). Nowhere is this imbalance more apparent than in his treatment of the various forms of thinking. Thus, in his first major statement about the primary and secondary processes in Chapter VII of *The Interpretation of Dreams*, Freud offered the beginnings of a structural conceptualization: "I propose to describe the psychical process of which the first system alone admits as the 'primary process', and the process which results from the inhibition imposed by the second system as the 'secondary process'" (Freud, 1900a, p. 601). After a little further discussion, however, one can almost hear the sigh of relief with which Freud says:

> It will be seen on closer consideration that what the psychological discussion in the preceding sections invites us to assume is not the existence of two *systems* near the motor end of the apparatus but the existence of two kinds of *processes of excitation* or *modes of its discharge*. . . . Let us replace these [structural] metaphors by something that seems to correspond better to the real state of affairs, and let us say instead that some particular mental grouping has had a cathexis of energy attached to it or withdrawn from it . . . (1900a, p. 610)

And thereafter, he usually equated primary process with condensation and displacement (see Gill, 1967), viewed as economic concepts, even offering as equivalent phrases "*primary process* (mobility of cathexis)" (Freud, 1915e, p. 187).

Thus, despite the fact that Freud continued to associate the primary process with the large structural units of his theories (the system *Ucs.* and later the id), even making it their principal defining characteristic (Gill,

1963), psychoanalysts have been most impressed by the economic formulation, and have considered the central property of primary process versus
secondary process to be the nature of the operative energy.[1] The economic
characterization of the primary process is that the energies involved are
uninhibited, free, and not neutralized, whereas those of the secondary
process are inhibited, bound, and neutralized. [See Chapter 4, this volume.]
"Inhibited" means that they do not press for or are restrained from immediate discharge; "bound" means that the cathectic charge of an idea stays
with it (as opposed to the unstable relation of free energy, which is easily
separated from the presentation it cathects); and "neutralized" means that
the motivational energy cathecting the presentation in question is relatively
aim-inhibited, socialized, sublimated, or otherwise remote from direct
expression in its most primitive form. Freud did not clearly differentiate
these three properties of the drive energy of thought, but I believe that this
formulation explicates and summarizes several developments in contemporary ego psychology.

In a number of ways, this sophisticated economic formulation has
advantages over Freud's initial structural formulation of the two types of
processes as the functioning of two systems, the *Ucs.* and the *Pcs.-Cs.* The
structural approach seems to demand an oversimple dichotomy, while the
quantitative concept of energy suggests a continuous series with the ideal
primary process as one logical extreme, the complete secondary process as
the other, and actually encountered thought processes somewhere in between. (I believe it would be possible to develop structural concepts that
would obviate these economic ones while retaining their desirable properties, but I shall not attempt to do so here.) The conceptual separation of
three properties of the energy allows for further differentiation, which also
promises to let the theory more closely approximate the great variety of
empirically observable cognitions. Thus, for example, I was able to follow
Hartmann (1950) in linking preoccupation with direct drive aims in the
content of thought with deneutralization as a criterion of primary process,
quite independent of condensation, symbolization, and related formal features which presumably indicate freedom of cathexis, and thereby to set up
separate content and formal indications of the primary process in Rorschach
responses (Holt & Havel, 1960). In practice, the totals of these separate
indicators have tended to be correlated to an extent ($r = .50$) that indicates a
strong common factor, yet with enough empirical independence to support
a conceptual separation.[2]

Because of such examples of good fit with empirical—usually clinical—
data, many people have considered the economic concepts of psychoanalysis to be among its most valuable theoretical resources, despite many unclar-
ities and inconsistencies on the methodological level. Since the working
analytic clinician does not often need to concern himself about metapsychological issues, psychoanalysis has been slow to undertake a reconsideration

of such apparently fundamental propositions as those embodied in the economic point of view of metapsychology (Rapaport & Gill, 1959). Within the scope of this chapter, I cannot undertake a general critique of the doctrine of psychic energy (see Rubinstein, 1967a, and Chapter 5 and 6, this volume). Instead, I shall present half a dozen lines of argument that what Freud wrote about the primary process presupposes and necessarily requires the postulation of structures that bring it about.

1. *General considerations.* To begin with, it must be conceded that [even in classical metapsychology,] *no* psychological phenomenon is susceptible of a *purely* dynamic–economic explanation; a complete explanation must include all the metapsychological points of view (Freud, 1915e; Rapaport & Gill, 1959) and thus, of course, the structural.[3] The concepts of force and energy originate in physics, where they do not exist *in vacuo*. In any concrete manifestation, they are always intimately linked with masses arranged in space and time, and in fact cannot be defined and measured except in terms of centimeters, grams, and seconds and the corresponding abstract terms. If cathexis, libido, and similar economic concepts are to keep the name of energy, and if metapsychology is to be the kind of theory that Freud had in mind when he modeled it on physicalistic physiology, it must contain some conceptualization of what it is that generates energy, transmits or conducts it, stores it, transforms it, and finally uses it to do work.

Psychoanalytic theory has been strangely silent about structures, laying most of its theoretical emphasis on energies without specifying much about the nonenergic arrangements necessarily implied. Part of the reason for this silence, I believe, is that in Freud's original theories, the structures were explicitly neurological; but when he decided to give up—at least temporarily—the attempt to neurologize, the psychic structures hypothesized in the topographic model of Chapter VII [of *The Interpretation of Dreams*] were uncomfortably vague, metaphorical, and unspecifiable. Rapaport (1951a, 1957, 1959) did more than any other theorist I know of to emphasize the theoretical importance of structure in psychoanalysis (see Gill & Klein, 1964), yet he did not provide a satisfactory definition either.[4] Rubinstein (1967a) is right, I believe, in arguing that psychoanalysis will ultimately have to develop new, protoneurophysiological concepts of structure. For the present, the essentially metaphorical concept implied by existing metapsychology can be used if it is interpreted protoneurophysiologically.

Wherever we observe functions, we must logically assume structures of some kind that do the functioning. In this very general sense, then, structures are implied by the functional concept of the primary process. Specifically, the term "mechanism" habitually applied by psychoanalysis to condensation and displacement in such phrases as "the mechanisms of the dream work" clearly implies not just functions but structures.[5]

But the most important way in which structure is implied lies in Freud's conception that the primary process is *not* a completely fluid, random chaos; it has a perverse logic of its own. Indeed, the whole enterprise of interpreting dreams, delusions, and other baffling forms of pathological cognition is based on the premise of a hidden order in apparent disorder, which is the essential "method in madness." For example, Freud wrote:

> No influence that we can bring to bear upon our mental processes can ever enable us to think without purposive ideas; nor am I aware of any states of psychical confusion which can do so. Psychiatrists have been far too ready in this respect to abandon their belief in the connectedness of psychical processes. . . . Even the deliria of confusional states may have a meaning, if we are to accept Leuret's brilliant suggestion that they are . . . unintelligible to us [only] owing to the gaps in them. (1900a, pp. 528–529)

Indeed, it is widely conceded that one of Freud's greatest achievements was this discovery that there was *meaning*[6] where the predominant view saw only random error. He was able to elucidate hidden intelligibility in what was proverbially considered crazy and senseless by discerning recurrent regularities, thus recognizable and interpretively reversible operations of thought. And it is difficult to imagine how an inner order can be achieved and maintained without enduring structural means.[7]

Paradoxically enough, however, when he conceptualized his clinical insights in the theory of the primary process, Freud's stress on the freedom of cathexis pointed directly back toward chaos. In this theory, the explanatory effort is concentrated on the forces that break down the laboriously achieved order of adult thought, rather than on the stable arrangements that bring about illogical but predictable and intelligible distortions. No doubt, from the standpoint of the ordinary citizen or the logician, to whom man is a naturally rational animal, what demands explanation is the abnormal—the bizarre breakdowns of thought, which phenomena seem consistent with the basic entropic model of an energy that tends toward a minimum of organization. Yet despite this emphasis, Freud gave a number of indications that he realized the need for structural concepts to account for irrational, magical, wishful, and symbolic as well as for realistic and adaptively effective forms of thought.

Specifically, when he came to describe and discuss the operations of condensation and displacement in dreams and jokes (well summarized by Gill, 1967), Freud made many statements that at least imply—if they do not positively require—some more differentiated structures than the general system within which the processes were taking place.

In opening his discussion of condensation (1900a, Chapter VI), Freud first pointed to the brevity of the dream as compared to the dream thoughts, from which, he said, "we might conclude that condensation is brought about by *omission* . . . [But if] only a few elements from the dream-thoughts find their way into the dream-content, what are the conditions which determine their selection?" (p. 281). Taking up his dream of the botanical monograph, he notes that

> the elements 'botanical' and 'monograph' found their way into . . . the dream because they possessed copious contacts with the majority of the dream-thoughts, because, that is to say, they constituted 'nodal points' upon which a great number of the dream-thoughts converged . . . (p. 283)

From this discussion we can extract the following general principle:

2. *The dream work, or the primary process generally, makes use of a structured network of memories: the drive organization of memories.* In analyzing a dream, Freud always made use of the assumption that its unconscious materials were not random flotsam, but were organized in an intelligible way. Their apparent or relative disorganization is attributable to their being organized in a way that is strange to conscious thought.

> If we regard the process of dreaming as a regression occurring in our hypothetical mental apparatus, we at once arrive at the explanation of the empirically established fact that all the logical relations belonging to the dream-thoughts disappear during the dream-activity or can only find expression with difficulty. According to our schematic picture, these relations are contained not in the *first Mnem.* systems but in *later* ones; and in case of regression they would necessarily lose any means of expression except in perceptual images. (Freud, 1900a, p. 543)

This passage implies that the first system of memories to be formed is one organized according to simple simultaneity of occurrence, and that in the young child there is no organization according to similarity—that is, no conceptual organization of memory. Rapaport expands this to the concept of the "drive organization of memory":

> . . . the primary organization of memories occurs around drives. All the memories organized around a drive, and dependent for their emergence in consciousness on drive-cathexis, are conceptualized as *drive-representations*. In this drive-organization of memories the following hold: . . . Any representation may stand for the drive; that is, the memory of any segment or aspect of experience accrued in the periods of delay, and around the gratification, may emerge as an indicator of mounting drive-tension. . . . Conceptions like "participation," "omnipotence of thought," "pars pro toto," all express consequences of . . . [the] "free mobility" [of cathexis in drive organization], and of its corollary, the complete interchangeability of the representations of a drive. This interchangeability is in turn the consequence of the fact that at this stage of memory-organization there do not yet exist discrete and well-delineated "objects" or "ideas," but only "diffuse" ones. . . . The thought-process based on drive-organizations of memory . . . [is] conceptualized as the "*primary process.*" (Rapaport, 1951a, pp. 693-694)

Some of the apparent arbitrariness of the primary process comes from regression to a drive organization of memories. But this *is* an organization; there are limits to the substitutions that can apparently be made freely [despite Rapaport's declaration that there is "complete interchangeability"], and these limits [help to] constitute the drive organization. Even though loosely organized, the memories themselves ultimately become highly stable and structural.

A further point is implied in Freud's discussion of the dream work and joke work:

3. *The nonarbitrariness of many condensations and displacements requires a structural explanation.* It is easily overlooked that not just any image or idea gets combined with any other in condensations. With rare exceptions (which stand out because the results are so bizarre), the condensations found in dreams, Rorschach responses, schizophrenic productions, and the like involve the fusion of only those images that have some common elements enabling a connection to be made. To be sure, sometimes these elements are extrinsic and accidental (as in Rorschach's example of a schizophrenic contamination [response], "grass–bear"; but here the area responded to was both green and bear-shaped, thus not wholly inappropriate as a bridge of common elements; cf. compromise formation). Mostly, however, it is not even obvious that condensation is involved. Images of persons are very often fused or composite, because they always have elements in common, sometimes many of them. Yet a screening process must go on, in which points of similarity are found and used.

Freud clearly implied an organization of this kind when he remarked: "The direction in which condensations in dreams proceed is determined . . . [in part] by the rational preconscious relations of the dream-thoughts" (1900a, p. 596). He described a "painstaking technique" of composition which "makes clever use of any similarities that the two objects may happen to possess" (p. 324). Again, when "a dream is constructed, . . . the whole mass of dream-thoughts . . . [is] submitted to a sort of manipulative process in which those elements which have the most numerous and strongest supports acquire the right of entry" (p. 284). Moreover, it is quite apparent in many of Freud's examples of verbal condensations that the words combined were similar in sound; and clang associations indicate displacement of thought along lines of a specifiable (if "nonessential") form of similarity. Any of these processes implies the existence of some structural arrangement to carry out similarity-finding operations according to stored programs or rules. Such structures may keep well in the background so that we are not aware of them, except when they break down as in acute schizophrenia, when the most bizarre, forced, and queer fusions and other distortions occur.

4. *The fact that the content of images is affected in certain types of condensation argues that a structural, and not merely an economic, explana-*

tion of the primary process is needed. Freud described a certain type of condensation that he called a "composition"—a composite image, in which elements of several individual and separate images, derived from memory traces, are fused. (An example is his dream of his uncle with a yellow beard; see Freud, 1900a, pp. 136 ff.) Such a composite image is a good example of the structural point just made; some conceptual mechanism is required so that it can carry out the purposes Freud attributed to it: "firstly to represent an element common to two persons, secondly to represent a *displaced* common element, and thirdly, too, to express a merely *wishful* common element" (1900a, p. 322). In addition, however, he likened their production to the means by which

> Galton produced family portraits: namely by projecting two images on to a single plate, so that certain features common to both are emphasized, while those which fail to fit in with one another cancel one another out and are indistinct in the picture. In my dream about my uncle the fair beard emerged prominently from a face which belonged to two people and which was consequently blurred. (1900a, p. 293)

In a way, such a composition resembles a compromise formation—a new image constructed to serve as a bridge between two ideas in order to receive their cathexes. But the economic explanation does not differentiate a composition from a condensation in which the presenting image is unchanged. In a composition, there must clearly be some kind of arrangement to bring the two or more images together, directly molding them and breaking down their perceptual identity. Again, what is needed is obviously a mechanism,[8] a structural explanation.

5. *The use of the primary process for defense requires that it include mechanisms (i.e., structures).* The disguising effect of the primary process on thought is so striking that from the beginning Freud spoke at times as if this type of working over was always defensive—especially with respect to displacement. As Gill (1967) demonstrates, the resulting confusion in the psychoanalytic literature has been pretty well resolved in favor of the view that the primary process is the main type of functioning possible to a regressed state of the organism and does not require defense to exist, though it can be used defensively. The distortions it gives rise to would have no value for defense, however, if the disguise could not be counted on to stay put. If condensations and displacements were simply the result of fluid, freely shifting cathexis, the original and threatening direct content could not reliably be disposed of: It might turn up again at any moment, which would require a hypervigilant censorship ready to repress it whenever drive energy happened to recathect it. It seems most economical, therefore, to assume that when condensation and displacement are used as defenses, they are the result of mechanisms producing and maintaining a *stable transfor-*

mation of the original, threatening material. Indeed, Freud (1916–1917, p. 174) may have had something of this kind in mind when he said, of displacement, "it is entirely the work of the censorship," which is a structural concept.[9]

6. *Dreams often contain repeated elements, which would be a remarkable coincidence without structured means of dream work.* It is a common clinical finding, even in young children, that whole dreams occur again and again in essentially identical form. Moreover, recurrent dream figures may prove, on analysis, to be the product of the usual processes of condensation or displacement, yet they crop up again and again. It would be remarkable indeed if such constancy could be attained by means of a chaotic primary process, without any structural constants to bring about the specific condensed or displaced products. It seems much more plausible to postulate not only stable memory schemes, but stable mechanisms of dream work channeling the impulse material into set forms.[10]

7. *Neurotic symptoms typically involve structuralized forms of the primary process.* According to Gill (1963, p. 113), an example of "a structure regulating an originally *ad hoc* primary-process discharge is repeated discharge by a mechanism of displacement, as in a phobia, for example. We can speak of this as a primary-process *structure.*" Or take the example of a conversion symptom: Freud taught long ago that a paralysis, for example, typically expressed both the wish and the defense against it, in what often strikes us as an ingeniously organized compromise formation or condensation. Such symptoms are, as we know all too well, highly stable and difficult to modify, which speaks for their eminently structural character. The same point applies to most defenses and to character traits, some of which involve structuralized mechanisms of the primary process—for instance, habitual displacement in a bullying, scapegoating person.[11]

8. *Symbolism.* So far, I have been speaking about condensation and displacement, and not about symbolization, though that is often considered a hallmark of the primary process. How does a symbol differ from a displacement?

When Freud first used the concept, in the form Strachey refers to as "mnemic symbol" (Breuer & Freud, 1895, pp. 71, 90), it was applied to any portion of an experience (usually a traumatic one) that later was used to stand for the totality; thus, a pain could be a "symbol" of a constellation of memories from the time at which the pain first occurred. A few months later, in the "Project," Freud explicitly equated symbolization in this sense with displacement: "Hysterical repression evidently takes place with the help of symbol-formation, of *displacement* on to other neurones" (1950 [1895], p. 352). By 1900, Freud was familiar with the existing literature on dreams, in which several authors (particularly Scherner and Volkelt) made much use of the idea that dream contents were symbols that could be interpreted; back in 1895, in fact, he and Breuer had spoken of symbolic relations in symptom formation and in normal dreams. He did not begin to add the long section on symbolization to Chapter VI of the dream book until 1914, however.

Meanwhile, in the context of comparing dreams and jokes, he had remarked:

> Among displacements are to be counted not merely diversions from a train of thought but every sort of indirect representation as well, and in particular the replacement of an important but objectionable element by one that is indifferent and that appears innocent to the censorship, something that seems like a very remote allusion to the other one—substitution by a piece of symbolism, or an analogy, or something small. (1905c, p. 171)

In the revision of the dream book in 1914, he repeated this thought with an added restriction and warning:

> It would therefore carry us far beyond the sphere of dream-interpretation if we were to do justice to the significance of symbols and discuss the numerous, and to a large extent still unsolved, problems attaching to the concept of a symbol. We must restrict ourselves here to remarking that representation by a symbol is among the indirect methods of representation, but that all kinds of indications warn us against lumping it in with other forms of indirect representation without [our] being able to form any clear conceptual picture of their distinguishing features. (1900a, pp. 351–352)

He went on to bring in the idea of the inheritance of acquired characteristics, very much in his mind that year after *Totem and Taboo*, and he apparently was so struck by the widespread use of some symbols today and in historical documents as to think that it constituted evidence of a kind of archaic language or prehistoric inheritance. In short, the issue of the "universality" of symbols caused Freud to go off on a tangent about a racial inheritance of innate ideas, where today we find it difficult to follow him. Perhaps it was partly for this reason that he was reluctant to state directly that symbols were displacements, which in other respects they clearly seem to be.[12] For a symbol is a cathected presentation standing in the place of some other, less neutral idea directly connected with drive aims; and empirically it is difficult to decide in the case of many dream contents whether to consider them symbols or displacements, if one tries to follow Freud's usage unquestioningly.

I propose, therefore, that we consider symbolism a special case of displacement, with the following characteristics: A symbol is a socially shared and structuralized displacement substitute. The first characteristic, its being used by a large number of people, implies the second one and helps explain it; if any particular displacement substitute were a purely *ad hoc*, transitory phenomenon, one would indeed have to assume some kind of "racial unconscious" or other type of pre-established harmony to account for the fact that many people arrive at the same displacement. In the case of some symbols, such as the use of elongated and penetrating objects as penis symbols, one need not assume much more than the fact that many people know of the particular object (say, a sword); the intrinsic formal resemblances are sufficient to account for the rest. "The so-called universal symbols . . . are created anew by each person out of his own perceptions and experiences. Their universality stems from the common experiences that all men share" (Beres, 1965a, p. 16). In other instances, it is harder to account for the sharing of the symbol on quite this basis, and easier to look to unconsciously (but *not* genetically)transmitted cultural elements like the linguistic and mythological examples to which Freud pointed (1916–1917, Chapter X; Freud & Oppenheim, 1957 [1911]). In any event, however, the stable recurrence of symbols is the clue to their structural nature. Indeed, Freud explicitly denied that symbols are freshly constructed each time they appear: ". . . there is no necessity to assume that any peculiar symbolizing activity of the mind is operating in the dream-work . . . dreams make use of any symbolizations which are already present in unconscious thinking" (1900a, p. 349).

At this point, a number of objections may legitimately be made to the line of argument I am pursuing, for it is easily prey to a number of fallacies: those of reification, personification, and "mechanomorphism" (Waters, 1948). It is all too easy to commit Whitehead's fallacy of misplaced concreteness, assuming wherever there is a namable function or a particular type of thought product that a corresponding structure must exist to bring it about.[13] The result is the *ad hoc* sterility of faculty psychology. Likewise characteristic of an earlier era in psychology is the fallacy of assuming the need to postulate a personified structure within a [theoretical conception of a human being], a prime mover to commit the acts of will or an ultimate knower to whom all information must be reported. The "apparatus"[14] postulated to operate between input and output *is* the knower, the willer, the actor, so no metaphysically mischievous homunculi need be invented in addition—a fallacy all too often overlooked by ego theorists.

Moreover, the promiscuous postulation of structures to take care of functions can result in an extremely unparsimonious theory and one that more closely resembles a clockwork mechanism than a human being. Köhler (1929) warned against this fallacy under the name of "machine theory," pointing out the fact that it is not necessary to assume that order and regularity can occur only in systems with fixed tracks and no degrees of freedom. Culbertson (1963) makes a similar point in demonstrating that it is theoretically possible to design an automaton with a determinate program that can successfully simulate any exactly describable sequence of behaviors, but that as soon as more than a few specific acts are called for, such a "complete robot" becomes impossibly cumbersome and its design requires many more units than the human being has neurons.

The burden of these cautionary statements is that we must not postulate a structure *ad hoc* for every identifiable function, but that we must parsimoniously set forth a general theory capable of flexible and vicarious functioning. If it is well enough designed, it can make use of such nonmechanomorphic structures as the steady states achieved by an open system. So far, so good; but when we come right down to specific issues, such rules are difficult to apply. Need we assume a separate structure to bring about every one of the many types of condensation and displacement that Freud described? Surely that would involve one or more of the above-noted fallacies. One, then, for all types of condensation? If so, it would have to be able to scan the drive organization of memories and select from them according to a variety of rules, eliminating some entirely and putting together collective and composite figures, again in conformity to a set of principles recorded somewhere. To attribute such a congeries of functions to a single structure in the name of parsimony would in no way banish arbitrariness and could hardly propitiate Occam.

I do not propose, therefore, any specific set of structural concepts; nor do I have a general theory of primary-process functioning ready to program on a suitable computer, much as I believe that Colby's (1963) attempt at the latter was a laudable failure that should not simply be abandoned. At present, two points seem salvageable from the discussion. First, there are enough specifiable and different functions involved in the operations of condensation and displacement as Freud described them to make it impossible for us any more to be content with the few very general structural concepts and operational rules he assumed, plus his economic concepts, as a sufficient explanation (see Gill, 1967). Any more adequate conceptualization will have to postulate more structures and more specific ones than he did. And second, it is difficult to anticipate any principles other than the general one of creative intuition to guide the selection and framing of specific structural concepts in any such theory building, so long as psychoanalysis clings to its present ambiguous type of psychic structure.

Despite the facts that Freud himself can be quoted in support of a structural conception of the primary process, and that recent writers have been arguing this point quite explicitly, the economic conceptualization does generally hold favor with psychoanalysts (see, e.g., Arlow & Brenner, 1964; Beres, 1965b), among whom the intimate association of the primary process with the id makes a structural explanation seem like a contradiction in terms. For did not Freud liken the id to "a chaos, a cauldron full of seething excitations" (1933a, p. 73)? In the same context are other familiar and similar characterizations:

> it has no organization, produces no collective will, but only a striving to bring about the satisfaction of the instinctual needs subject to the observance of the pleasure principle. The logical laws of thought do not apply in the id, and this is true above all of the law of contradiction. (p. 73)

There is no negation, no concept of time. "The id of course knows no judgements of value: no good and evil, no morality. . . . Instinctual cathexes seeking discharge—that, in our view, is all there is in the id" (p. 74).

Could anything be less ambiguous or more clearly antithetical to a view that seeks to attribute the very defining characteristic of the id, the primary process (see Gill, 1963), to the operation of structures? Before agreeing, recall Freud's characteristic style of theorizing (Chapter 3, this volume). No other writer is easier to misrepresent by quoting him out of context, for he characteristically states his points "as it were, dogmatically—in the most concise form and in the most unequivocal terms" (1940a, p. 144) and then later on puts in the reasonable qualifications that take the harsh edge of extremity off the original formulation. Recall, moreover, his famous statements about concepts and their definitions (1914c, p. 77; 1915c, p. 117): His failure to propose and adhere to formal, comprehensive definitions for his terms was a deliberate strategy, a policy of conceptual flexibility that could allow maximal freedom to remain responsive to the facts as he observed them, rather than binding himself indefinitely to the level of wisdom he had attained when it seemed desirable to introduce a term.

In this light, it should be no surprise that Freud's later writings also contain less famous passages in which a far-reaching amount of structure is attributed to the id. The latter has, for example, "a world of perception of its own. It detects with extraordinary acuteness certain changes in its interior" (1940a, p. 198)—changes in need tension. As Freud had said in 1923, "The id, guided by the pleasure principle—that is, by the perception of unpleasure—fends off these tensions in various ways" (1923b, p. 47). The id must contain memory traces, or schemes, for it includes the repressed, and we know that such buried memories may persist unchanged for many years ("impressions . . . which have been sunk into the id by repression, are virtually immortal" [1933a, p. 74]). Moreover, it must have trace-like structures embodying the heritage of symbols and other residues of ancestral experience, which Freud relegates to it, since "It contains everything that is inherited, that is present at birth, that is laid down in the constitution" (1940a, p. 145), and this "archaic heritage of human beings comprises . . . memory-traces of the experience of earlier generations" (1939a [1937–1939], p. 99). (It is interesting to note among Freud's final jottings in 1938 one dated July 20: "The hypothesis of there being inherited vestiges in the id alters, so to say, our views about it" [Freud, 1941f [1938], p. 299].) These last statements attribute to the id a truly astonishing amount of structure, if taken literally. My point, however, is not to demonstrate that various statements seem mutually contradictory, nor to urge that we take any one set of them at face value while ignoring others, but to recognize Freud's fondness for bold, striking formulations and his preference for leaving the synthesis of his ideas to the future. As Freud noted with respect to another ego–id issue: "The apparent contradiction is due to our having taken abstractions too rigidly and attended exclusively now to the one side and now to the other of what is in fact a complicated state of affairs" (1926d, p. 97).

Moreover, if we take seriously Freud's repeated insistence that "The ego is not sharply separated from the id" (1923b, p. 24), we may come to realize that the contradictions may be as much our own doing as Freud's. For if id and ego did, in his view, shade imperceptibly into one another, then it was reasonable to assume that some parts of the id were much more highly structured—more ego-like—than others. Gill (1963) has taken this stance in approaching an improved definition of ego and id, "a definition in which id and ego are conceived of as a hierarchical continuum of forces and structures existing at all levels of the hierarchy" (pp. 146–147):

> . . . the id is the most primitive level of a continuum, but a level at which there is already some advance toward secondary-process organization, some reality principle, some structure. The ego . . . would not include the most primitive levels: these would be called id. . . . In the undefined "border" region . . . behavior would be called "id" in relation to behavior higher in the hierarchy but "ego" in relation to behavior lower. (pp. 145–146)

One of the merits of such an approach is that it removes the apparent paradox and makes it quite reasonable that there should be structures located toward the id end of the apparatus to mediate the various manifestations of the primary process, overlaid by increasingly adaptive and efficient counterparts toward the ego end.

THE DEVELOPMENT OF THE PRIMARY PROCESS

As Rapaport (1960a) noted, the conception of an undifferentiated phase at the beginning of life implies an undifferentiated form of cognitive function that is not yet either primary or secondary process; for if the primary process existed at birth, there would have to be an id, since the primary process is the defining criterion of the id. It therefore follows that there must be a development of both the primary and the secondary processes; indeed, this may be the central aspect of the differentiation of ego and id. The writers whose advocacy of the undifferentiated-phase conception is best known (Hartmann, 1939; Hartmann et al., 1946; Rapaport, 1960a) make no particular point of the implication that the primary process undergoes development, probably because their purpose was to emphasize the early development of ego rudiments, the apparatuses of primary autonomy, which subserve the secondary process. It is, I believe, indisputable that such anatomical "apparatuses" as the sensory organs and the associated neural structures are innate and that they function at birth, but it can be quite misleading to speak as if the function of perception were an apparatus of primary autonomy: One can easily overlook the many kinds and aspects of perceiving, and the fact that they go through many developmental stages involving qualitative as well as quantitative changes. Academic developmental psychology has learned a great deal about this and related aspects of growth, which psychoanalysts can allude to so summarily as "the development of the secondary process"; it is a story far too complex to be reviewed here.

The position I wish to develop is that primary-process thinking (or ideation) is not present at birth, and does not arise from the undifferentiated phase by a simple process of bifurcation,[15] but that it presupposes many of the stages of what Piaget (1937) has called the development of "sensorimotor intelligence." Until the infant can attain perceptual object constancy and the capacity to conceive of an object that is not immediately present in its perception, nothing worthy of the name of thought can go on. The basic facts of cognitive development, therefore, lay the groundwork for the primary and secondary processes alike.

One circumstance that makes this position seem a perverse or paradoxical one is the ambiguity of the term "primary process," for it is used by psychoanalysts to refer to modes of acting and experiencing affect ("processes of discharge") as well as to a kind of cognition. The distinguishing feature of the primary process as compared to the secondary process in the realm of action is the seeking of immediate gratification; in the realm of emotion, it is an unmodulated, crude experience that suffuses the entire organism. Since both of these characterizations fit the conative and affective functioning of babies quite aptly, and since psychoanalytic theory generally deals with "*the* primary process" in an undifferentiated way, it is no wonder that most of us accept unquestioningly the familiar passages in which Freud says that the primary processes are the oldest ontogenetically, and no wonder we assume that the cognitive life of the baby is as well conceptualized by "the primary process" as by the more directly observable infantile inability to tolerate much delay of gratification and total abandonment to tears or glee. As I shall try to show, however, the cognitive primary process fits what we know about the first months of life far less well.

In the rest of this chapter, I shall use the term "primary process" to refer exclusively to a type or system of thinking, with autistic or magical as well as wishful properties. It is only in this sense that I mean that the primary process is the product of development. For that matter, observations about action and emotion in early infancy do not particularly call for the hypothesis of an undifferentiated phase. Here is another instance in which overemphasis on the economic point of view, involved in speaking about the primary process as a type of *discharge*, may have confused the issues.

The Origins of Primary-Process Ideation

What is the justification for the position that the infant is incapable of any kind of thinking? My basis is the observations and theoretical reflections on them published by Piaget (especially 1937) and Wolff (1960, 1967). Piaget shows, to begin with, that a long period—about a year—of sensorimotor development must elapse before the infant can develop a world of stable, permanent objects. At the earliest stages, he writes,

> . . . the child does not know the mechanism of his own actions, and hence does not dissociate them from the things themselves; he knows only their total and undifferentiated schema . . . comprising in a single act the data of external perception as well as the internal impressions that are affective and kinesthetic, etc., in nature. So long as the object is present it is assimilated in that schema and could not therefore be thought of apart from the acts to which it gives rise. . . . None of this implies substantial permanence . . . The child's universe is still only a totality of pictures emerging from nothingness at the moment of action, to return to nothingness at the moment when the action is finished. (1937, pp. 42–43)

What general psychology knows as the perceptual constancies, making possible our familiar world of recognizable objects that do not seem to change radically in shape, color, size, and so forth with movements of eye or head, or changes in illumination—all this is clearly the result of a slow process of learning.[16] No doubt, as these most basic types of cognitive development are taking place, there is a great deal of perceptual fluidity, with displacement-like fragmentation and condensation-like flowing of momentary impressions into one another.

Might this not, however, be called the primary process in pure culture? The question is obviously one of definition and not a factual issue about which one can legitimately argue. I submit, however, that it is more useful, and more consistent with general usage and definitions of the term "primary process," to look on such perceptual experiences as merely some of the raw material out of which the primary process is fashioned in the course of development.

Without stable objects, in an amorphous world of swirling flux, it is hard to imagine that anything we could call ideation goes on. Remember that at first the cortex is typically not fully myelinated, the eyes often move independently—in short, the somatic perceptual apparatuses of primary autonomy are not yet fully functional—and the senses are not entirely differentiated one from another, so that the world must indeed be what James (1892, p. 29) called a "blooming buzzing confusion." Under such conditions and before the development of object constancy and permanence, the (to us) stable world of a quiet nursery provides a never exactly repeated kaleidoscope of constantly changing impressions, of physiognomically assaultive colors, of mixed-up and fused elements from all the senses.[17]

Certainly nothing like the primary process in the sense of a primitive but meaningful language, susceptible of being interpreted, could be going on. If ever psychic life approaches the truly chaotic, it must be at the beginning of life; and the central point of my argument is the proposition that primary process is not synonymous with chaos, with random error.[18]

Wolff (1967) has summarized well the slow process of growth during the first months of life, when the functioning of the innate sensorimotor schemes enables the infant to order its impressions and expand a bit its small island of preadaptation to an average expectable environment (Hartmann, 1939). During this time, the consciousness of the child presumably consists entirely of perception, and objects exist for it solely as "things-of-action," which cannot be conceived or imaged separately from action on them, a process which Bruner (1964) calls "enactive representation."

After about four months, the baby enters what Piaget describes as the third stage of sensorimotor development. At this point, the permanence of objects is far from attained, but the infant recognizes familiar faces and is beginning to act as if he had a reasonably stable world. In Piaget's observations of his own children, not until the eighth month did he report an observation that rather directly suggests the primary process. The child makes a movement that is followed by an interesting, novel result without, however, having directly caused that result. Nevertheless, ". . . the action . . . is promoted to the rank of a magic-phenomenalistic procedure and is used in the most varied circumstances" (Piaget, 1936, p. 204). As Wolff summarizes it,

> The coincidence of his effort and a chance event is apparently sufficient for the child to link the event as effect to his action as cause, as though all events which occurred simultaneously with his activity were assimilated to the procedure and became a part of it. Without regard for objective causality the child generalizes his procedures to all interesting events, and behaves *as if* he believed in the magical efficacy of his actions . . . *as if* his effort had 'magical phenomenalistic' causal powers. (1960, p. 89, italics added)

Before we agree to call such instances of *post hoc ergo propter hoc* magical and thus primary process, let us pause to note for a moment that very similar behavior has been observed in experiments on conditioning and learning in lower animals. Guthrie and Horton (1946) described this kind of thing in the behavior of cats learning to escape from puzzle boxes; and Skinner (1948) even spoke of such behavior in pigeons as "superstitious." In Guthrie's box, the trap door could be sprung by the pressure of a paw in a certain spot, which the animal would usually encounter accidentally in the course of more or less wild efforts to claw its way out. After a number of trials, some animals develop ritualistic-appearing sequences of postures, which happen to coincide with their stepping on the release button and which are adopted *as if* they had a kind of magical efficacy. In this instance, however, the experimenters were not willing to assume that the cat engaged in magical thinking.[19]

With respect to the baby, too, therefore, I suggest that we go slowly in assuming much of a thought process accompanying this piece of learning that is called "magical phenomenalism." Again, it looks to me like one of the bits of experience that form the raw material for the primary process, but nothing more. The magic gesture remains isolated and rather easily extinguished; the Land of Oz is still several years away. And as Wolff pointed out, "Despite these magical characteristics, the sensorimotor behaviors of the third stage are the basis for later objective reality adaptation" (1960, p. 98). A little later, he continued:

> the magical procedures of the third stage are reality-adaptive for the child, who conceives of the environment as being "at the disposal of his action," and these procedures appear magical only from the observer's point of view. The adaptive value of such procedures is indicated by their transformation into reality-adaptive means during the fourth stage . . . Psychoanalysis . . . has not so far explored the possibility that primary-process functions may play a role in reality adaptation, and has not shown in a systematic fashion how the primary-process functions may actually prepare the way for later secondary-process functions. (1960, pp. 116–117)

This last possibility appealed to Wolff, for in the course of his integration of psychoanalytic and sensorimotor formulations relevant to this stage, he suggested that "The apparatuses subserving the reality principle would operate at first according to primary processes, and would gradually become more reality-oriented and conform to secondary-process regulations" (1960, p. 122).

If we assume, instead, that at the third sensorimotor stage no true primary process is yet present, and emphasize the point that the magic is largely contributed by the observer's point of view, it becomes possible to see how the same elements can follow two lines of development: one leading to adaptation and the secondary process, and another to a different type of ideation that will indeed eventually be systematized into magical or primary-process thinking.[20]

The Consolidation of the Primary Process

One of the means by which such consolidation can take place is temporary regression.

> Piaget . . . reports many observations which show that the transition from magical phenomenalism to objective causality is slow and painful. Long after the child has acquired an objective conception of spatial, temporal, and causal relationships, he tends to revert to magical phenomenalism whenever he is confronted by insoluble tasks which he intends to solve. (Wolff, 1960, p. 140)

This passage strikes me as quite important, since it suggests that a regressive return to an earlier operation as a result of frustration cannot be the same as the first occurrence of the allegedly magical procedure. Just as the hypnotically age-regressed adult is structurally incapable of acting much like a baby, the child who has developed to the sixth sensorimotor stage has attained a sophistication and power of thought in the context of which an act that earlier hardly differed from a conditioned response can begin to take on a new type of meaning. He is now capable of more truly internalized thought (free from the immediate embeddedness in action on external objects) and goal-directed striving, coordinated processes that began in the fourth stage.

Moreover, the child is now beginning to be able to delay gratifications:

> Sensorimotor theory attributes the capacity for delay to the acquisition of mobile schemata [i.e., those that are freed from their concrete, action-bound context], and to the conservation of objects independent of ongoing action. Because the child can now conserve the object without acting on it, he is also able to institute goal-directed actions which entail a delay of the consummatory act. . . . By means of the delay mechanisms, he can search for and discover the means to achieve his end. (Wolff, 1960, p. 117)

Wolff (1967) reasons from these findings of Piaget's that Freud's account of the origins of ideation cannot be true. Freud (1900a) speculated that when the infant was hungry and frustrated in his need for immediate gratification, there would occur a hallucinatory cathecting of memory traces of a previous experience of gratification. Rapaport, who called this "the primitive model of cognition," remarked: ". . . all that is assumed here is that the sequence *restlessness* → *absence of breast* → *hallucinatory image* occurs *in infancy*. It is irrelevant[21] for the model whether or not it does occur" (1951c, p. 411). This is, however, Freud's account of how the primary process comes into being; presumably (though he did not specify it) condensation and displacement are involved in the process by which drive cathexis raises the memory trace to hallucinatory vividness. Wolff (1967) and Paul (1967) agree on the untenability of the conception of essentially veridical memory traces implied in this account, and Wolff rejects the possibility of early infantile hallucination on the additional ground that it implies the capacity to conceive or represent an absent object without some kind of action on it.

Even less satisfactory is Freud's further proposition that the repeated frustration ensuing upon barren hallucinatory attempts at immediate gratification causes a turning to reality and a search for the need-satisfying object by adaptive means. I believe that this is an implausible account of how the secondary process might develop, and suggest an almost diametrically opposed proposition: It seems more reasonable to suppose that the *primary process* develops out of frustrated goal seeking, which can much more plausibly bring about regression than advance in mental organization.[22] To be sure, my formulation follows the general outlines of Freud's, except that it does not include hallucination as the resulting type of primary process, and it does of course assume that a fair amount of cognitive development would necessarily have occurred.

Once such advance to the sixth sensorimotor stage has taken place, the regressively revived magical procedures, fluidity, and other primary-process-like aspects of sensorimotor behavior can take on new meaning: They are re-experienced in the context of a growing coherence and internalization, so that they now have the possibility of coalescing into what can be plausibly conceived of as a process, a different *system* of ideation.

It was from Rapaport that I learned to recognize that the primary process in general, and the various types of regressed states in which we expect to find it, are characterized by synthetic functioning, which is another way of saying that the modes of primitive cognitive functioning in regressed states have their own peculiar systematization. Yet this systematic character of the primary process clearly cannot be present at the beginning of life, but must be developed, in large part by the same experiences and by the growth of the same structures [schemes] that produce the successive versions of the secondary process, each one more efficient and adaptive than its predecessor.

Rapaport came rather close to these formulations in his important developmental paper (1960a), when he brought out at considerable length the organized and systematic nature of primitive, mythic thought. He in turn based his exposition on Freud's *Totem and Taboo*, in particular Freud's point that taboos are part of a "system of thought . . . . which gives a truly complete explanation of the nature of the universe," formed under the influence of synthetic functioning (Freud, 1912-1913, p. 77). "Freud's formulation," Rapaport wrote, "implies that there are various such synthetic functions which differ from one another: we observe these in, for instance, paranoia, dream, phobias, animism, religion, and science" (1960a, p. 842), as well as in different states of consciousness (see Rapaport, 1957). But Rapaport followed Freud in attributing the organized part of such thinking to the secondary process. Thus, he concluded that ". . . all thought forms involve both primary and secondary processes, but differ from each other in the kind of synthetic function they involve; that is to say, they differ in the degree of dominance the secondary process achieves over the primary" (1960a, p. 843).

Though he recognized that there were diverse syntheses of thought, some of them at a low level and characterizing cognition that in most respects partook of the primary process, Rapaport did not question Freud's assumption that any kind of organizing or synthesizing was *ipso facto* an aspect of secondary process. Possibly he stopped at this point because he was only beginning to consider the idea that the primary process involved the functioning of structures.

I propose, instead, that we consider some kind of synthetic functioning[23] to be an inevitable consequence of the structure of the intact and relatively mature central nervous system, unless it is functionally crippled in a specific way. Such crippling can occur; I am impressed by the suggestion of Wynne and Singer (1963) that in some families there is a pervasive climate of meaninglessness which artificially hampers the development of synthetic functions. With persuasive examples, they demonstrate how certain patterns of intrafamilial communication convey a sense that experience is not connected, that clear-cut causal relations do not exist, and that therefore it is useless to seek order and intelligibility in the world. These are the families in which there develop schizophrenic children whose thought disorder is marked by vagueness, amorphously wandering attention, and abortive inconsequentiality. Many simple schizophrenias are of this type; nothing clearly resembling the primary process is seen, I believe, because it cannot develop or is not allowed to.

Let us look more closely at the role of synthetic functioning in the primary process, returning to the example of magic. When we see it unmistakably in the play of children in the early verbal stages, magical ideation is characteristically *causal,* implying a cognitive expectation that certain forms of behavior may be used as means to attain specific ends. But this is already a kind of synthetic function! It is a way of organizing experience into meaningful sequences; no matter that it does so fallaciously, or that its rules of inference are invalid—that is what makes it primitive and childish. Take away the synthetic aspect of a false integration and you have only disjointed fragments, or aimlessly meandering, woolly thought. Consider the predicative reasoning called the hallmark of schizophrenic thought disorder by von Domarus (1944) and Arieti (1955). It is a kind of autistic logic, which leads to the maddest tangles of psychotic thinking; yet it too is intrinsically synthetic, another form of groping for meaning, a way of trying to reach conclusions.

When even such basic units of primary-process thinking as these prove on examination to be synthetic, it seems artificial in the extreme to claim an admixture of secondary process for every evidence of synthesis that can be found. It is a possible position, but a strained one indeed.

Assume with me, therefore, that the various forms of synthetic functioning are not necessarily an exclusive characteristic of the secondary process, but constitute something more elemental and inescapably human. If an immature organism has insufficient information and imperfect tools of thought, but an insistent need for some kind of closure—especially in the service of the quickest attainment of pleasure—it has the necessary raw materials for the development of a primary process. The very prematurity of an attempt to make sense out of the world will guarantee that it will generate false modes of thought, short-circuited logic, and a crude kind of purposiveness in which primitive ("drive") aims elide the realistically necessary, intermediate steps to gratification.

From the beginning of his life, a child is also exposed to culture, and to a special child's subculture, which contains numerous crystallized and far-reachingly organized primary-process systems. Myths, legends, fairy stories, and other simple types of fiction incorporating recognizable forms of the primary process seem to be the favorite fare of young children in other societies besides our own. Despite their casual sadism and the terrifying archetypes that people them, these magical tales offer a comfortingly oversimplified view of a world that is within the child's grasp. I find it a fascinating possibility that they also comprise an indoctrination into consolidated and extended forms of the primary process, a cultural transmission of ways to dream—to fantasy consciously and unconsciously, even to construct delusional systems and other kinds of symptoms—ways that are culturally viable because rooted in certain kinds of world views, as Erikson's studies of some American Indian tribes have so beautifully shown (1939, 1950; see also 1954). Here may be a new horizon for functional anthropology: *cultural styles* of primary process. I suspect that it will be possible to go beyond the demonstration of characteristic contents and to show preferences for certain specific variants of the formal mechanisms Freud described—modes of magical and autistic thinking which will be meaningfully related to other themes and traits in the culture concerned.[24]

Just so, within the broad outlines of culturally imposed limits, there ought to be individual styles of primary-process thinking as well. The first attempts of some of my students (Eagle, 1964; Kafka, 1963) to demonstrate the existence of such idiosyncratic patterns in dreams and projective-test data have not met with much success. We do not as yet have instruments of sufficient delicacy to identify such styles, but I believe that the tools can be developed once we know what we are looking for. The discovery of stable individual patterns of primary-process thinking would, of course, be excellent evidence for the structural theory I have been advancing here.

DREAMS, HALLUCINATIONS, AND
THE ORIGINS OF THOUGHT

Let us return to the problem of hallucination, and see what the observational evidence might be for hallucination in the infant.[25] To begin with, impressive physiological evidence has been adduced in recent years for very early onset of the dream cycle. The rapid eye movements (REMs) accompanying an activated or "paradoxical" stage of sleep, which in the adult and verbal child accompany hallucinatory visual dreaming with a high degree of reliability, occur throughout the preverbal stage of infancy, along with other physiological indicators of dreaming like the cycle of penile erection (Fisher, Gross, & Zuch, 1965). Yet it is as difficult to accept the inference that the neonate has anything resembling the adult type of visual dream as it would be to accept the observed erections as evidences of "phallic wishes," which Fisher does *not* propose. And the fact that premature infants spend even more of their sleep in this dreaming-like phase (Parmelee & Wenner, 1964, 1965) makes it seem more plausible that the physiological sleep-and-dream cycle is another innate given (like Wolff's "categories") into which content can be put when and only when the capacity to represent absent objects develops. Otherwise, the dream life of the fetus and neonate would have to consist exclusively of preformed archetypes!

The typical observational evidence for hallucination in the infant is the following kind of sequence, which I saw in my own month-old son: Near the end of a period of sleep, just before a feeding was due, the baby would stir, whimper, and then start to make sucking movements with his lips, whereupon his abortive outcries ceased while the lids remained closed over his moving eyes. It is tempting to jump to the conclusion that he was going through something very much like the primitive model of cognition, hallucinating the postponed gratification. Reflect, however, that during the *actual* experience of satisfactory nursing the same infant's eyes were either closed or relatively quiescent, and it seems altogether doubtful that the visual part of the total nursing experience is at all salient. Was a cluster of oral sensations being hallucinated? Hardly; if the baby does not have a fist, bit of bedclothes, or other object to suck on, he always has his own tongue and lips to furnish him with *real*, not simulated (hallucinatory), afferent input. The behavior can thus be accounted for simply by assuming a learned connection between the enteroceptive sensations of mounting hunger and the activation of the sucking scheme in a kind of "vacuum activity," as Wolff (1967) suggests, giving rise to pleasurable sensations. The fact that just the pleasure afforded by non-nutritive sucking is calming and can help delay the child's urgent demands to be fed is well known to mothers and the manufacturers of pacifiers. As far as the hunger contractions are concerned, they are cyclical anyway and will spontaneously subside for a while, regardless of the type of distraction that gets the child through a bout.

Nevertheless, sooner or later true hallucinatory dreaming does begin, for it seems well established by the time the child has enough powers of verbalization to describe it. Is it not possible that when it does begin, it follows the primitive model of cognition and constitutes a relatively pure expression of the primary process? Let us reconsider the arguments just cited. On the matter of the capacity of the infant's schemes to mediate iconic representations, the primitive "model" has been rejected on the grounds of ignoring the sensori*motor* nature of the earliest type of memory records, the schemes.[26] Yet these very motor components can persuasively suggest the inference that phenomenological content is involved quite early in the "REMming" of babies.

Consider the following observations on my son at eight weeks:

After a large and apparently satisfactory supper, the baby was put on a pillow in a reclining infant-seat in a lighted room with his parents, where he indolently sucked his pacifier and dropped off to sleep. After about 20 minutes of calm, deep sleep, he went into a prolonged REM period, which contained numerous episodes such as these: his eyes moved toward the right (his preferred direction of gaze, where accordingly he usually saw his mobiles and toys); he began to suck on the pacifier as his breathing became loud and accelerated; then he smiled briefly a couple of times and relaxed.—His eyes moved two or three times toward the left while he frowned, breathed heavily and irregularly, nostrils occasionally distended, looking and sounding anxious.—There were frequent movements of fingers and toes, once a coordinated extensor movement of both arms and legs accompanied by facial signs of distress, the eye movements including some vertical as well as horizontal components.—Once, a series of three deep sighing inhalations and exhalations, followed by a smile.

Though these observations were not as systematic and complete as would be desirable, what is impressive about them is the extent to which the observable components of behavior are orchestrated, linked together into affectively convincing sequences.[27] The most obvious hypothesis to account for this highly organized pattern is that there was some subjective experiential content. Notice, moreover, that these observations are *not* well conceptualized by the assumption that memory traces of experiences of gratification are being cathected. Rather, chained sequences of sensorimotor schemes seem to be activated, and since the motor part is clearly in evidence it seems quite reasonable that the perceptual aspect should be hallucinatorily present too.

Notice also that the eight-week observations above do not fit the primitive model of hallucinatory cognition in one other respect, which is crucial for the issue of whether the hypothetical infantile dream is to be thought of as prototypical primary process: It did not occur in the context of an active, frustrated drive. Rather, hunger had been sated at the breast, and the infant had also been given plenty of opportunity to enjoy as much additional non-nutritive sucking as he wished. Nevertheless, the sucking scheme was active during parts of the REM period, accompanied by a smile and by apparently experienced gratification. Data of the kind just cited are additional reasons (beyond the ones cited in earlier chapters by Rubinstein, (1967a) and by Klein, (1967) for rejecting the conception that the central process in motivation is the buildup of accumulated energy or tension, which is then "discharged" in consummatory behavior.

True, there are anatomical and physiological bases for supposing that the dream cycle and the cyclic nature of motives may be directly related (Jouvet, 1961, 1962). Quite possibly the dream, whenever it does first appear, is organized by active motivational processes of some kind. The motivational conception implicit in recent neuroanatomical and neurophysiological work is far from any of Freud's various theories of instinctual drives, however. Notice, also, the apparent presence of unpleasant episodes in the two-month-old baby's "dream"—abortive or fragmentary "nightmares." Unless one adopts the mythological preformism of a Melanie Klein, it is difficult to reconcile such inferred contents with the primitive model. It looked to me as if my son's dream experience was composed of re-enacted, fairly representative samples of his waking life. Most of the sensorimotor schemes whose operations presumably made up his daytime experience were plainly operating during his REM period, for better or for worse so far as the pleasure principle is concerned. There is no reason to think of the putative dream as pure-culture primary process, therefore, any more than the waking, perceptual experience of the infant.

The unique situation of activated sleep makes it possible for the baby to use his only available means of "conserving objects," the enactive one of exercising his sensorimotor schemes, in the actual absence of the real objects. The loss of muscular tonus accompanying this stage of sleep means that the motor aspect will be fairly minimal, especially so far as large muscles are concerned. The small movements involved in the sucking and looking schemes, however, seem to go on unimpaired by the state of sleep. The state of relative deafferentation brought about by sleep probably plays a major role in enabling the realistically absent objects to be conserved or represented in a partly iconic manner. In the waking state of consciousness, the infant of a few weeks is almost wholly lacking in autonomy from the environment: He is captured by objects, has no means for gaining any distance from them, but is totally involved to the extent that they have any actuality for him at all (Rapaport, 1957; Erikson, 1964). It is therefore quite easy to understand the late appearance of the capacity to imagine something that is not perceptually present in addition to the insistent inputs that do persist; this capacity does not seem to develop until the second year.

But it is an unwarranted extension of Piaget's observations to conclude that hallucination is not possible during the first year *in sleep*. Studies of visual attention in infants during the first weeks of life (Frantz, 1964; Hershenson, Munsinger, & Kessen, 1965; see Wolff, 1967, fn. 9 for a brief review of some of this evidence) show that the looking schemes develop a good deal more rapidly than had been supposed, and are capable (at least under ideal, controlled conditions) of sustaining enough perceptual identity so that the infant can discriminate familiar from novel presentations. However vague and schematic the images that could be generated in sleep by such structures, there is every reason to assume that they do occur along with the enactment of their motor components. According to this way of conceiving it, there would be no identifiable moment at which hallucinatory dreaming begins: Dreaming would be, from its inception, a *sensorimotor* matter with a gradually increasing phenomenal component. It may well be that in dreaming, as well as in waking life, action and experience are not yet differentiated for the preverbal infant. As schemes become more mobile, the motor component of dreaming gradually diminishes.

Yet dreaming probably becomes more purely perceptual and less motor *before* its waking counterpart does, because of the lack of external input. In this way, it may serve as a bellwether for the developing mobility of schemes—their ability to function without motor action on the immediately present object. The innate capacity to dream may therefore be an important influence in the development of the secondary as well as the primary process. Once it has occurred passively, the separation of the cognitive from the motor functioning of schemes can be achieved actively and in a waking state. At first, there may be a spillover of dream-like phenomena into states of consciousness approaching that of sleep. The dozing child may have hypnagogic images; the resting baby who lies quietly in a still nursery with eyes closed may have dreamy reveries or fantasies. It seems to me a good deal more plausible that the first waking images detached from simultaneous sensorimotor functioning might occur in these transitional states of consciousness, rather than in the kind of situation where Piaget first observed the conservation of objects: the child wide awake, in full perceptual contact with a rich array of stimuli, and in the midst of purposive interaction with objects. That is the time when the child is most likely to be stimulus-bound, enslaved to the impressive perceptual reality of objects he is in contact with; no wonder that Wolff (1967) dates the time of this accomplishment—the beginning of true thought—as late as 18 months. By then the child is likely to have started the learning of language and to have made a beginning in differentiating a self, both of which related achievements may be necessary to enable him to get the required distance or autonomy from his perceptual environment.

But here we are getting into a host of complicated problems: the issues of autonomy, activity, and passivity, the development of the self, the learning of language and concepts, the growth of the capacity for focal attention, and the orienting reflex, all of which are vitally involved in the development of more realistic and adaptive forms of thinking—in short, the secondary process. And while it is difficult and artificial to stop the account of an intricate developmental process at any particular point, I hope that the discussion above suffices to indicate ways in which extensive development takes place within the realm of what can loosely be called the primary process.

In conclusion, let me restate my central points. When Freud proposed the radical conception that dreams, neurotic and psychotic symptoms, and other such primitive and seemingly incomprehensible forms of thought and behavior could be interpreted, he pitted his new theory of the primary process against the prevailing view that such phenomena were essentially random, stochastic, and intrinsically meaningless. Freud's view was not only that determinism must be assumed to apply to all corners of psychology, but that the functioning of the unconscious or the id was something like an ancient, secret language. Its grammar was strange and perverse, yet it did follow rules that he could formulate, and with the aid of a symbolic dictionary to its vocabulary he taught us to translate so that sense could be made out of what others had considered inherently senseless.

Yet when he came to fit these discoveries into his metapsychology, Freud gravitated to an explanation in terms of energies which paradoxically but necessarily denied all the stability he had so painstakingly elucidated. The more explicit he was in stating the economic theory of free (or mobile) cathexis, the more it regressed toward the entropic image of "a chaos, a cauldron full of seething excitations" (Freud, 1933a, p. 73).

If, however, we turn from dynamic and economic to a structural emphasis in our theory, we can conceptualize the primary process as a special system of processing information in the service of a synthetic necessity. It must therefore presuppose the operation of stable structures, and it must be the product of a considerable development.

CHAPTER 11

The Present Status of
Freud's Theory of the Primary Process

Almost 10 years elapsed between the writing of the preceding chapter and the present one. During that time, the scoring manual for primary process attained its final form, and it was applied in numerous researches in many parts of the United States, Canada (particularly at the University of Montreal), Italy (at the University of Rome), and several other countries. There were many encouraging signs that the method had clinical utility, and clear statistical evidence that its scores predicted important aspects of behavior.

Meanwhile, I had had ample opportunity to reflect on the theory in light of this empirical experience. The present chapter is an attempt to summarize what I have learned about a major aspect of ego psychology: the psychoanalytic theory of thinking.

THE OBSERVATIONAL BASE OF THE CONCEPT
OF THE PRIMARY PROCESS

Whatever the gaps in his philosophical training, Freud saw certain issues in the philosophy of science with extraordinary clearness. In his paper *On Narcissism*, speaking of basic concepts such as instinct and libido, he wrote:

> . . . these ideas are not the foundation of science, upon which everything rests: that foundation is observation alone. They are not the bottom but the top of the whole structure, and they can be replaced and discarded without damaging it. (1914c, p. 77)

The situation in which we find ourselves today is worse than these sensible words imply, however: Not only do we lack a satisfactory high-level theory, we cannot even be sure of what our facts are. A fact is not merely an observation; it is an observation reported or recorded—that is, formulated—transferred from an experiential to a symbolized status, encoded into semantic symbols (words), presentational symbols (Susanne Langer's [1942] term for graphic or plastic representation), or purely conventional ones like those of mathematics. In psychology, we work almost entirely in the semantic realm, so we record most observations in words. But a word is a concept, and it therefore entails a theory, tacit or explicit.

Thus, I might claim that our task is to replace Freud's energic theory of the primary and secondary processes with a more defensible and satisfactory one; and indeed that is part of the task. But what *are* these processes that need an alternative explanation? Are they simple observables, like the rising of the sun or the running of the deer? As Freud used the terms most of the time,[1] the answer must be negative. They are remote from direct observation in two ways. First, they are inferred intervening variables that account for an observed output as the transform of assumed or inferred input, all of which implies a developed theory of cognitive functioning. Both the primary and secondary processes involve transformations of meaning, but in different ways: The secondary process is a type of information processing according to rules that are (at least to a first approximation) not difficult to specify; but the primary process covers a wider, more diffuse realm—impulse, affect, and behavior as well as thought—and operates by less easily specifiable rules. Second, in the way their boundaries are set much more is implicitly assumed, which needs to be explicated.

SOME ORIGINS OF FREUD'S CONCEPT[2]

Let us look at the latter issue first. It is not an easy point to make clear. If we tried to put ourselves in the position of a naive observer who had never heard of Freud's ideas, and if we were exposed to the phenomena in which he discovered some unity, would we come up with the same groupings? Freud did not approach experience with any fewer preconceptions than anyone else. Language, common-sense psychology, and the formulations of psychologists and philosophers to whom he was exposed all tended to encourage him to assume that thinking as we usually encounter it is a more or less unitary process: orderly, logical, realistic, proceeding in coherent ways from clear, definitive percepts and sharply formed concepts to specific conclusions or decisions. To be sure, the more you consider such thinking and attempt to describe precisely what you mean by it, the more complex it becomes and the more idealized; it begins to resemble less and less the actual cognitive processes of people like you and me in most of our everyday waking lives. Nevertheless, it was easy for Freud to believe that the learned professors who wrote the books on thought—men like Herbart, Brentano, Mill, and Lipps—knew what they were talking about so confidently and authoritatively, and so he could take it as established that this secondary process, as he called it, was a unitary system of thought so well known that he had little more to do than to allude to it. Before we turn our attention to the neglected night side of human cognition, on which Freud so quickly focused, let us take notice of his silent assumptions that conscious, waking, intelligible cognition forms a single system, and that everyday fallible deviations from the ideal type of scientific thinking are only quantitatively, not qualitatively, different from it.

Freud's letters to his fiancée show that in his late 20s he was already interested in dreams, before he had any exposure to psychiatric or even neurological patients. From adolescence he had been an avid reader of poetry and imaginative literature, and a devotee of the visual arts whose taste was not satisfied by the common man's demand for a good likeness. Dreams, poetry, nonphotographic art—these human productions have in common a rich strangeness: All allude to the forms and contents of realistic experience without simply reproducing them. They are *strange* in that they are not faithful copies of what the assumed secondary process would yield, but still bear a resemblance to the latter, and *rich* in that so often they are elaborated, with as much added as has been taken away, and in that they have a mysterious[3] power to evoke emotional responses. It was a short step to the assumption that an allusive cousin of a prosaic waking cognitive product must be a transform of it; hence the result of some *process of transformation*, which Freud came to call the primary process.

We know also that Freud had an excellent sense of humor, enjoying and collecting jokes and witty sayings long before he thought of writing a book about them. As he so aptly demonstrated, much verbal humor depends for its effect on allusion; hence it is not difficult to assimilate it to the same hypothesis that a distorting process has transformed an originally sober, straightforward thought.

At this point, I want to emphasize particularly the naive *realism* that Freud implicitly assumed in his concept of the primary process. Paradoxically, it implied a realistic, straightforward, veridical cognition prior to the primary process. If the primary process distorts reality or logic, its theory requires the pre-existence of something veridical to be transformed. Is this odd implication merely the result of logic chopping, or is there any basis in the Freudian canon for it? Consider the following:

> . . . we are driven to conclude that two fundamentally different kinds of psychical processes are concerned in the formation of dreams. One of these produces perfectly rational dream-thoughts, of no less validity than normal thinking; while the other treats these thoughts in a manner which is in the highest degree bewildering and irrational. . . . this second psychical process . . . [is] the dream-work proper. . . . We have found from [the study of hysteria] that the same irrational psychical processes, and others that we have not specified, dominate the production of hysterical symptoms. In hysteria, too, we come across a series of perfectly rational thoughts, equal in validity to our conscious thoughts; but to begin with we know nothing of their existence in this form and we can only reconstruct them subsequently. . . . we discover by analyzing the symptom which has been produced that these normal thoughts have been submitted to abnormal treatment: *they have been transformed into*

> *the symptom by means of condensation and the formation of compromises, by way of superficial associations and in disregard of contradictions, and also, it may be, along the path of regression.* (Freud, 1900a, p. 597)

The "perfectly rational" and valid dream thoughts are the text that is reconstructed after the interpretation, which runs the distorting primary process backwards, as it were. It is quite evident in this remarkable passage that Freud conceived of the results of his therapeutic reconstructions of both dreams and neurotic symptoms as actually having existed unconsciously before the disguising work of the primary process came to bear on them.[4]

Elsewhere, he makes it clear that whenever a dream contains something that seems to be "a product of some . . . higher intellectual function,"

> . . . *these intellectual operations have already been performed in the dream-thoughts and have only been* TAKEN OVER *by the dream content.* A conlusion drawn in a dream is nothing other than the repetition of a conclusion in the dream-thoughts; if the conclusion is taken over into the dream unmodified, it will appear impeccable. . . . a calculation in the dream-thoughts . . . is always rational. . . . [When] speeches made, heard, or read [are] revived in the dream-thoughts . . . [their] wording is exactly reproduced. (1901a, pp. 667–668)

At first, when I noticed these passages, I thought that Freud was only trying to contrast the obscurity of the dream with the intelligibility of its latent meaning; and no doubt that was part of what he was saying. Yet he does consistently speak as if the dream thoughts contain the most primitive wishes and are the products of unconscious mental functioning, which nevertheless is veridical, rational, and "impeccable."

Very well, you may say, it was not so bizarre of Freud to assume that a grown person might have a thought that was clearly and logically formulated but so abhorrent in its wishful content that he would have to disguise and transform it to make it consciously tolerable. But then why did Freud call "this second psychical process" the primary process? Doesn't the term contain a genetic hypothesis? Indeed it does. By the choice of this name, Freud tells us he meant to imply

> . . . not merely considerations of relative importance and efficiency [efficacy?]. I intended also to choose a name which would give an indication of its chronological priority. It is true that, so far as we know, no psychical apparatus exists which possesses a primary process only and that such an apparatus is to that extent a theoretical fiction. But this much is a fact: the primary processes are present in the mental apparatus from the first, while it is only in the course of life that the secondary processes unfold, and come to inhibit and overlay the primary ones; it may even be that their complete domination is not attained until the prime of life. (1900a, p. 603)

This is one of the key passages establishing the fact that Freud conceived of the primary process not only as a process of defense by means of cognitive distortion, but as a primitive mode by which the immature psychic apparatus functions. Another is the following conclusion to an extended an explicit discussion of this issue (about which Jones and Silberer had a controversy) in his book on jokes:

> If we did not already know it from research into the psychology of the neuroses, we should be led by jokes to a suspicion that the strange unconscious revision [i.e., primary-process transformation] is nothing else than the infantile type of thought-activity. (1905c, p. 170)

As Gill comments, ". . . in this explanation he appears to equate infantile and even early childhood mental activity with primary-process functioning" (1967, p. 285). What remains unclear is whether this developmental interpretation implies one or the other of the following two explanations for the fact that, in the beginning, children's thought has "archaic" characteristics: (1) In its crudest developmental forms, the psychic apparatus subjects veridical perceptions and correct logical thoughts to distorting transformations and does so naturally, sometimes in pursuit of pleasure, but without being defensively motivated to do so; or (2) the earliest versions of the structures that underlie cognitive–affective functioning are crude and function crudely. At times, Freud does sound as if he might have had something like the latter formulation in mind, but he never made it explicit and probably never confronted the issues in just these terms.[5]

Recall, also, that Freud began theorizing about thinking in the attempt to understand the dreams and the neurotic symptoms of adults (notably himself), not as a part of a program of research on infants and young children. Indeed, he never mounted any such program, not even on his own children; he wrote to Fliess (on February 2, 1897): "Why do I not go into the nursery and experiment on Annerl [on the question of whether there is a period in infancy when disgust is absent]? Because working for 12½ hours I have no time for it, and the womenfolk do not support my researches" (Freud, 1985 [1887–1904], p. 230). His observations on his children's cognitive processes were quite incidental and unsystematic, therefore, and there is no record of his ever studying any others; he never analyzed a young child himself. His contributions to our understanding of childhood must seem all the more remarkable for having been the result mainly of retrospective reconstructions based on memories and fantasies supplied by adult patients.

One of the limitations of such a method, however, is an inescapably adultomorphic cast to the conception of the primary process. As I have argued in Chapter 10, there are many reasons for supposing that primary-process thinking itself undergoes considerable developmental change, though Freud's cognitive-developmental theory is well summarized in the last-quoted passage: The (presumably unchanging) primary process is gradually replaced, in conscious thought, by the secondary process (also conceived as essentially unchanging).

One piece of internal evidence that, even when he conceived of the primary process as the primitive mode of psychic functioning, Freud modeled it on adult dream work is the fact that he does not mention diffuseness, vagueness, or fluidity among its defining properties. Most students of children's thinking are impressed by these qualities, and by the slippery flightiness that makes it so difficult to approach the young child by methods that are designed for work with adults—including the Rorschach test. Freud was of course quite familiar with these elusive structural properties in dreams, even though his own, as reported in *The Interpretation of Dreams*, rarely have much vagueness or fluid unspecifiability. Where he does discuss such properties, he says that they are a means of conveying a content—for example, that it is *unclear* who is the father of a baby (1900a, pp. 329–333)— or that they indicate a failure in the synthetic function of secondary revision, which he usually interprets as being motivated by resistance and defense: "*. . . there is an intimate and regular relation between the unintelligible and confused nature of dreams and the difficulty of reporting the thoughts behind them*" (1901a, p. 643). The more obscure and confused a dream appears to be, the greater the share in its construction which may be attributed to the factor of displacement (1901a, p. 655). Finally, ". . . in the case of obscure and confused dreams . . . The wish . . . is either itself a repressed one and alien to consciousness, or it is intimately connected with repressed thoughts and is based upon them" (1901a, p. 674). To the best of my knowledge, nowhere does he say that vagueness or confusion are simply properties of primitive thought or of the primary process itself.

A DIGRESSION ON PERCEPTION AND COGNITION

It is important at this point for us to focus on a difference between Freud's and contemporary usage and theory. When Freud spoke about thinking or thought processes, he did not include perception, whereas we are likely to use the more general term, cognition, which often is construed to include perceptual processes, since in practice they can hardly be distinguished from thinking. Like his contemporaries in psychology and psychiatry alike, Freud assumed as a matter of course that perception is a simple matter of coming into contact with reality. We owe to Piaget (e.g., 1937) the phrase "the *construction* of reality," and so successful was the "New Look" movement in cognitive psychology during the years following World War II that psychologists now take it for granted that perceiving is an active process in which a person's motivational and structural properties play an intrinsic part. Ironically, the earliest and most extreme version of the New Look "viewed perception as expressing solely wish or need fulfillment. . . . This guideline was based on a vulgarized version of Freud's message" (Klein, 1970, p. 7). The enthusiasts for a dynamic theory of perception did not notice that Freud made the prevailing assumption of "immaculate perception," that distortions are introduced subsequent to a veridical input of sensory images.[6] Those who tried to make experimental demonstrations of "perceptual defense" rarely quoted Freud directly, even though he had described denial (or "disavowal," as it is translated in the *Standard Edition*) in ways that made it sound like a perceptual process. No one seemed to notice that when he discussed "disavowal of reality," he usually made it not a part of seeing but subsequent to it. For example, "when a little boy first catches sight of a girl's genital region . . . he sees nothing or disavows what he *has seen*" (1925j, p. 252; emphasis added); and "They disavow the fact and believe that they *do* see a penis, all the same" (1923e, pp. 143-144).

This position was quite consistent with the one he had earlier adopted toward the perceptual disturbances of hysterics, which were among the most prominent symptoms of that condition in the earliest years of Freud's practice: ". . . hysterically blind people are only blind as far as consciousness is concerned; in their unconscious they see" (1910i, p. 212). That is, there is no disturbance in their basic processes of contacting reality, only in their becoming conscious of the input.

Even when he discussed the disavowal of reality by psychotics, Freud did not consider the possibility that the perceptual process itself was distorted. He began his paper *The Loss of Reality in Neurosis and Psychosis* (Freud, 1924e) by noting that in psychosis the ego "withdraws from a piece of reality," a metaphorical statement that leaves the nature of the process as unclear as it had been in his earlier paper on the same topic (Freud, 1924b). He ended that brief note by asking what was the "mechanism, analogous to repression . . . by which the ego detaches itself from the external world. . . . such a mechanism, it would seem, must, like repression, comprise a withdrawal of the cathexis sent out by the ego" (p. 153). That was equivalent to saying that the psychotic loses interest in, not perceptual contact with, external reality; in the later paper he added: ". . . neurosis does not disavow the reality, it only ignores it; psychosis disavows it and tries to replace it" (1924e, p. 185). The replacement takes place "by the creation of a new reality which no longer raises the same objections as the old one" (p. 185). It becomes clear that this "new reality" is not perceptual but a delusional construction when he says: "Thus the psychosis is also faced with the task of procuring for itself perceptions of a kind which shall correspond to the new reality" (p. 186), adding the probability that "in a psychosis the rejected piece of reality constantly forces itself upon the mind. . . ." Thus, in the one context where he talks about the "creation" of a reality, it is clearly a "new, imaginary external world" (1924e, p. 187) defensively put in the place of the real world, which nevertheless continues to intrude via the (presumably still functioning) perceptual apparatus.

In his paper *Fetishism*, Freud (1927e) makes it crystal clear that disavowal is not a perceptual process. He considers the situation in which "the boy refused to take cognizance of his having perceived that a woman does not possess a penis" (p. 153). First, he distinguishes *Verleugnung* (disavowal) from *Verdrängung* (repression) by limiting the latter to affect and applying the former to "the vicissitude of the idea." He goes on to criticize Laforgue's (1926) term "scotomization" as

> particularly unsuitable, for it suggests that the perception is entirely wiped out, so that the result is the same as when a visual impression falls on the blind spot in the retina. In the situation we are considering, on the contrary, we see that the perception has persisted, and that a very energetic action has been undertaken to maintain the disavowal. (pp. 153–154)

(Again, in the *Outline*, Freud spoke of the "*disavowal* of the perceptions" [1940a, p. 204]. He even postulated a splitting of the ego in cases of extensive disavowal, such that one part maintains the original perception and related ideas while the other maintains a contrary belief system (1940e).

Let me summarize the conception of perceiving that is implicit in Freud's various incidental remarks, after noting that only in the unpublished "Project for a Scientific Psychology" (1950 [1895]) did he undertake any substantial theorizing about this topic. A fundamental consideration, which Freud returned to many times, was his conviction (following Breuer, in his theoretical chapter in their joint book [Breuer & Freud, 1895], and the generally received scientific opinion of the day) that consciousness and memory must be attributed to separate parts of the brain, since if neurones retained permanent records of their patterns of excitation (necessary for memory), they could not subserve the observable openness of perceptual consciousness to constant change. Indeed, this physiological/anatomical argument may have been responsible for Freud's persisting assumption that perception is a complete process antecedent to the involvement of memory, motivation, or other influences.

Anyhow, here is his notion of how perceiving takes place: An external stimulus in the form of physical energy impinges on a sensory surface, which reduces it in quantity but transmits its other properties (of which Freud spoke mostly about its "period" or vibratory frequency, but which presumably included its patterning or information content in other respects also) to the nervous system. After 1900, he tended to replace references to nerves and neurones by the term "system *Pcpt.*," partly because of the tangle he got into in 1895 and the following year or two in attempting to specify a neurological theory of perception and of consciousness. Some of the time, he postulated separate systems for the latter two functions; for example:

Excitatory material flows in to the *Cs.* sense-organ from two directions: from the *Pcpt.* system, whose excitation, determined by qualities, is probably submitted to a fresh revision before it becomes a conscious sensation, and from the interior of the apparatus itself [systems *Ucs.* and *Pcs.*], whose quantitative processes are felt qualitatively in the pleasure–unpleasure series . . . (1900a, p. 616)

At other times, he identified them (e.g., in the footnote to p. 541, added in 1919: "*Pcpt.* = *Cs.*"; ". . . the system *Pcpt.-Cs.* . . . is turned towards the external world, it is the medium for the perceptions arising thence, and during its functioning the phenomenon of consciousness arises in it" [1933a, p. 75]). The inconsistency was characteristic, as was Freud's tendency to speak at times as if perceptions arise in the sense organs themselves. The separation is implied in his conception that perceptions could exist in a veridical but nonconscious form, as in hysterical anesthesia.

In one of Freud's earliest unpublished discussions of these matters (the letter to Fliess of December 6, 1896), he takes from the beginning a developmental standpoint:

> . . . I am working on the assumption that our psychical mechanism has come into being by a process of stratification: the material present in the form of memory-traces being subjected from time to time to a *re-arrangement* in accordance with fresh circumstances—to a *re-transcription.* . . .
> I should like to emphasize the fact that the successive registrations represent the psychical achievement of successive epochs of life. (1896, pp. 233, 235)

Then he sets up the precursor of the picket-fence model of Chapter VII, a linear diagram proceeding from *W* ("neurones in which perceptions originate, to which consciousness attaches"), through *Wz* ("the first registration of the perceptions; it is quite incapable of consciousness, and arranged according to associations by simultaneity"), *Ub* ("the second registration" arranged perhaps according to causal relations, perhaps corresponding to "conceptual memories"), *Vb* ("the third transcription, attached to word-presentations and corresponding to our official ego"; unlike the preceding, these can attain a "secondary *thought-consciousness* . . . probably linked to the hallucinatory activation of word-presentations") and finally to *Bews* (evidently *Bewusstsein*, consciousness, though he does not say so).[7]

Perception is too evanescent to give us an integrated picture of reality; that must be attained through an organization of memory traces. It is easy for us to overlook this fact about Freud's thinking when he speaks about the "loss of reality" in neurosis and psychosis, for example; the reality that is disavowed is this internal construct within the realm of verbal memory, not reality as directly perceived. As Schimek (1975) points out, here is where Freud located the distorting effects of drives, not in perception. It is important to grasp this distinction between a veridical or autonomous perceptual process and a vulnerable process of forming an inner world (Hartmann, 1939) or vision of reality (Schafer, 1976). If Freud was a child of his time in retaining the "conflict-free" notion of perception, he led the way to our greatly broadened and deepened contemporary view of cognition in recognizing the distorting effects of wishes and defenses on this second stage of constructing an enduring picture of reality. And notice that Freud assumed some such construction of a reality in memory early in (preverbal) development, though he implied more than he ever explicated about the changing nature of the world of the child corresponding to the several systems of registrations ("at least three, probably more" [1896, p. 234]). Here is a basis in Freud's words for a Piagetian conception of successive stages in the child's construction of reality. But Freud, unlike Piaget, treated perception as invariant, undergoing no such successive developmental changes as memory.

It should not surprise us, therefore, to find Freud attributing clear, differentiated, veridical, adult perception to the infant, which could supply the baby with the grist for his distorting primary processing in the *Mnem.* [memory] systems, the *Ucs.*, or the id. And indeed he did very plainly assume precisely that—for example, in the "Project" when he was discussing wishful memory in the nursing infant:

> Let us suppose . . . that the mnemic image wished for . . . is the image of the mother's breast and a front view of its nipple, and that the first perception is a side view of the same object, without the nipple. In the child's memory there is an experience, made by chance in the course of sucking, that with a particular head-movement the front image turns into the side image. The side image which is now seen leads to the [image of the] head-movement; an experiment shows that its counterpart must be carried out, and the perception of the front view is achieved. (1950 [1895], pp. 328–329)

Not only did Freud think of the infant as capable of highly differentiated and realistic perception, but he attributed to the nursling a reversibility of thought processes that Piaget, by actual observations, found only in children several years older. But then, Freud was willing to attribute adultomorphic secondary-process thinking even to a simple, primitive organism:

> Let us imagine ourselves in the situation of an almost entirely helpless living organism, as yet unoriented in the world, which is receiving stimuli in its nervous substance. This organism will very soon be in a position to make a first distinction and a first orientation. On the one hand, it will be aware of stimuli which can be avoided by muscular action (flight); these it ascribes to an external world. On the other hand, it will also be aware of stimuli against which such action is of no avail and whose character of constant pressure persists in spite of it; these stimuli are the signs of an internal world, the evidence of

instinctual needs. The perceptual substance of the living organism will thus have found in the efficacy of its muscular activity a basis for distinguishing between an 'outside' and an 'inside'. (1915c, p. 119)

I want to underline the fact that, in thinking of perception as a straightforward, almost mechanical process by which any percipient organism comes into contact with the objective structure of reality, Freud agreed with the prevailing psychological outlook of his time.[8] Before approximately the last 50 years, psychologists were remarkably uninterested in perception and slow to go beyond the astonishingly varied discoveries of Helmholtz. As to child psychology, as recently as 40 years ago an authoritative manual (Carmichael, 1946) not only contained no chapter on perceptual development but had only a couple of index references to any aspect of perception. One of these is to the hypothesis that childish mispronunciations of words are attributable to "crude perception," not further specified (p. 493); the other is to a section on perceptual learning, which turns out to be a summary of experiments on problem solving, some of which required perceptual reorganization. None of the research cited antedates Köhler's (1917) celebrated demonstration of insightful learning in apes, which seems to have been its principal stimulus, and the major focus of all this subsequent research seems to have been on learning, not perception. Surely during Freud's scientifically formative years, the last quarter of the 19th century, developmental psychology paid no attention to the seemingly inaccessible perceptual worlds of children. And that was the era of anthropomorphic comparative psychology, in which it was a prevalent assumption that other animals perceived the world essentially as we do (Boring, 1929, pp. 472-476).

To go back a moment: When I began this bit of hypothetical reconstruction of how Freud may have arrived at the concept of the primary process, the point was to demonstrate that some preconceptions guided Freud in his choice of its limiting and defining properties. So far we have seen the following implicit assumptions: (1) the assumption of naive realism—that all percipient organisms naturally and easily form phenomenal copies of external reality merely by being exposed to it, though young human beings, at least, also tend to distort the veridical input, for reasons yet to be discussed; (2) the assumption of a single kind of reality, namely the kind Freud himself and his mentors reported—a notably Euclidian, Apollonian world of pellucid air, clean sunlight, and crisply articulated, differentiated forms moving against stable backgrounds (in which the real always had the property of simple location, and object constancy was complete and reliable); (3) the assumption that young children, psychotics, and all of us in course of constructing dreams subject these veridical inputs to distortions in processing them internally, through operations Freud denoted as primary process.[9] Finally, I am suggesting also the possibility that a kind of latent esthetic criterion may have directed Freud's attention differentially to attractively interesting transforms (or what appear to be transforms) of adult percepts, concepts, and trains of thought.

THE PHENOMENAL REFERENTS OF THE TERM "PRIMARY PROCESS"

Part of what I hope to have shown is that the factual basis for the concept of the primary process was quite diffuse, being *any cognitive or perceptual product that seemed for whatever reason to be the result of a distorting transformation.* That is, wherever the inferred cognitive processing fell short of the secondary-process ideal *and* any of the output seemed to violate reasonable expectations by appearing in some way unrealistic, quantitatively and—especially—qualitatively changed, Freud's first insight was to notice a similarity with other such products and to group them together. The collection became highly diverse, to say the least: dreams, delusions, and hallucinations; the peculiar or even bizarrely incomprehensible speech and drawings of insane persons and those suffering from deliria due to fever or drugs; the unrealistic myths and folk tales of "primitive" peoples; the play and imaginative chatter of children; works by the creators of all types of plastic and literary art; all sorts of neurotic symptoms—alloplastic as well as autoplastic; jokes and witticisms; slips of the tongue and a whole range of other parapraxes or errors; and almost any manifestation of psychological defenses.

Moreover, as time went on, Freud included even more in his concept. A thought product might appear quite ordinary, logical, and realistic; but if its producer were submitted to psychoanalysis and furnished the analyst with "associations" (further thoughts or other products stimulated by elements of the material under scrutiny), Freud could often find exactly the kinds of linkages he had originally traced in analyzing dreams as the defensive distortion of wishful fantasies, fears, or longings. Just as the work of secondary revision (the only secondary-process part of the dream work) at times smoothed out every telltale indicator of condensation and displacement in the manifest dream, so in the silent, subsurface phase of its generation a thought might have undergone primary condensations and displacements and still end up as unimpressively ordinary and reasonable. Freud and other analysts (notably Kubie, 1954) came at last to believe that there is an incessant stream of unconscious or preconscious ideation, often accompanying conscious secondary-process thought and lending it color, idiosyncrasy, and emphasis even though it might not transgress the socially defined bounds of rationality and realism. Such a conception, attractive though it may be in its bold sweep and its capacity to explain many observations, cannot be given satisfactory empirical test. It can neither be proved nor disproved, which state of affairs relegates it to the status of a scientific curiosity or even that of a wholly negligible triviality.

Where, then, are we left in our search for the *facts* about the primary process? If it is entirely inferred, susceptible only of being constructed to fill a felt gap in a scientific theory of thinking, then we seem to be in hard straits. For the sad fact is that we never know and never *can* know all the inputs to this hypothetical process. We must construct most of them, as well as the nature of the transformations they have assumedly undergone, from meager and in many ways suspect data: usually a cognitive product such as a dream text or the recountal of a pattern of acting out, plus whatever else the patient says in some conjunction with the critical material (e.g., occurring in the same analytic hour) or as a response to the request, "Tell me what you think of next." At times, but not often enough, the analyst has some independent corroboration of facts as alleged by the analysand, or may even offer his own hypotheses about presumably related or contributory data when the patient is notably silent about facts known to both of them. (For example, an analysand's dream may contain classic birth symbols, while he fails to mention the analyst's obviously perceptible pregnancy.) Even the Pötzl experiment or other experimental attempts to influence dream imagery by precisely known presleep presentations fail to provide satisfactory information about input (see Fisher, 1960a). Fisher's papers (e.g., 1954, 1957) contain many plausible and ingenious reconstructions of his subjects' dreams, the day's residues for which included far more than the briefly exposed slide (e.g., things seen on the trip from the ward to the experimental room), but also far less than the full contents of the slide itself. Sometimes pictorial content expressly chosen for its suitability to the safe indirect or allusive depiction of the patient's known problems gave no sign of having ever been admitted to preperceptual processing, much less used in constructing the dream's imagery. Clinical research would be much easier if people only weren't so ornery!

I think it is safe to hazard that in the ordinary, reasonably successful psychoanalysis, most dreams are analyzed either not at all or in the most fragmentary way. If an analyst can find a single useful linkage or hypothetical connection between something in the dream and anything in the rest of what the patient says, he or she is doing well enough, and training analysts generally warn against zealous attempts at complete analysis of any dream.

Let me press this point home quite sharply: If you cannot independently establish what all the inputs and outputs of a hypothetical process are, you can have *no* certainty that any one theory of the intervening processes is superior to any of a great many others. Formally, the situation is analogous to the attempt to solve a set of simultaneous equations with too many unknowns. Or consider the famous black box problem. You are given a black box with some wires leading in and others leading out. You may not open the box or do anything other than put signals in and measure what comes out, but must determine how it is wired inside. A hard enough task, but think how much more difficult if your data consist of a large number of values, *some* of which probably are a subset of the inputs, and you have to decide even that from a study of the outputs! This is indeterminacy with a vengeance.

A SCHEME FOR SCORING
PRIMARY-PROCESS MANIFESTATIONS

Fortunately, however, Freud did not restrict his usage of the term "primary process" to inferred transformations, but also used it to refer to certain kinds of thought products. As Gill put it:

> Consistent with his distrust of formal definitions, Freud was not concerned to provide even a complete theoretical or conceptual definition of primary process, much less an explicit operational definition. Yet in his writings about dream work, joke work, and symptom formation he was concrete enough to enable the clinician to know how to use the concept of primary process in regard to specific thought products. (1967, p. 265)

As I noted earlier, I used these works in setting up rules for identifying specific kinds of thought products—Rorschach responses—that might be called manifestations of the primary process. Because I was working with ordinary Rorschach protocols, without the benefit of "associations" from which to attempt a reconstruction of the processes by which each came about, I excluded all categories that implied such highly judgmental inferences. Nevertheless, I was able to find 60 specific types of primary-process manifestations. One-third of them define various types and levels of wishfulness, as I now call it, though my original intent was to write operational definitions of degrees of neutralization. That last term was Hartmann's (1964) generalization and extension of Freud's idea of sublimation of libido, as a qualitative change in the psychic energy generated by the sexual instinct. He also linked this economic concept to the secondary process, as did Rapaport (1951a), making explicit what was implied but never baldly stated[10] by Freud, that marked wishfulness of thinking was a hallmark of the primary process. Freud came this close: ". . . *a normal train of thought is only submitted to abnormal psychical treatment* [i.e., the primary process] *. . . if any unconscious wish, derived from infancy and in a state of repression, has been transferred on to it*" (1900a, p. 598). Taking Freud quite seriously, I have proceeded as if the presence of verbally expressed wishes of the kind usually considered to be infantile or repressed is a criterion for calling the thought product primary process in nature. I made the simplifying assumption that the libidinal and aggressive wishes Freud described in his writings on instinct theory were all I needed to worry about. (It has recently occurred to me that the wishes to be taken care of and to be a grownup without having to wait are probably good candidates that were omitted; but no great harm has been done by their omission because they are rarely perceptible in Rorschach responses, except in overtly oral forms, which *are* picked up.) Finally, it seemed evident that something more than a dichotomy (infantile vs. adult) was called for, particularly since there were so many socially acceptable, relatively unthreatening, and therefore not repressed manifestations of orality, anality, voyeurism, sadism, and the rest of them. So I called the more primitive, raw, and blatant forms of these wishes, which one would ordinarily expect to be repressed, Level 1 primary process, and the more socialized forms Level 2 primary process.

The other 40 categories are structural or formal manifestations of the primary process: types of condensation, displacement, symbolization, contradiction, and other miscellaneous kinds of distortion of perception or verbalization. My scoring manual requires 37 pages to define and exemplify these formal indications that the primary process has been at work; here I can hope to do no more than suggest the organization of the manual and the nature of the scoring by the following extract, which presents about half of the material concerning one category, Composition. (Its scoring symbol is "C-co 1"; the first letter indicates that it is a form of Condensation, and the final digit classifies it as one of the more blatant, unsocialized, or direct manifestations of the primary process, which are called Level 1.)

COMPOSITION: Freud (e.g., 1900[a], p. 320) used this term to refer to one result of condensation—an image that is a composite of parts that do not actually belong together in nature. We distinguish two types, depending on whether there is some external social support or precedent for the resulting unrealistic image. Distinguish carefully from C-a-c 2, Arbitrary Combination: in both types of responses reality is violated in that they bring together what does not belong together in literal reality. The difference, however, is that when this combination results in something with an organic unity or an unbroken boundary, it is considered a Composition, and when the incongruous elements are merely brought into juxtaposition, it is an Arbitrary Combination. Theoretically, it requires more violation of the integrity or object constancy of an image to invade its natural boundaries with a foreign element that is grafted on than merely to bring them into an unusual or even bizarre arrangement, which still respects the identities of the separate images. . . .

   a. *Impossible fusions* (often cross-species): parts from two or more percepts are combined to make a new, hybrid organism. Score *only when* the composite image does *not* have some existence in a common cultural reality (usually people with animal parts or vice versa).
     "Witches—they seem to have tails for some reason"; "dogs—kind of antennae for a tail"; "lady with a paw"; "a rabbit with bat's wings" . . .

   b. *Improbable* (though theoretically conceivable) *fusions*: persons or animals with more parts than necessary (e.g., "a two-headed lobster"; "animal skin, a head at each end"; two-*bodied* caterpillar"). Also, deformities or freaks that can occur in nature, e.g., "female form with hands sticking out of shoulders"; "baby with a moustache"; "men with long, pointed heads" . . .

c. A percept of a face with *parts organized in an unrealistic way*: mouth going vertically, horns next to nostrils, etc.; "face—but the mouth is where the nose should be"; "a mask, with the eyes upside down" (Holt, 1969, pp. 26-28)

I have introduced this much about my scoring scheme to make the following points: (1) It is possible to derive an extensive operational definition of the primary process from Freud's writings, thus to delimit a realm of empirical observations. (2) Since this operational definition is highly differentiated, not global, it is possible to ask how much empirical unity there is in this realm. Otherwise put, do the various specific varieties of the primary process form anything like an internally coherent system of thought?

In search of an answer to that question, let us consider the empirical relationship of the wishful to the structural indications of the primary process in Rorschach responses. If we add together all of a person's scores on the 20 types of wishful content, and all of his scores on the 40 types of structural or formal signs of the primary process, using a miscellaneous assortment of subjects, we can correlate the two arrays of scores. In a group of 305 Rorschachs, from 121 college students and other normals, 81 schizophrenics, and 103 neurotic and organically ill persons, the correlation between these two sums was .71. That is suspiciously high; but even when the inflating influence of the number of Rorschach responses is held constant, the partial correlation is still .50—not only highly significant, but large enough to indicate that it makes sense to consider wishfulness and such structural characteristics as condensation and displacement all part of one concept, the primary process.

Two factor analyses (summarized in Holt, 1966) have been done on some of my principal Rorschach scores, with remarkably congruent results. Heath (1965) analyzed data from a sample of 24 students at Haverford College; Kahn (1965) obtained his data from 43 convicted murderers. Both samples would ordinarily be considered too small to give replicable results, but despite differences in the kinds of other tests besides the Rorschach, in statistical method, and in subjects, the first two factors in each analysis are nevertheless recognizably the same. The first principal factor each time is most highly loaded with percentage of Rorschach responses containing Formal indications of the primary process, and with measures of the amount of the more extreme (Level 1) Content indications (wishfulness). The second factor is mainly defined by measures of intelligence, but also includes a percentage of the more socialized (Level 2) indications, mostly of wishfulness. The implication, I believe, is that Level 1 scores more defensibly indicate the primary process, while I may have encroached on the realm of the secondary process in my definitions of Level 2 scores, particularly those of Content indications. Otherwise, however, the statistical explorations of the various categories and scores derived from them support the proposition that Freud's descriptions of the empirical varieties of primary-process products (as applied to Rorschach responses) describe something unitary. His intuition seemingly enabled him to discern in his extremely variegated observations a single conceptual entity, which we might as well continue to call the primary process.

Thanks to the efforts of many of my students and colleagues, there now exists a considerable body of research using my scoring manual as a way of measuring primary-process thought and relating it to an impressive range of other variables. For example, in ten independent studies (most of which are summarized in Holt, 1970), as many different experimenters have used my scoring system and the measures it yields of capacity for regression in the service of the ego to test Kris's (1952) hypothesis that that capacity is a necessary condition for artistic creativity. In a variety of different samples, using several criteria of creativeness, male subjects have yielded fairly consistently positive results, though female subjects have not.

I am glad to be able to say that there has been some theoretical yield, too, from about a quarter of a century of part-time empirical work on the problem of measuring the primary process, though it is of a rather negative kind. I am not speaking now about metapsychology, but about what might be called the clinical theory of thinking—lower-level statements about the primary process and related matters. Time and again, I sought in vain for theoretical guidance about decisions that had to be made: What kinds of wishes should be included in the content measure of what I originally called "drive-dominated thought"? As long as I didn't question the dual-instinct theory, it seemed easy enough: anything sexual or libidinal in terms of the classical stages of psychosexual development, plus anything aggressive. Now that I have taken a hard look at the motivational theory of psychoanalysis and have found it wanting (see Chapter 7, this volume), I do not believe that it can any longer be considered a reliable guide.

The two degrees or levels of primary-process scores, alluded to above, embody a distinction that has proved useful, though it is quite without theoretical backup of more than the most general kind. These two levels dichotomize a continuum of control or socialization, concepts about which psychoanalytic theorists have written, though seldom relating them to the primary process. Indeed, the whole issue of the relation between the primary process and controls and defenses leaves a great deal to be desired in terms of clarity and specificity in the ways it has been discussed, except for a few books and papers like Schafer's (1954, 1958). This issue is important both practically and theoretically, for it is at the heart of the major distinction between adaptive and maladaptive regression: primary-process thinking used "in the service of the ego"—creatively, humorously, playfully, and so on—and the primary process as an indicant of pathological thought disorder.

The lack of specificity in the theory plagued me at every step of constructing the manual, for writing scoring rules means setting boundaries in a world of continuous gradation, and only rarely have I been able to appeal to any criterion other than my own largely intuitive judgment about where to draw lines of definition that say, for example, when an image indicates a homosexual wish. "Two men dancing" is scored as an indication of the primary process if it is social or ballroom dancing, but not if the dance is part of a cultural ritual. If that decision appears arbitrary to you, let me confess that, though I can defend it, it feels all too arbitrary to me also.

When Joan Havel and I were first setting up the categories of formal manifestations of the primary process, we drew heavily on Rapaport's "pathological verbalization" scores from his chapter on the Rorschach (Rapaport et al., 1945–1946), on the grounds that schizophrenic pathology of thought was to be understood as a breakthrough of the primary process into consciousness. Many of his scores correspond nicely with the phenomenological varieties Freud described in his discussion of the dream work and joke work; thus contaminations and fabulized combinations were pretty clearly aspects of condensation, and clang associations were displacements. But what about peculiar, queer, and incoherent verbalizations? These specifically linguistic categories were among the best indicators of schizophrenic thought disorder, yet Freud said nothing about them. They are well correlated with other formal variables, even in samples that exclude schizophrenics, so I have continued to include them, although without theoretical backup.

The relation between the primary process and defenses is a ticklish and difficult one to handle. Gill (1963) showed that some defenses themselves functioned according to principles of the primary process (e.g., displacement in projection), but that they form a hierarchy corresponding to the continuum from the primary to the secondary process. How, then, should we handle a Rorschach response like this one: "Why do you show me these disgusting sexy pictures?" I think that most analysts would entertain the hypothesis that the subject is projecting his sexual wishes onto the blots or the examiner while strongly disclaiming them. I have followed the practice of scoring the remark as an indicator of the primary process because of the sexual wish (scored L 1 S), treating the rest of it as indicating a pathological attempt at control of that wish (Prj–) and letting the implicit displacement go unscored. Again, I can defend the decision, but wish that theory provided clearer guidelines.

Despite its premier status in defining the primary process, not all displacement should be scored because of the fact, so well developed by Gill (1967), that there are manifestations of displacement and condensation all along the continuum from the primary to the secondary process. This theoretical development was initially a shock to me, though I quickly recognized in it my familiar problem of distinguishing different levels of condensations and displacements, and of setting limits. It also reminded me that for a long time the only signs of displacement I could find in Rorschach responses were the Control categories of Remoteness, several ways in which a person can make wishful content less close to home (e.g., distant in time, space, level of reality). Such an operation seemed to be the replacement of a crude and direct wishful content by a more socially acceptable, safely controlled one—clearly an instance of secondary-process displacement. But if Freud's own fundamental definition of the primary process were thus to be overturned, what guidance was available?

In the foregoing, I have tried to demonstrate that the term "primary process" has two somewhat different meanings. As an explanatory concept, it employs the apparatus of Freud's metapsychology—psychic structures, forces, and energies—and with the collapse of that conceptual edifice, the corresponding meaning of the primary process has lost its utility. As a descriptive concept, it retains promise and usefulness, even though its empirical referents are in some ways accidental, being based on Freud's personal predilections and on traditions of intellectual culture. Empirical demonstrations (just cited) of a moderate level of interrelationship among its identifiable subparts suggest both that there is something like the separate system of prelogical and wishful thought Freud described, and that more than one such system may exist.

Freud intended his conceptualization of thinking to be mainly a developmental one, but he did not follow through and elaborate it by systematic observations of children at various developmental levels. Overvaluing the economic or energic point of view as he did, he tended to minimize the conception of various developmental stages or systems of thought without entirely abandoning it, and simultaneously put forward the incompatible conceptualization of a continuum of thought from an ideal type of the primary process to an opposite, secondary-process pole. In doing so, he was wavering between two very general developmental models: the *phasic* (the conception that growth takes place mainly through a succession of internally integrated stages) and the *linear* (the conception that growth is mainly a matter of steady, small increments).

I believe that internal requirements of psychoanalytic theory make the following definition—which entails the linear model—the most satisfactory, and it is the one on which my scoring system for the Rorschach is based. It starts from the position that the primary process must be defined in terms of Freud's (1911b) two principles of mental functioning.

> Thus, the more thought (and also affect and behavior) can be characterized as an unrealistic seeking for immediate gratification, the more it is to be considered primary process . . . And the more thought or behavior is organized by adaptive considerations of efficiency in the search for *realistic* gratification, the more it approximates the ideal of secondary process . . . (Holt, 1967d, p. 294 n.)

The logic of the system seemed to leave this as the most consistent definition, but it does raise difficult questions. Does the reality principle actually imply clear logical structure as well as respect for the consensually established structure of reality? If the primary process is a joint function of wishfulness and unrealism, what do you do with discrepant cases—thought products that contain manifestly wish-related content but that are neither illogical nor inconsistent with reality? What about the reverse case, when a thought product shows no sign of wishful content but does fall short of secondary-process standards of logic and realism? In general, I have treated either criterion as sufficient, but once again drawing boundaries has been problematic.

In particular, several difficult issues are raised by the lack of clear theoretical guidelines for the classification of thought products as primary process on the basis of their formal properties, though they boil down to one question: Just because a form of thought is *not* unimpeachably secondary process in nature, is it necessarily primary process? Gill (1967) put it in the form of this question: Are there other mechanisms of the primary process besides condensation and displacement? He was able, to his own satisfaction, to reduce to condensation or displacement all other possibilities that had been suggested, including plastic representation, concretization, contradiction, symbolization, autistic logic, fragmentation, and timelessness. More precisely, he said:

> If condensation and displacement as Freud described them in the dream work are seen as the characterization of id functioning from the economic point of view, the "other" characteristics of id functioning are the result of looking at such functions from the several other metapsychological points of view. (1967, p. 294)

At the time, that seemed to me a good resolution. Since then, however, I have realized that it leaves us with only two distasteful alternatives in defining the limits of what is to be considered primary process: We can stick to the argument by authority, accepting everything that Freud said in describing unconscious and id functioning and nothing but what he said, or we can open the floodgates to all possible deviations from perfection. Partly, the hidden villain in the piece is the innocent-appearing proposition that the primary process and the secondary process are not really systems of thought, but hypothetical endpoints of a continuum. The trouble with that comes when you start describing real thought products and try to locate them with any degree of precision on the continuum. There turn out to be at least two continua to begin with, one of wishfulness and one of efficiency or realism; and the attempt to formulate the latter suggests that it be divided into at least two more continua, consistency with reality (as consensually defined) and logical clarity.

Just as soon as you go from the theoretical level to the practical one of classifying actual thought products, you find that even three continua are not enough. For example, I have felt the need for four rated continua: Defense Demand [the degree to which a response is unacceptable as a social communication], Defense Effectiveness, Form Level, and Creativity of Response. And none of the last three correspond directly to realism or clarity of logical structure! Further, consider Defense Demand: Is it tenable to take the position, as I have in my scoring manual, that a response should be considered a primary-process manifestation merely because it contains evidence of wishfulness that is so socialized and attenuated as not to raise an eyebrow at a polite tea party? "Please, may I have a cup of tea?" is surely such a remark, yet it obviously meets the scoring criteria for the expression of an oral wish, for rather immediate gratification.

You may counter that the problem here is that I am not taking the continuum idea seriously enough, but insisting on applying an outmoded dichotomy. Is it really outmoded? Do we not constantly see clinical and research evidence that there is something like a special system of thought that operates in dreams, symptoms, and disordered thinking generally? I believe that we do, and that the situation is exactly analogous to another paradox, the antithesis between typology and dimensional scaling in the field of personality assessment. Consider Loevinger's (1966, 1976) developmental types for a moment: They consist of configurations of traits, many of which have been traditionally measured as separate continua, and which can continue to be so treated despite the evidence that they are empirically clustered in a theoretically intelligible fashion. When she proposed meaningful and factually based developmental types or clusters, that introduced a welcome order into the bewildering diversity of personality description, with its hundreds of continuously varying, arbitrarily bounded traits. Is not something of the same sort possible in the realm of thought?

Surely there is a great need for a typology comprising *several* systems or forms of thought in addition to the primary and secondary processes. The concept of the primary process was eagerly seized by psychopathologists, since it seemed to formulate so well the thought disorder of schizophrenia. Yet, as Rapaport et al. (1945-1946) showed empirically, Freud's concept did not provide any help in clarifying theoretically the differences among various kinds of thought disorders in mania, in depression, and in schizophrenia, or even in distinguishing psychosis from neurosis: All are "breakthroughs" of the primary process. Similarly, it is all very well to say that "the child" thinks with the primary process, "the adult" with the secondary; but does that mean that only quantitative differences may be found in thinking at different developmental levels? Psychoanalytic theory provides for nothing more.

In the first attempt to apply my scoring scheme to thought products other than Rorschach responses, Goldberger (1961; see also Goldberger &

Holt, 1958) found it possible to use the manual's criteria of the primary process in rating the free verbal productions of subjects kept in perceptual isolation (sensory deprivation) for eight hours. His ratings and mine attained a satisfactory degree of interjudge reliability, however, only after we made a further distinction. We were troubled by the fact that much of what his subjects said was vague, or concrete, or substandard in terms of grammar or rhetoric, or incomplete, or otherwise intellectually *déclassé*, without meeting any standard criteria of the primary process. We decided, therefore, to classify and scale these as forms of *regressed secondary process*, which we were able to distinguish from both well-controlled and poorly controlled primary process, and then to rate all three with reliabilities of about .9.

Once I had admitted the idea that there was regression from the secondary process not to the primary process but to developmentally earlier forms of everyday thinking, I began to have doubts about some of my "miscellaneous" formal signs of the primary process, like physiognomic responsiveness or the intrusion of irrelevancies—were they primary process or regressed forms of the secondary process? Psychoanalytic theory again gave no guidance, and the question remains unanswered.

From what I have presented so far, I hope to have made it clear that, in its present state, the theory of the primary process is in sad disarray. Its empirical referents are only generally specified, too imprecisely to give firm guidance to concrete attempts at measurement. Taken either as a low-level clinical theory or in its higher-level metapsychological guise, it is fundamentally lacking. As usual, Freud's clinical intuition had a good deal of validity, and his ideas about thinking have had both clinical and research utility, but they badly need reformulation.

PART V

Critical Reflections on Psychoanalytic Theory as a Whole

CHAPTER 12

The Death and Transfiguration
of Metapsychology

This overall critique of metapsychology was first presented as the Sandor Rado Lecture to the Center for Psychoanalytic Training and Research of Columbia University, New York City, on April 20, 1978. I began it, therefore, with a brief review of my own relationship to psychoanalytic theory and the remark that Rado, whose memory was being honored, had gone through something of the same kind of odyssey—

from an initial orthodoxy to a phase of increasing criticalness to an attempt at a radical revision of the theory while holding fast to the basic discoveries and fundamental insights. How much more difficult it must have been for him, who was Freud's friend, colleague, and spokesman! Yet even before his master's death he was able to give public voice to a dissatisfaction with the theory of instincts and its scientific shortcomings, and stated his conviction that the factual findings of psychoanalysis needed to be disentangled from non-empirical, speculative elements. He went on to formulate in broad outlines an alternative conceptualization, adaptational psychodynamics, marked by a common-sense organismic orientation and a strong sense of the person's biological rootedness. All this he managed to achieve without the kind of dramatic break with mainstream psychoanalysis that characterized so many others who began by criticizing from within the movement and ended by attempting to set up rival schools that repudiated much of the factual substance of psychoanalysis. To the end of his life Rado proclaimed himself an adherent of Freudian psychoanalysis while attempting "to prepare the ground for a comprehensive theory of the dynamics of human behavior that will correlate psychodynamics with physiology and genetics" (Rado, 1962, p. 107).

I added that I had "prepared these remarks in that same spirit," and continued:

Theoretical work in psychoanalysis presents many difficulties and frustrations. It takes much time and a surprising amount of effort. One has to stay for long times at an uncomfortably high level of abstract thinking. It cannot be done at all by committees, and the number of productive collaborative pairs of theoretical workers in psychoanalysis and psychology is extremely small. Therefore, theorizing gets bound up with individual ambitions and struggles for recognition, which leads to polemical attacks and angry defense; often the level of debate sinks, beneath the weight of so much emotion and threatened self-esteem.

No wonder, then, that progress is slow. The latent emotional content of many theoretical positions again and again causes antagonists to caricature one another's positions and waste time trouncing synthetic opponents. Alternatively, how vulnerable we are to wishful belief that novel proposals may be at last embodiments of Truth! I confess to having embraced psychoanalytic metapsychology, as presented by David Rapaport, in this spirit, and after a long, painful disillusionment to have come near to committing the same kind of error in overestimating the potentialities of general systems theory. Elsewhere (Holt, 1978b) I picture it not only as the embodiment of an emerging scientific world view that is replacing the reductionistic mechanism of scientific materialism, but as perhaps the hoped-for alternative to metapsychology. A year after having written it, I believe that my enthusiasm was excessive, and that my eagerness to believe was too much determined by a longing to discover that someone already has the answer. Instead of adopting a ready-made theory, we have to tailor our own, and that means starting with a re-examination of basic theoretical issues. So, instead of presenting a new theory now, I mean to discuss some fundamentals. (Holt, 1981a, pp. 129–130)

A decade later, I still do not have a comprehensive new theory, but the need for a critical re-examination of fundamentals seems as necessary as ever.

The present situation of psychoanalytic theory is, in two words, confused and confusing. Many people consider metapsychology dead or at least in a terminal phase with no hope of recovery, while others maintain that it is as clinically useful as ever and that they have every intention of continuing to use it. Still others concede the need for some revisions, though not of a very radical kind. Within the camp of the theory's severe critics, there is a sharp split between one group who are at work on a variety of possible substitutes for metapsychology and another who are content to be rid of it and who see no need for a replacement.

Beneath all this diversity may be discerned some strikingly different positions on basic methodological issues: Is psychoanalysis a science or one of the humanities, like history? If a science, is it or can it be a natural science or should it be a social/behavioral science, and what is the difference? Does it have one theory or two? If two, how do they differ and what is the relation between them? What relations should obtain between psychoanalysis and adjacent sciences—the biological disciplines on one hand, the social and cultural ones on the other? Some perplexity about how to proceed with our common theoretical task may be alleviated if we can sort out the grounds of disagreement, determine the varieties of unspoken premises along with the declared programs, and eliminate disagreement based on mutual misunderstanding or on clearly fallacious starting points.

THE DISCIPLINARY STATUS OF PSYCHOANALYSIS

I shall begin by stating in rather bald outline the major contemporary answers to two questions: What kind of discipline can and should psychoanalysis be? Should it be one theory or two? There seem to be four major positions on the first issue:

One group of theoreticians says that psychoanalysis is and should remain a natural science. Freud believed that, I think, and generally wrote about it that way. Since he never discussed the possibility that there might be more than one kind of science, he did not specifically classify it as a natural science, though I believe it clear from context that that is how he thought of it. Hartmann (1964) explicitly aligned psychoanalysis with the natural sciences, as do many other conservative analysts today; among the innovators, Peterfreund (1971) clearly takes this stance.

A second group holds that psychoanalysis is a science, but of some other sort than the objective, natural sciences, perhaps one of the social/behavioral sciences. Gill (1976, 1977) is a prominent spokesman for this viewpoint; he writes, for example, "to argue that psychoanalysis is not a natural science is not to argue that it is not a science. Natural-science dimensions are not the only ones in which the canons of science can be employed" (Gill, 1977, p. 594).

A third position is that psychoanalysis is one of the humanistic or hermeneutic disciplines, not a science at all—clearly the position of Home (1966). Schafer (1976) comes very close to such an assertion, though he mostly contents himself with denying that psychoanalysis can be a natural science without explicitly locating his alternative, action language, among types of intellectual disciplines. Binswanger and other existential analysts, he points out, did proclaim that psychoanalysis was one of the humanities, as do a good many contemporary self-styled humanistic or "third-force" clinical psychologists.

Finally, there are various mixed or combinatory positions, to the effect that psychoanalysis is and should be some combination or amalgam of natural science, social science, and/or a humanistic discipline. Gedo and Pollock's (1975) monograph asserts that Freud's psychoanalysis was a "fusion of science and humanism." In various ways, such theorists as Modell, Brenner, and Wallerstein assert that psychoanalysis should be a comprehensive discipline, refusing to give up either the experiential or the nonexperiential realm and adapting its theories and methods to the peculiar demands of all relevant data.

The question, "Two theories or one?" as my late friend George Klein (1976) posed it, is evidently another way of approaching many of the same issues, at least in part. Even more answers to this question are being voiced today.

There are three kinds of one-theory positions, as I see it.

1. Psychoanalysis is a single theory, in which metapsychological terms are the technical concepts in terms of which clinical observations are conceptualized; or they are merely concepts on a higher level of generality or with broader scope, not different enough from the clinical concepts to be called a separate theory.

2. Psychoanalysis *should* be one theory, a clinical one, even though it is currently saddled with an unnecessary intrusion from natural science, metapsychology. According to Klein and Gill, we should just let metapsychology fade away and get on with the job of extricating the clinical theory from its dying clutches, developing and systematizing our theory of neurosis and treatment into a science of subjective meanings.

3. By abandoning metapsychology and replacing it with a new framework based on information processing and systems theory, we can construct a unitary theory that will encompass the phenomena of body and mind, structure and meaning. The theorists (e.g., Rosenblatt & Thickstun, 1977; Rubinstein, 1975) who go this route deny explicitly or implicitly that differences between meanings and other kinds of data require separate theories.

I am familiar with two groups who maintain that there should be two theories: the followers of Rapaport, who see nothing wrong with maintaining a special or clinical theory *and* a general or metapsychological one; and the followers of Ricoeur (1970), who maintain that psychoanalysis needs a hermeneutics to deal with meanings and an energetics to deal with man's instinctual life—about which more shortly.

IS PSYCHOANALYSIS A SCIENCE?

At this point, I will abandon my posture as impartial outside observer and enter the fray with some opinions and arguments. The underlying difficulty, I believe, is metaphysical: The more one tends, consciously or not, toward a dualistic position on the mind–body problem, the more one will feel that there is an unbridgeable gulf between the subjective and the objective world, between the realm of external physio-chemical fact and that of inner meanings, and thus between science and the humanities. Descartes, who if nothing else was clear and unambiguous, was forthright about it: All of being had to be divided into two fundamentally (i.e., ontologically) different and incommensurate halves—a world of matter, characterized by simple extension in space, which he assigned to science, and a world of the soul, which became the proper province of religion and philosophy. All conscious phenomena were attributable to the activity of man's soul, the *res cogitans* which he considered a substance, too, but without spatial extension. [See also Chapters 6 and 14, this volume.]

Common sense and the lofty authority of Aristotle had agreed for a millennium on a kind of unitary organismic view, pervaded though it was with animism and other primitive conceptions. But no one should underestimate the formidable old French genius and the hold of his ideas on the minds of most generations since his (the 17th) century. Even today it seems obvious to the man in the street that mind and matter are utterly different categories, so that we often hear the incredulous question, "Do you really think you can make a *science* about the human mind?"

Quite a few people since Descartes have thought that they could, notably Fechner, that common father-figure for such diverse disciplines as Freudian psychoanalysis and experimental psychology. Inspired by the surge of *Naturphilosophie*, Fechner saw in the little-known experiments of E. H. Weber a key to unifying matter and mind mathematically. Despite the dichotomous thinking of those who saw quantity and quality as the hallmarks of different worlds and who proclaimed that subjective, qualitative experience could never be quantified, he set about measuring sensations in precise ways and trying to prove them to be quantitatively related to physical dimensions of stimuli. By now psychophysics is one of the most austerely secure enclaves of psychology's conservative establishment, where it is an accomplished fact that a hard-nosed discipline in the natural-science tradition can deal with purely subjective phenomena.

Most psychologists and psychoanalysts I have read and talked to give little thought to the mind–body problem and just can't take it very seriously. "That's metaphysics; leave it to the philosophers," they say. "*We* are concerned with the real world of our experiments or our patients." Under the influence of a vulgarized logical positivism, psychologists may openly declare metaphysics meaningless, or psychoanalysts who have read some of Freud's scornful remarks may join him in confessing that they do not respect this alleged discipline. Nevertheless, and despite the undoubted fact that metaphysics offers no secure answers and no empirical way of settling its disputes, it takes its revenge on those who ignore it. It is of the very nature of the questions metaphysicians tackle that everyone must take some implicit stand on them, and it is dangerous to remain unaware of that fact. Philosophy cannot give you one true solution to the mind–body problem, but it can show you the range of proposed solutions and the implications of each. Psychoanalysts—of all people—should respond positively to the idea that what you don't know *can* hurt you, and that there is a clear gain in expanding our consciousness of matters we are not usually aware of.

As Whitehead (1925) has so persuasively argued, the sciences underwent a rapid growth starting shortly after Descartes and in part freed by his having bifurcated reality. Overwhelmingly, scientific materialism prevailed throughout the 19th century in all the sciences, rather quickly suppressing the romantic scientific trends that were stimulated by *Naturphilosophie*.

Freud absorbed the prevailing scientific ethos at the University of Vienna, despite his earlier love of the humanities and his attraction to the idea of *Naturphilosophie*, which were largely transmitted to him through their literary expression. Thus, though Goethe had been an influential figure in the nature-philosophical movement and had carried out scientific studies in that spirit, it was primarily as a poet that Freud knew and loved him.

In the years when Freud's major orientations were being laid down, the intellectual resources simply did not exist to integrate his interests in natural science on the one hand, and in literature, philosophy, cultural anthropology, and similar disciplines on the other. Instead, in Germany the last couple of decades of the 19th century saw the rise of a serious and extended attempt to develop a separate methodology for the humanities as compared to the sciences. We do not know whether Freud was aware of it; he never mentioned any of the participants (Dilthey, Windelband, and Rickert are the best-known names). They were understandably repelled by the harsh reductionism of contemporary spokesmen for the mechanistic discipline they conceived natural science *necessarily* to be, a conception at once suffocatingly narrow and imperialistic in its arrogant claim to be the only valid way of attaining truth. They proclaimed that the cultural disciplines have their own approach, a fundamentally different one. It sought the *understanding* of *individual* persons, events, and works of art (hence they called it "idiographic"), while science was concerned only with *explaining* by the discovery of *general laws* (hence, it was "nomothetic" or "nomological"). Understanding is an intuitive, empathic process, they wrote. They did not feel it necessary to document their assertions by making any actual study of the working methods of real scientists or humanistic scholars, and failed to distinguish between what many scientists claimed to be doing and what was centrally necessary to science. Thus, asserting that science cannot study an individual, they failed to note that science is defined by its methods, not its subject matter—not to mention overlooking the fact that individuals were being studied in a good many contemporary sciences. Many philosophers of science (notably Polanyi, 1962; see also Sherwood, 1969) have subsequently attacked the false dichotomy between understanding and explaining, showing that these are complementary aims of all scientists and many humanists as well.[1]

In the end, then, the late-romantic reaction against 19th-century scientism failed either to develop a well-reasoned set of logical distinctions between scientific and humanistic disciplines or any distinctive idiographic methods—much less any separate logic—for the humanistic scholar. Yet, to the best of my knowledge, this remains the only major effort to develop a separate methodology for the humanities and/or social sciences. It is easy to find assertions that such a methodology exists, but never with specific citations. For example, "the logic and method of the humanities is radically different from that of science, though no less respectable and rational, and of course much longer established." So writes Home (1966, p. 43), a British philosopher–psychoanalyst whose slight paper would be worth hardly more than a passing glance if it had not been taken seriously and quoted approvingly by a surprising number of recent psychoanalytic writers (e.g., Barratt, 1976; Guntrip, 1967; Klein, 1976; Schafer, 1976; Wallerstein, 1976). I carefully reviewed Home's paper and prepared a summary and rebuttal of his arguments for that reason, but have decided to hold my fire. It is full of undocumented and unargued assertions, some so absurd that I had to struggle with the impulse to ridicule someone who may be a decent person and good analyst even if surely a bad philosopher. Patently, this paper gets cited so much not because of any cogency, but because it says what a lot of our colleagues want to believe. I stress the wishful aspect because in various small ways there are indications that Home believes that the allegedly different, humanistic methods are going to be less exacting, less tedious, and altogether more fun than those of science. Home says, for example, that scientific method demands "that a clear distinction always be maintained between observation and inference, whereas in a humanistic study a clear distinction is demanded only in respect of who is saying what" (pp. 43–44). (Try to sell *that* to any good historian!) And he proclaims that an "interpretation is a new kind of fact," though "Unlike a scientific fact, it cannot be demonstrated." Home seems to reassure those analysts who fail to distinguish observation from inference that they need not worry—the interpretation itself is a basic datum, and empathy is a sufficient method and ultimate criterion for establishing what a patient feels or wants.

One reason this blurry kind of thinking succeeds in being so persuasive, I suggest, is that the 19th century's narrow misconception of a rigorously objective, nomothetic science persists to this day, among some of the loudest self-appointed spokesmen for scientific psychology like Skinner (1971) and Eysenck (1954). They would have us believe that science is a wholly objective business, cold and completely rational, requiring only quantitative precision, with meticulous handling of cut-and-dried facts which are either directly perceived or established by the operation of automatic machines, and put together by unambiguous rules of logic. We clinical psychologists have to live with condescending colleagues of this kind who maintain that science is—can be!—nothing more than the shrunken thing they do, and that psychoanalysis surely cannot be construed as part of it. Polarized oversimplifications are so much easier to make convincing than inherently more ambiguous, middle positions! Even as sophisticated a writer as Schafer (e.g., 1976) falls into this dichotomizing error; he portrays the world of natural science as exclusively dominated by mechanistic, deterministic, reductionistic theories, the only alternative to which is a theory of action in which the actors are spontaneous and their acts uncaused.

In actuality, natural scientists are not lifeless, superobjective, rational machines. They are real people, not so different from you and me, who are passionately and stubbornly devoted to their hunches, which sometimes transparently arise from sources in infantile fantasy and body language, who deeply respect and rely on intuition, whose wishes and feelings and expectations at times intrude on the way they observe and theorize and process data, but who have a method of great power to help them muddle through to an approximate truth.

Listen to this introspective report on his working methods by no less a natural scientist than Einstein.

> Man seeks to form for himself . . . a simplified and lucid image of the world, and so to overcome the world of experience by striving to replace it to some extent by this image. This is what the painter does, and the poet, the speculative philosopher, the natural scientist, each in his own way. . . . To . . . elementary laws . . . there leads no logical path, but only intuition, supported by being sympathetically in touch with experience. (Quoted in Holton, 1973, p. 377)

Some years ago, I made as conscientious an effort as I could to seek out just what were the methods used by colleagues in the humanities and those in the sciences (Holt, 1961). I had to conclude that the similarities were many and striking, and that the few differences I could find were more of degree than of kind.

If we turn from the unprofitable arguments based on a misunderstanding of what scientists actually do, the main arguments adduced by Home and others of his persuasion, including Ricoeur, proceed as follows. Scientific method was developed for the study of objects that cannot communicate with us, and with which we cannot easily identify. It explains in terms of causes, external forces acting on bodies. The psychoanalyst must deal with human beings, who are as alive and human as he is, and he must use his empathic ability to construct hypotheses about why they act the way they do—hypotheses which must be in the form of motives or *reasons* for acting, not external causes. Reasons are meanings; causes are the operation of impersonal agencies without the mediation of understanding and decision. Therefore, there can be no science of meanings.

First, is it true that natural scientists don't deal with meanings? Look over the shoulder of a high-energy physicist at the raw data of observation he deals with—for example, photographs of tracks left in a bubble-chamber by colliding elementary particles. To the untrained mind, they might as well have been left by a gaggle of geese on a barnyard; they are as hard to make sense of as an X-ray or an EEG tracing or a Rorschach test psychogram—to anyone who lacks the requisite technical training. With it, meaningless marks take on a great deal of meaning, and distinctions the layman cannot perceive may become good or bad news.

Some may object that those are not primarily verbal meanings, and still question that the latter can be the data of a true science. Such a position seems to be based on simple ignorance. There are in fact several partly quantitative, relatively rigorous, well-established sciences that take as their data verbal meanings or subjective sensations or both: for example, psychophysics, structural linguistics, and a good deal of social and personality psychology. Before seriously studying psychoanalysis, I worked in survey research, where I learned the demanding discipline of content analysis, the quantitative and qualitative analysis of verbal meanings. Fortunately, the pioneers of that branch of social psychology and sociology did not realize that it had been declared impossible to use the scientific method on verbal meanings, so they went right ahead and did it.

I realize that when many people say that "science doesn't deal with meanings," they do not intend to deny that such operations as recognizing, classifying and counting verbal meanings can be carried out, or even the quantification of information via Shannon's information theory. What they have in mind, I believe, is not such relatively elementary operations, but the *interpretation* of dreams and free associations to elucidate their unconscious meanings. Let me call to your attention that several flourishing research groups are working with exactly this kind of data, and showing that with careful definition of terms, and training at the task, psychoanalysts can independently agree well enough on unconscious meanings. I am thinking particularly of Rubinstein and Dahl, Merton Gill and his colleagues, and the team in San Francisco headed by Weiss and Sampson. Even a list without claims to comprehensiveness must mention the pioneering work of Bellak, and Luborsky, and research teams in Chicago and Topeka. The scientific study of psychoanalysis is not only possible, but has been actively under way for quite some years. If psychoanalysts made it a routine part of their professional training to work on attaining consensus, as workers do in other sciences concerned with ambiguous and demanding kinds of data, such research could make faster progress.

In the end, then, the case against psychoanalysis as a science rests on the distinction between causes and reasons. I could not begin to do justice to all the subtle arguments in the considerable philosophical literature on this topic, even if I had mastered it (which, as the philosophers like to say, is a counterfactual conditional; [see Eagle, 1983]). The very size of the literature shows that what at first seemed a striking and basic difference between science and the humanities, to which one needed only to allude to make a telling point, is not self-evident at all and is indeed highly controversial.

I will content myself with offering my version of one point of view. I am impressed by the great structural similarities in the concepts of reason and cause, enough so that in everyday language we frequently use the terms interchangeably—indeed, dictionaries give each as a synonym of the other. For years, I have operated on the assumption that a reason is one kind of cause, a *psychological* cause, and that various types of causes can be handled in the same study without confusion. Anyone who does clinical work, or teaches students how to gain enough understanding of a person to be able to help him, knows that just because one is a psychoanalyst or a clinical psychologist one is not restricted to a person's reasons for his behavior, whether stated or empathically sensed or rigorously inferred. How can a responsible clinician ignore contributory *causes* of psychiatric disorders, such as poverty, malnutrition, brain damage, genetic defect, or the effects of pharmacological agents—shying away from any such determinants as "somebody else's business" because they are not subjective meanings, or even taking the quixotic position that they can affect mental status not directly but *only* as they are meaningfully interpreted by the patient? Whenever psychoanalysts are confronted by a new patient and have to make realistic predictions of prognosis or analyzability, they probably consider the person's motives for seeking treatment, fantasies about what psychoanalysis is, intellectual limitations, financial situation, place in a family configuration, and state of physical health, and treat this mixture of reasons and causes together in one informal predictive system with no difficulty in principle. So let us stop worrying about the alleged impossibility or logical incoherence of something we do all the time!

It is evident, I hope, how fully I believe that psychoanalysis can be and should be a science as well as a healing art, and perhaps a humanistic discipline also. We do not need to be so particular about specifying just what kind of science it has to be, partly because many of the categories people use are anachronistic, and because philosophers of science by and large do not find deep-going differences between, say, natural and social sciences.

ONE THEORY AND ONE MODEL

As to whether psychoanalysis is or should be one theory or two, I think that the question is wrongly posed. Psychoanalysis is one theory, but sooner or later any good theory needs to be supplemented by one or more models, which are easily mistaken for supernumerary theories. I will expound this position further in just a while, after an attempt to clarify the distinction between "theory" and "model."

First, however, a brief aside about Paul Ricoeur (1970), a French philosopher who has a considerable following among psychoanalysts. His position and his arguments roughly resemble those of Home, and though that really does not do him justice, I will confess that his writings strike me as a great deal more impressive on hasty reading than after close study. He does not consider psychoanalysis a science, repeating the same tired old arguments. He too believes that since we are dealing with meanings, not observations in the centimeter gram–second system, scientific method is simply inapplicable, quantification is inappropriate, and psychoanalysis is freed from the necessity of trying to predict anything or of being subject to any substantial constraints. If true, that would be its death knell: When anything goes, nothing goes anywhere.

I was disappointed to find that when Ricoeur is faced with difficult problems, he retreats into evocative verbalism with no clear content. Psychoanalytic hermeneutics, he says, should be directed toward "the conditions of possibility of a semantics of desire" (1970, p. 375). Ricoeur is gifted at the old trick of mystification by metaphor. Thus, since genetic reconstruction has some similarity to archeology, a conveniently multisyllabic word for a discipline that fascinated Freud, Ricoeur speaks always about "the archaeology of the subject" when he means a genetic analysis. Following John Ciardi, I call such inappropriate use of figurative language in the service of self-congratulation, obfuscation, and intimidation "poesy." What could, in a suitable context, be imaginative use of evocative language easily degenerates into poesy when the writer uses it instead of defining terms, confronting issues, and either undertaking onerous conceptual analysis or admitting that he is stumped.

Nevertheless, Ricoeur manages to sound convincing to many a psychoanalyst who feels that there must be some alternative to either the inhumane mechanism of hard science or the boneless stuff of literature and speculative philosophy. When Ricoeur maintains that hermeneutics is a relevant and autonomous intellectual discipline with its own methodology, arguing his case at great length in a book of satisfying heft and occasionally stupefying unreadability, many a student is convinced. If he seems to represent a whole school of allegedly distinguished intellectuals, with the extra prestige (for Americans) of a European provenance, then the nonrational aura of legitimacy becomes difficult to resist. A skeptic finds himself beset with nagging self-doubts: Do I just miss the point? Is something essential lost in translation? He reminds himself that there have always been bad writers of impenetrable prose, like Kant and Piaget, who nevertheless are profound and creative thinkers. He may even, after undergoing some identification with an aggressor like Ricoeur or Lacan, ask himself: Are we confronted merely by an etiolated arborization of a Hegelian logos, or is this a veridical ascent to a dessicating but authentic tessitura of abstract apodicticity?

Let us not forget that Ricoeur's training is not in the philosophy of science, but in religious hermeneutics, an outgrowth of biblical exegesis with the dubious distinction of being the oldest attempt to treat verbal meanings in a disciplined way. Dubious, because its methods are prescientific, set in an era when scientific method did seem to have nothing to offer. Not only does it therefore lack any means of generating testable propositions, but Ricoeur shows no interest in doing so. I have yet to see any evidence that it is an arcane source of wisdom that we should all proceed to study. (See, in this connection, Rubinstein, 1976a, for a valuable analysis of hermeneutics as an alternative to the pursuit of psychoanalysis as a science [and Grünbaum, 1984].)

The Distinction between "Theory" and "Model"

Before turning to a consideration of the kinds of relationships that may obtain between metapsychology and the rest of psychoanalysis, I think it will be useful to introduce and discuss briefly some terminology from a prominent modern school of the philosophy of science. Any science has a *domain*, a *language*, and at least one *theory*; it often also has *models*. The domain of a theory is the body of phenomena it treats and should account for. We need consider it only briefly; the main point I want to make is that some programs for the development of psychoanalytic theory explicitly or implicitly presuppose much narrower domains than we are accustomed to considering. Ricoeur (1978, p. 836), for example, wants a sharp restriction of psychoanalytic theory to "the codification of what takes place in the analytic situation and . . . in the analytic relationship"—further, only to what can be expressed in words. Advocates of psychoanalysis as a "pure psychology" would have us eliminate from our purview all bodily phenomena, including psychosomatic symptoms; all hormonal, pharmaceutical, and other biochemical influences on mood, thought, and behavior; and any other direct consequences of the fact that we all have bodies. Personally, I think such a restriction of realm is too high a price to pay, as well as being unnecessary.

As to the language of a science, I want to underline only a couple of points. First, notice that it is logically distinct from theory and model; thus, working on the deficiencies of a language does not take care of all theoretical issues. Roy Schafer (1976, 1978) did psychoanalysis a service, I think, in pointing out many of the inadequacies of the metapsychological language of psychoanalysis, and some of his suggestions for its improvement seem to me well worth trying out.[2] But metapsychology is much more than a language, and by not considering the role of theory and model in a science, Schafer has left the mistaken impression that they may be dispensed with if only one's language is adequate.[3]

What, then, is a *theory*, and how does it differ from a *model*? With deceptive simplicity, philosophers of science tell us that a theory is a set of sentences about the domain of a science in its language. Evidently, in the hypothetical early or natural-history phase of a science, which Freud said was devoted to "describing phenomena and . . . proceeding to group, classify and correlate them" (1915c, p. 117), scientists might work almost entirely with directly observable variables, establishing statistical findings or empirical generalizations. We usually say we have a theory, according to

Hempel (1965, p. 178) only when we can state "comprehensive laws, in terms of hypothetical entities, which will account for the uniformities established on the first level." And Hempel gives as examples of this theoretical level, "general statements that refer to electric, magnetic, and gravitational fields . . . ; or to ego, id, superego, libido, sublimation, fixation, and transference" (p. 178). (Notice that he includes concepts both from metapsychology and from the clinical theory.) Logicians and philosophers tend to define theories in terms of an ideal case, complete with axioms, theorems, and a comprehensive set of valid laws. In practice, theories grow in a more disorderly fashion, and do not have to have all these properties to be considered theories. By and large, however, they seek a simple kind of order in the diversity of nature by the use of abstractive or hypothetical terms, related to each other in law-like propositions. They are linked to reality, and are thus made testable, by sets of correspondence rules which define empirically at least some key concepts.

A theory is often quite abstract and formal, ideally taking the form of a set of mathematical equations (like Newton's laws of motion). To be understandable, it needs a *model*, which interprets or "realizes" it in a set of different but familiar terms, often visually concrete ones. Illustrating this distinction, Nagel (1961) cites Bohr's theory of the atom, which was framed in bare mathematical equations, and his model, which describes a visualizable structure somewhat like a solar system. This distinction, which may seem innocent and simple enough, is not universally accepted, unfortunately, which is one reason for the confusion both in the usage of the terms "theory" and "model" and in some thinking about conceptual problems of psychoanalysis. I will have more to say about it later, therefore.

The Relationship between Metapsychology and Clinical Theory

Let us turn at last to the long-deferred task of considering opinions about the ways metapsychology may be related to the clinical theory of psychoanalysis. Many people have been puzzled by their coexistence and have offered various interpretations of their relationship.

1. Klein, Gill and others have said that the relationship is that between a theory and a metatheory: Metapsychology is a theory about the clinical theory. Let us clear up this misunderstanding right away: "Metatheory" (a term introduced by Carnap) is "a theory concerned with the investigation, analysis, or description of theory itself" (Gove, 1981, p. 1421). It is thus a branch of the philosophy of science, and whatever else metapsychology may be, it is not that.

2. Perhaps the relationship is that between a theory and a model. Clinical psychoanalysis—for example, the first six chapters of *The Interpretation of Dreams*—is the theory, and metapsychology (the seventh chapter)

is the model. This is an appealing possibility, for the last chapter contains the visualizable topographic conception of the psychic apparatus, actually pictured in schematic diagrams, which seem to satisfy some of the definitions of "model" I have just given. This interpretation also accounts for the patent physicalism of many metapsychological terms—their property of being a borrowing from outside psychoanalysis or psychology, which has so outraged some recent authors (among whom I might easily be included, for the insight is new to me). All the talk of forces, energies, reservoirs, and pathways in the seventh chapter and elsewhere is an extended analogical realization of a *psychological* theory in presumably more familiar terms.

Consider the situation in physics during Freud's formative years: The theory of electricity was abstract and formal, extremely difficult to grasp without the aid of a concrete realization, so such writers as Lord Kelvin and Sir Oliver Lodge published books in the 1880s containing a great many visualizable models drawn from other branches of science. One of the best known is the model of the behavior of electrical currents in a circuit in terms of the flow of water in a set of pipes. Most of us rely on that model to this day in an attempt to grasp the meaning of electrical concepts. Using this model does not *reduce* electricity to hydrology, or explain it in foreign terms, but puts the phenomena within our intuitive grasp.

Hempel (1965) comments sympathetically:

> Considering the great heuristic value of . . . structural analogies, it is natural that a scientist attempting to frame a new theory should let himself be guided by concepts and laws that have proved fruitful in previously explored areas. But if these should fail, he will have to resort to ideas that depart more and more from the familiar ones. (p. 445)

He goes on to give an example from atomic physics of a model based on macroscopic electric charges, which had to be modified to suit the new set of facts. A good precedent, I thought, for Freud to have followed in taking a system of physical forces and energies as a model and then altering their properties as needed, so that, for example, psychic energy is directional unlike physical energy. The justification for such a procedure, however, is that it should provide "increased scope and greater explanatory and predictive power" (Hempel, 1965, p. 445), but Freud never developed any means of generating and testing predictions. He too used the model of interconnecting water pipes, but with this important difference: In physics, both the phenomena modeled and the model itself yield measurements, and thus empirical laws connecting directly measurable variables.[4]

The misfortune of psychoanalysis is that Freud never developed any means of generating and testing predictions, mistakenly believing that there was scientific value in spinning out theoretical speculations that could not be falsified by any kind of data. If metapsychology had been a true model, it would have been possible to use the known laws of forces and energies in circuits or systems of pipes to generate clinically testable propositions; without that disciplining from data, the changes in the original properties of concepts from physics became mere *ad hoc* tinkering.

Actually, metapsychology has some properties of a language, some of a theory, and some of a model, but is not fully or clearly any of these. That fact in itself accounts for much of the confusion about what metapsychology is and what to do about it. Let me remind you, however, that psychoanalysis has lots of company in its theoretical misery: "The emptiness and shallowness of many classical theories in the social sciences is well brought out by the attempt to formulate in any exact fashion what constitutes a model of the theory." So says the philosopher Suppes (1969, p. 18).

And to those of my collegial friends who think we can do without a metapsychology, let me remind them that a highly developed theory does need a model, the terms of which are *not* the terms of the theory itself. In this sense, I think we should be open-minded about the attempts of Peterfreund (1971; Peterfreund & Franceschini, 1973), Rubenstein (1974, 1976b) and Rosenblatt and Thickstun (1977) to construct models of clinical theories using block diagrams, information-processing systems, and other such outlandish-seeming resources from other sciences. True, they are not framed in terms of meanings, but perhaps they can make useful predictions about the meanings people produce in psychoanalysis. The real question then is, do they generate anything empirically testable? If so, they are a big advance over metapsychology. And if so, are these predictions clinically valid? If the model is not adequate to represent the *relationships among* meanings, the results will be distorted. But note that the models do not need to consist of meanings, any more than a computer model of the economic system has to consist of brokers or bankers in order to predict these people's behavior.

3. A third possible relationship is that between a descriptive and an explanatory theory, clinical theory presumably being descriptive, metapsychology explanatory. It is not surprising that this view has many adherents, for it is a plausible approximation, though one that breaks down rather quickly under scrutiny. Clinical psychoanalytic theory *is* closer to observation; it does contain some empirical generalizations; and some parts of it are evidently more descriptive than metapsychology. The latter clearly does not describe what psychoanalysts observe, and does attempt to explain. So far, so good; but there are two important objections: Much of clinical theory is truly explanatory, and metapsychology is not, as Rubinstein (1967a) and Swanson (1977) have convincingly shown in two complementary papers.

4. And now, a fourth and last type of relationship between metapsychology and the clinical theory—the special case of model versus theory in which the model serves a bridging function between two sciences with two different subject matters. It is possible in principle to imagine the following

happy state of affairs, which strikes me as an ideal possible outcome. Suppose we could construct a faithful model of purely psychological events and transactions, such as the laws of actions, wishes, fantasies, dreams, symptoms, and other familiar meaningful phenomena of our everyday clinical lives. By calling it "faithful," I mean that it operates quite far-reachingly in the way our clinical theory does, and that it enables us to make predictions which repeatedly are verified. Please notice that logically it *just does not matter* what the terms of such a model might be, though preferably they should be easy to work with and to imagine visually; I am assuming that such a model would *not* use psychological terms, and that it would not use anatomical or neurophysiological terms either. But entertain with me the following real possibility: It might *also* be a good model of neurophysiological theory! Then we would be in the enviable position of being able to use the same model to generate and test two quite different and independent sets of predictions—some about psychological events, some about measurable events in the human organism (notably in the brain).

One reason I have become so attracted to systems theories is that they seem to offer just such an exciting possibility. Very briefly, the idea is as follows: We begin by treating the human person as a psychobiological system, a natural unity in which it is possible to discern and abstract out a psychological subsystem and a biological subsystem. Each of these, being part of the same larger system, should follow generally parallel or analogous rules or system principles. General systems theory is an attempt (not completely successful so far) to develop a model of the nature and functioning of all systems, or, somewhat more narrowly, of living systems (Miller, 1978). Its terminology and concepts are those of cybernetics, operations theory, communications engineering, and mathematics—not reassuringly familiar stuff,[5] like water in the pipes, but surely not either the terms of neurophysiology (e.g., neurons and neurotransmitters) or of clinical psychoanalysis (e.g., motives and situations). What makes systems theory seem to be worth exploring is that it does have some properties of both contemporary psychoanalytic and neuroscientific theories. Despite its own considerable deficiencies (Berlinski, 1976), I believe that it can serve as a starting point for attempts to construct just such a bridging model as I have described.[6]

But whether that turns out to be a fruitful lead or a false one, there is no reason in principle that such an intermediary or Janusian model might not be found, with one face turned toward biology, one toward psychology. I believe that this is what Rubinstein has been calling for since 1967 with the perhaps misleading term "protoneurophysiology." The point is that the model should not itself be either neurophysiology or psychoanalysis; it can serve a valuable function for both disciplines by giving them a common language and a common set of propositions, perhaps rendered graphically in flow charts or the like—a *lingua franca* through which they can engage in mutually stimulating dialogue and trade of ideas. It does not mean, either, that psychoanalysts would be expected to give up their own language and theory and start talking about feedback circuits instead of Oedipus complexes. It would still be necessary for many of us to concentrate on refining and developing our distinctively psychoanalytic theory, which is basically the clinical theory. The progress of model building will be limited by the achievements of our own in-house theoretical effort, though there can be useful exchanges of ideas between the two enterprises and convergent efforts, just as there can be between the modeling project and workers in the neurosciences.

The final contribution of the systems outlook is that it provides an intelligible rationale for the cooperation and interrelation of all the sciences [as we saw in Chapter 9]. With this understanding, we can stop fearing that chemistry could ever take over psychiatry or that the growth of neuropsychology could threaten social psychology or psychoanalysis. Instead of withdrawing, remaining insulated and isolated from other sciences as psychoanalysis was for too many years, we can confidently cooperate, both learning and teaching in our contacts with colleagues in the biological and social sciences.

SUMMARY

Let me recapitulate briefly what I have tried to do. First, I examined the perennially arising question, "Can psychoanalysis be a science, and if so, of what kind?" and found that modern philosophers of science see no real difficulty here. No methodological issues of special importance hinge on the question of where to classify it among the sciences, either. Like psychology, its methods are akin to those of its neighbors on both sides, natural science and social science. The logical structure of empirical inquiry and theory construction is widely conceded to be essentially the same throughout all the sciences.

I concluded next that the relationship between metapsychology and the clinical theory is not a simple one, a fact that is understandable in light of the history of our discipline. The distinctions now made among elements of a science—its domain, its language, its theory, and its model or models—are of recent origin, and there is not even full consensus among philosophers of science about the definitions of these terms, not to speak of the babel of interpretations and usages of such key terms as *model* among psychological and psychoanalytic writers. What we call metapsychology is at once a distinctive vocabulary or language, a set of theoretical propositions, and at least one explicit model (Freud's diagram of the ego, superego, and id). Moreover, to a considerable degree, it is possible and perhaps illuminating to look on much of it as an attempt to model clinical theoretical propositions by use of analogous concepts drawn from physics. But since Freud did not have just this task in mind when he wrote his metapsychological works or even the Project, we should not be surprised that he did not accomplish it in a way that is easily corrected or supplemented. Other branches of non-psychological science today offer more attractive and potentially fruitful possible models than the closed systems of mid-19th-century electricity and hydrology.

The important issues raised by George Klein (1976) by his question, "Two theories or one?" might be rephrased thus: "How shall we go about improving psychoanalytic theory?" and "What is the appropriate relationship between psychoanalysis and the other sciences?" Rather than continue polemical disputes about metapsychology and clinical theory, let us go about clarifying, simplifying, and organizing clinical psychoanalytic theory undistracted by several prevailing misapprehensions. Let us not be so afraid of committing the methodological sins of reification and personification, which contemporary philosophers consider relatively venial, that we sacrifice the power and the fecundity given by theoretical terms (cf. Schafer, 1976). We should keep in mind the dangers of slipping into regressive modes of theoretical thinking, and also the fact that any theory must be eventually testable, but otherwise may feel free to postulate any theoretical abstractions or hypothetical entities that seem necessary. With regard to the matter of testability, most of us who (like myself) got our grounding in the philosophy of science some decades ago, when logical positivism was riding high, need to become better acquainted with the progress that philosophers have made in clarifying the nature and role of correspondence rules (or operational definitions, as I was taught to call them). By and large, contemporary philosophers of science take a much more relaxed and permissive stance than formerly seemed necessary, having discovered that the rigid application of the stern strictures of the midcentury outlook would strait-jacket if not totally forbid some of the most fruitful work that has been done in the physical sciences. It still remains true that Freud defined many terms in ways that made metapsychology by and large untestable, and that we have to resist the temptations of a style of theorizing that gives the illusion of explaining everything because no possible state of affairs can embarrass it.

When I take a second look at such diverse theoretical enterprises as Schafer's (1976, 1978) action language, Rubinstein's (1975, 1976a) explication of clinical theory, Dahl's (1979) theory of emotions, the monograph by Rosenblatt and Thickstun (1977), and my own attempt to clarify the psychoanalytic theory of motivation (see Chapter 7), I have the distinct impression that all of these are promising beginnings but that they need to be further elaborated by being applied to extensive clinical material. Dahl and Rubinstein are currently showing one good way to proceed, by making a highly detailed study of the transcribed text of two hours from a completely recorded psychoanalysis. The clinical case is still the bedrock of psychoanalysis; though as soon as I say that, I wish for a more organic, vital, productive kind of metaphor. Let me say it directly: It is best not to get too far away from the details of specific people's lives and problems. Not just in the form of clinical vignettes, valuable as those may be for rhetorical and expository purposes; the fiction writer's freedom to select is exactly what we need to forego in favor of the constraining discipline of having to account for the concrete particularities of extended sequences of events in individual lives. Otherwise, it is just too easy to overlook the implications of one's assumptions, or to avoid having to grapple with inconvenient complications, or to paper over difficulties by inadvertently vague or metaphorically imprecise language.

If metapsychology is dying from impalpability and inconsistency, let it be reborn into a vital psychoanalytic science by the effort to account for our original and always most stimulating data, the transactions of the psychoanalytic hour. And, to the extent that it has been a model, let it be transfigured into an effort to achieve the kind of intermediation I have just described between psychoanalysis and the biological sciences of the human organism. Psychoanalysis may be a relatively young science, but perhaps we are mature enough to have outgrown sibling rivalry!

CHAPTER 13

The Current Status
of Psychoanalytic Theory

Now that we have reviewed the travails and failings of metapsychology in its three traditional divisions, the economic, dynamic, and structural points of view, it is time for a summary overview. I was spurred to prepare just such a survey and summing-up in the summer of 1984, when the Division on Psychoanalysis of the American Psychological Association invited me to give a lecture on the present status of psychoanalytic theory. It was part of a general plan for the convention to have invited addresses on the current state of all the principal psychological theories. In expanded form, the paper appeared in Division 39's official journal, Political Psychology *(Holt, 1985); it has been only slightly retouched.*

If one surveys the field of psychoanalytic theory in the mid-1980s, three major trends seem to preoccupy most of the recent literature: First, the decline if not the actual death of metapsychology, accompanied by a small rise of interest in the clinical theory. Second, the question of what kind of discipline psychoanalysis should be, scientific or hermeneutic. Third, the rise into increasing prominence of object relations theory and self psychology. All these trends are interrelated, but I will consider them one at a time.

THE DECLINE AND FALL OF METAPSYCHOLOGY

Almost all of the previous chapters were first published as a series of papers (Holt, 1962, 1965a, 1965b, 1967a, 1967b, 1967c, 1974, 1975, 1976a, 1976b, 1981, 1982; see also Holt, 1968, 1972a, 1978b), which I began with the hope of clarifying and systematizing the theory, along the lines Rapaport (1959) had begun. I am, of course, far from being the only or even the first critic of metapsychology. Kubie (1947) perhaps has the honor of priority; at least, he was the first I know of, and important critical contributions have been made by Applegarth (1971), Basch (1973), Eagle (1984), Galatzer-Levy (1976),

Gill (1976), Grossman and Simon (1969), Holzman (1976, 1985), Klein (1976), Leites (1971), Rosenblatt and Thickstun (1977), Rubinstein (1965, 1967a), Schafer (1976), Sulloway (1979), Wilson (1973), and Yankelovich and Barrett (1970), among others. I shall summarize the collective critique of metapsychology in a series of separate statements, mostly without attribution.

• *The relationship between metapsychology and the clinical theory has not been clarified.* Thus, the limits of each and the borderline between them are matters of dispute, and there is no consensus on what is the total body of clinical theory and of metapsychology.

• *Concepts are poorly defined.* Existing definitions are so vague, imprecise, and multiple that much of the theory cannot be pinned down enough to test it empirically, and different writers are free to use the same term in quite different ways. Consequently,

• *Concepts overlap one another partly or completely.* More than just the confusion of the neophyte is at issue when such a variety of terms exist, all referring to more or less the same subject matter, as, for example, "instinct," "libido," "drive derivative," "cathexis," "excitation," "id," "sexuality," "pleasure principle," and "tension reduction." One result is a needless complication by surplus levels and layers of theory. Another is:

• *Concepts are often reified*, abstractions treated as if they refer to substantial entities. The worst form of the error is personification or anthropomorphism, treating concepts such as drives or structures as if they were persons or had attributes such as striving and insisting that properly belong only to whole people.

• *Metapsychology contains many self-contradictions*, because Freud never went back over it, pulled it all together, and explicitly renounced ideas that had been superseded. The effort by Rapaport and Gill (1959) to do so is only a beginning, and has the further problem of incorporating two points of view not included by Freud and not universally accepted by other psychoanalysts.

• In developing its propositions, *Freud committed a good many logical errors and fallacies of reasoning.* Further,

• *Freud made extensive use of metaphor and other figures of speech at points of theoretical difficulty*, a practice that tends to conceal or divert attention away from the fact that problems were left unsolved.

• *Much of metapsychology is a translation into other terms of outdated physiology, anatomy, and early evolutionary biology.* Freud's first effort to go beyond clinical theorizing, the Project, was an explicitly mechanistic, biological model of the organism with particular reference to the structure and functioning of the brain. Though in many ways an astonishingly brilliant *tour de force* containing many anticipations of modern views of the nervous system, it was clearly a failure. Yet its anachronistic and erroneous notions of how the brain is organized and works, and of Lamarckian and

Haeckelian evolution, were revived (with slight terminological changes) in the metapsychology, by means of a metaphysical transformation.

After suppressing his early love for philosophy, Freud avoided facing philosophical aspects and implications of his theory. Therefore,

• *Metapsychology fails to take clear and consistent stands on basic philosophical issues*—for example, on the mind–body problem, or the problem of freedom and determinism, or the nature of reality. Much of the time,

• *Psychic energies, forces, and structures are assigned a metaphysical status separate from the world of material realities* such as measuring instruments. Therefore, propositions involving these central terms cannot be tested, nor can any of the key entities be measured. Hence,

• *Metapsychology is a closed system*, which Rubinstein (1967a) has shown can be translated into a purely formal model devoid of any content. But because it does not generate new propositions, as scientifically useful formal systems can, metapsychology has neither explanatory nor heuristic value.

In the course of studying the problems of metapsychology, I became aware of Freud's unique style of thinking and writing (see Chapter 3), and for a while thought that *it* might be the main source of trouble. A number of its features—for example, his tolerance for self-contradiction, his hyperbolic tendency to state generalizations in the most sweeping and universal form, and his fondness for figurative language—did make psychoanalytic theory a good deal messier, more difficult to understand, and harder to defend than it might have been. For a long time, I clung to the hope that if one could simply purge metapsychology of these stylistic defects, it would prove to be not only helpful to the clinician but a fertile source of testable propositions for the experimenter and other systematic researchers in personology as well as clinical psychology. But after a couple of decades spent in studying metapsychology and attempting to make it scientifically useful, I reluctantly concluded that the task was impossible. Moreover, metapsychology's defects are intrinsic, not simply products of Freud's personal style of thinking and writing.

At present, I think it is fair to say that metapsychology is virtually dead. Fewer voices defend it explicitly, and more join the chorus of those who find it wanting. To be sure, most practicing analysts have not paid much attention to the demise, never having put much stock in "that abstract stuff" anyway. What they do not realize is that they are far more committed to it than they know. For everyday terms like "ego," "id," "instinct," and "psychodynamics" are integral parts of metapsychology rather than the clinical theory. They share with more outlandish terms like "anticathexis" and "defusion" the fatal property of not referring to anything even indirectly observable and of contributing nothing to discourse beyond the nonrational gratification many of us get from speaking a recognizably psychoanalytic jargon. Eagle (1984) has demonstrated in some detail that those who, like

Kohut, claim to work solely within the terms of the clinical theory actually go beyond it into metapsychological territory—as indeed they must, unless they are willing to be as austerely atheoretical as Schafer (1976).

I recognize the harshness of the indictment above, but do not make it lightly or with any pleasure. It is anything but a comforting reflection to realize that most of one's career has been devoted to as worthless a theory as metapsychology has proved to be. Nevertheless, Rubinstein (1976a) is quite right, I believe, in stressing the fact that something like metapsychology is necessary to supplement the clinical theory.

A PHILOSOPHICAL CRITIQUE OF THE CLINICAL THEORY

A number of theorists, including my late friend George Klein (1976), reacted to the realization that metapsychology was bankrupt by counseling that we simply discard it and concentrate on systematizing and developing the clinical theory, claiming that it is capable of becoming a self-sufficient discipline on its own. Schafer (1976) meanwhile went a similar route, but produced his alternative, action language, which is not so much a theory in the usual sense as it is a controlled language for discussing clinical phenomena without falling into the fallacies of reification and personification that bedevil Freud's writings. After making a preliminary effort to extract the clinical theory from metapsychology, I withdrew in some discouragement, reporting (see Chapter 8) that the two were much more closely intertwined than Rapaport had suggested, and that there was no simple or obvious way to produce a set of excerpts from Freud's writings that would give the clinical theory definitive exposition.

Fortunately, a leading philosopher of science, Adolf Grünbaum, became interested in the problem of the scientific status of psychoanalysis in 1976 and began studying its literature. In the seven years since then, he has published a series of papers (Grünbaum, 1976, 1977, 1979, 1980a, 1980b, 1981, 1983a, 1983b, 1985) and a book (Grünbaum, 1984), in which he thoroughly reviews the question of whether psychoanalysis is a science, and how good a one (see also von Eckhardt, 1985). Here at last is a philosopher who has done his homework before criticizing Freud. Happily, Grünbaum has concentrated his efforts on the clinical theory. For in his own words,

> when Freud unswervingly claimed natural science status for his theoretical constructions . . . he did so first and foremost for his evolving clinical theory of personality and therapy, rather than for the metapsychology. . . . [He claimed] the *scientificity* of his clinical theory *entirely on the strength of a secure and direct epistemic warrant from the observations he made of his patients and of himself.* (Grünbaum, 1984, p. 6)

It happens that one of the great figures in contemporary philosophy, Karl Popper (1963), had attacked psychoanalysis as unfalsifiable, therefore no better than a pseudoscience. Grünbaum (1976, 1977, 1979) has earned the gratitude of all of us by taking Popper down a peg, showing that his arguments not only are based on ignorance of what Freud actually said, but have logical flaws as well. Citing several of Freud's propositions that can clearly be tested empirically and several passages in which Freud explicitly said that a single case running counter to one of his theories (e.g., that of paranoia) would refute it, Grünbaum has unanswerably established the claim of psychoanalysis to a place among the sciences by Popper's own criteria, as well as demonstrating that the serious challenge to the scientific credibility of psychoanalysis comes instead from the so-called eliminative inductivism. That is well known to psychologists as the underlying principles of experimental design and other forms of empirical research (Grünbaum, 1984, pp. 279–280). Plainly, psychoanalysis *is* testable inductively, though its record of genuine inductive validation is discouraging.

If much of the clinical theory is testable, how has it stood up? Are Freud's theories supported by the available evidence? Recall that Freud was benignly indifferent to attempts to test his theories experimentally, stating that they had been confirmed so many times clinically that such laboratory exercises as those of Rosenzweig (1938) were unnecessary. Meeting this claim head on, Grünbaum (1980b, 1984, 1985) argues that clinical data are so epistemologically contaminated as to be virtually useless for the purpose of testing or providing support for any of the theories. This is an important point, so let us look more closely at the way he reached such a discouraging conclusion.

Wilhelm Fliess seems to have been the first to point out the possibility that Freud's method left him wide open to the charge that when he interpreted the patient's productions, he was reading his *own* thoughts into them instead of discerning the *patient's* unconscious meanings. The very data of the patient's productions are suspect, because in so many subtle ways as well as through the more obvious means of interpretation, the analyst steers and shapes what the patient reports in his or her mislabeled free associations. Add the motivation to please the analyst (the positive transference), and it is easy to understand why Freudian patients produce classical Freudian dreams, while Jungian patients' dreams are full of mandalas, wise old men, and other Jungian symbols.

Freud was aware of such influences under the general name of suggestion, and his main argument against it was that the patient's "conflicts will only be successfully solved and his resistances overcome if the anticipatory ideas he is given tally with what is real in him" (1916–1917, p. 452). And to the extent that psychoanalysis is therapeutically successful, according to this Tally Argument, as Grünbaum has dubbed it, the interpretations *must* be valid. That would be all right, he concedes, if it were in fact the case that neurotic conflicts and symptoms could *not* be overcome in any way other than by giving correct (Freudian) interpretations. Besides, it assumes that genuine cures *are* achieved by psychoanalytic treatment reasonably often, and that spontaneous remissions do not occur. But comparative studies of the therapeutic efficacy of psychoanalysis and other forms of therapy for neurosis unfortunately have not supported Freud's claim. The burden is definitely on psychoanalysts to prove that their treatment is better than any other; the *best* construction one can put on currently available data is that psychoanalysis may be no worse than nonanalytic therapies. All offer slightly better recovery rates than spontaneous remission. But what all psychotherapies have in common may be nothing much more than the familiar placebo effect; hence, there is *no* support for Freud's assumption that neurosis cannot be cured except by accurate interpretations based on a true theory—his.

Another possible source of clinical evidence, the introspective testimony of analyzed patients, cannot come to the rescue, for there is no evidence that anyone—even after analysis—has direct introspective access to the kinds of internal processes postulated by Freud or to the causal linkages he asserted.

Thus, clinical data do not have the "probative value that Freud claimed for them," Grünbaum (1984, p. 245) argues. That by no means implies that analysts' interpretations are automatically false, he adds; they may sometimes be true, but there is no reliable way to distinguish the grain from the chaff among them.

But he has gone further, demonstrating that even if clinical data had no such liabilities and could be taken as perfectly trustworthy, they would not validate one of Freud's principal theories—the pathogenicity of repression. It is surely a cornerstone of the clinical theory, Grünbaum (1983b, 1984) says, that repressed material (memories of traumatic experiences, fantasies, and wishes) cause neurotic symptoms, dreams, slips, and the like. At first, it looked as if Breuer and Freud had an excellent method of testing this hypothesis, for it seemed that separate symptoms could be removed, one by one, through the undoing of specific repressions. Unfortunately, as Freud later put it (1925d, p. 27), "Even the most brilliant results were liable to be suddenly wiped away if my personal relation with the patient became disturbed." And with this discovery of the transference, Freud lost interest in the attempt to find any other proof for his hypotheses about the effects of repressed memories and wishes, took them for granted as somehow established by his clinical experience, and failed to adduce *any* confirmatory data.

I believe that Grünbaum somewhat overstates his point concerning the contamination of clinical data, which is not an all-or-none affair, and overlooks the possibility that fruitful use may be made of data gathered by therapists who have other theoretical and technical persuasions. With enough recorded treatments from a sufficient variety of analysts of all schools, it should be possible to find out just how far their patients' dreams, fantasies, childhood memories, and so on do systematically differ, and to what extent hypotheses of Freud's clinical theory hold, regardless of the nature of the treatment. If positive findings occur disproportionately more often in classical psychoanalyses, we are in trouble, for that would imply that they are a consequence of suggestion or Rosenthal (1963) effects. But until the research is done, *we just don't know.*

Grünbaum, von Eckhardt (1982), and some other critics on whom I am now going to draw agree that the large part of the clinical theory dealing with *genetic* hypotheses cannot be satisfactorily tested by means of the data available to psychoanalysts for yet another reason. All such retrospective clinical research falls afoul of one basic flaw, the lack of adequate controls to establish casual connections.

Take the simple case of Freud's early theory that hysteria was caused by so-called seduction—better called child abuse [that far I will go with Masson, 1984, but not much further]. Let us make the obviously implausible assumption that he *was* able to ascertain the true facts about childhood traumas by analyzing adults, and that he uncharacteristically had kept careful statistics about all his patients over a decade; he would have had an inadequately small sample. Very well; assume that he had been able to train a group of equally skillful analysts, scattered about in other major cities to be sure it was not just a Viennese phenomenon, and with a large enough clientele to provide a couple of hundred well-diagnosed cases of hysteria. Let us assume highly positive findings—convincing evidence of child abuse in 85% of the cases. The question next arises: How does that compare to the base rate, which was unknown? Even if it could have been discovered, he still would not have known what he needed to know: What are the chances that if a child is sexually assaulted, she or he will *develop* hysteria? There is no substitute for a prospective design to test such hypotheses, which are readily enough *formed* retrospectively: You have to get two samples of children, about half of whom are victims of abuse and half are in other relevant respects the same but are never assaulted sexually. Then you must follow them to adulthood and have them diagnosed by qualified clinicians who are blind to the childhood history. Incidentally, because such a study has never been done (and it would be extraordinarily expensive and difficult to do it), we still do not know for sure what the answer would be. Some recent research that approximates the above design indicates that child victims do suffer serious mental health problems in adolescence, but not classical hysteria. Even so, that near-miss is actually about as good a record of validation as any of Freud's other clinical hypotheses possesses.

Psychoanalysts must begin to face the fact that their primary and typical form of research, the uncontrolled clinical case study, is devoid of scientific value *except* as a source of hypotheses. A good deal can be done to

test nonetiological hypotheses with the undeniably rich data of psychoanalyses, but only if they are fully recorded (of course, with the informed
consent of the patients, and with the data carefully if minimally censored to
prevent recognition) and made available to all qualified researchers. Then
at last we will have public and replicable data; then the researcher can be
someone other than the therapist, and therefore truly disinterested and
uncontaminated. Thanks to pioneers like Dahl (1972), Gill (1982; Gill &
Hoffman, 1982), Luborsky (1977, 1984), and Weiss, Sampson, and the
Mount Zion Psychotherapy Research Group (1986), such work is under
way. We know how to reduce, order, and systematize the overwhelming
masses of data to make it possible to process them, though it takes lots of
willing workers who have both psychoanalytic and research training to
make the necessary judgments in controlled and replicable ways. Work is at
last beginning on clarifying rules of inference, the processes of clinical
judgment and interpretation, for the first time.

It is good to be able to report this progress. It shows that the situation is
not hopeless, but it *is* grave. Psychoanalysts have been living in a fool's
paradise, believing that the clinical theory was soundly established when in
fact very little of it has been, and virtually all of that thanks to the efforts of
nonpsychoanalysts. It is not enough merely to reassure oneself that psychoanalytic theory has great clinical value. The theory is, indeed, indispensable,
but to affirm that does not release us from the obligation to test, purge, and
improve it.

Let us turn next to the other most valuable body of work on the
validation of the clinical theory—the papers of Benjamin Rubinstein. Rubinstein is as unusual among analysts as Grünbaum is among philosophers in
having a deep and thorough knowledge of the philosophy of science as well
as of his own field. Both have the special merit, also, of thinking and writing
with great clarity.

Grünbaum relies entirely on direct quotations from Freud and from
other analysts when he considers propositions from the clinical theory.
Rubinstein, however, *reconstructs* the fundamental propositions of the theory, on the basis not merely of his psychoanalytic scholarship and many
years of clinical practice, but also of his participation in a long-term empirical research project on the process of clinical inference. Working closely
with Hartvig Dahl and a group of cooperating clinicians, he has undertaken
the task of logically reconstructing the inferential processes involved (1) in
many concrete instances of interpretations offered by the participating
analysts who all study the typescript of a recorded psychoanalysis, and (2)
in their selections of evidence for a variety of clinical hypotheses.

In the mid-1970s, Rubinstein (1975, 1976a) published a pair of remarkable papers, laying out the clinical theory's basic propositions or hypotheses,
and specifically addressing the question of whether it could be made self-
sufficient. He begins by distinguishing, within the realm of the clinical

theory, between the psychoanalytic theory of therapy (which he does not address) and what he calls its cognitive theory.

All of the clinical theory, he notes, is made up of abstract hypotheses, which of course do not refer to particular persons. When you analyze someone, however, you construct as it were a theory of that person, made up of *particular* clinical hypotheses. Each of them is a statement about events in the person's life history and their consequences; typically, they employ theoretical terms such as "unconscious wishes" and translate the abstract hypotheses of the clinical theory into concrete terms pertaining to one patient. Those are testable, but there are complications.

One of Rubinstein's most notable theoretical insights is his demonstration that, when properly reformulated, all the hypotheses of the clinical theory are *probabilistic*, despite Freud's deliberate attempt to give them universal formulation.

So what *is* the distinction between a "probabilistic" law and a "universally valid" scientific law, also sometimes called "nomothetic" or "nomological"? It makes a great deal of difference to the way we write about theory and to the kinds of research we do, whether we believe we are working with one kind of theory or the other. Take one of Rubinstein's formulations of a special clinical hypothesis: "If insulted, a person is likely to feel hurt." Had Freud said it, he might have put it thus: "The person who is insulted feels hurt"; in fact, he would not have recognized the probabilistic formulation as a scientific statement. Yet in nuclear physics, though we can specify to a tiny fraction of a second the half-life of any given radioactive element, all statements of this class are probabilistic. About any particular atom, it is impossible to say more than that it is somewhat likely that it will undergo radioactive decay at any time (just how likely is expressed in the half-life, essentially a formulation of a probability).

True, some physicists hope someday to discover a "hidden variable" that causes a specific atom to decay at just the moment it does. Science advances to some degree by the discovery of unknown determinants of events which otherwise can be expressed only as more or less probable. No doubt it will be possible to learn a great deal more about what kinds of persons do and do not feel hurt (and to what extent) when insulted to specifiable extents in specifiable ways, and in situations the parameters of which also remain to be described and measured. Obviously, however, the relevant research will not be done if no one realizes that it is needed. We do not even have any measurements of the degree of likelihood for most clinically observed behavioral sequences—how frequently we can expect to find them, the analogue of the half-life measurement.

The predominant tendency in psychoanalytic writing is to follow Freud's explicit or implicit claim for the universal validity of statements, but then to formulate them so vaguely that they are immune from the swift refutation that would otherwise so easily be their fate. The big difference in implications for research is that a universal hypothesis can allegedly be disproved by a single clear exception; hence, "crucial experiment" is the ideal form of research in this kind of science. If hypotheses are formulated in probabilistic terms, however, they call for *statistical* research. Right away, that raises a question of which most traditional analysts have never even heard: What is the *power* of your statistical tests? Briefly, statistical research demands large samples, which are extremely difficult to obtain in psychoanalytic research.

THE STRUCTURE OF THE CLINICAL THEORY

To return to Rubinstein's argument, here is the basic scheme of the clinical theory, as he outlines it:

> (a) . . . all activities in which a person engages . . . are motivated even if on the face of it they may not seem to be; (b) . . . within limits people respond to external situations in more or less specific ways; and (c) . . . the presence in a person of certain motives and response dispositions may be explained, at least in part, by events early in that person's life. (Rubinstein, 1975, pp. 10–11)

From these three major points he draws three classes of *general* clinical hypotheses:

1. *Motivational* hypotheses (e.g., the hypothesis of the persistent manifestation potential of unconscious motives).
2. *Situational* hypotheses (e.g., the hypothesis of in part functionally equivalent situations).
3. *Genetic* hypotheses (e.g., the hypothesis of the development of situation-specific responses into more or less permanent dispositions).

There remains a group of *miscellaneous* general hypotheses (e.g., those involving the concept of unconscious fantasy and that of context fragmentation—i.e., that the material of experience may be broken into separate fragments detached from their contexts, and then recombined as in dream condensations).

Then, Rubinstein includes a large set of *special* clinical hypotheses.[1] These are rather general too (e.g., "When faced with an obstacle, most people will try to overcome it"), but they differ in being less abstract—they are statements about people, not processes. Other special clinical hypotheses are those concerning the specific types of defense mechanisms and the Oedipus complex. They too may be divided into motivational, situational, genetic, and other hypotheses. As Rubinstein comments, they are statements about people, or can easily be transformed into such statements. I refer you to his text for the full catalogue (which he says is incomplete) and his explanation of the details; I hope the preceding suffices to give some of the flavor of this effort.

Many of the generalizations of the clinical theory, when made explicit, sound almost embarrassingly commonplace—a property that led Sherwood (1969) to dismiss them as "platitudes." In my own effort to explicate the clinical theory implicitly used by Freud in the Dora case (briefly described in Chapter 8 of this volume), I too found that a great deal of it is common-sense psychology; and I agree with Rubinstein, *contra* Sherwood, that such generalizations play a critical part in psychoanalytic explanations. For the general and special clinical hypotheses, which together form the clinical theory, may be regarded not only as ways to explain behavior, but "as entailing certain rules of inference by the application of which particular clinical hypotheses are inferred" (Rubinstein, 1975, p. 28). And the latter, you will remember, include the interpretations that make up the explanation of individual neuroses.

CAN THE CLINICAL THEORY BE CONFIRMED?

Now we are ready to come to Rubinstein's ideas about how the clinical theory may be tested. He first addresses the confirmation of *particular* clinical hypotheses (those dealing with single cases), noting that since they too are probabilistic, in approaching their validation we must ask not for a true/false answer but about the degree to which each hypothesis is proba-ble. Second, he points out the fact that many particular clinical hypotheses contain theoretical terms—unobservables like "unconscious wish" or "re-pression." Therefore, they cannot be tested *directly*, only indirectly. Yet, "It is part of the logic of scientific procedure that only a hypothesis that is directly testable, or in some way logically connected with directly testable hypotheses, can be confirmed or refuted" (1975, p. 34).

Statements about unconscious wishes or fantasies can give rise to di-rectly testable hypotheses, however, though those are predictions concern-ing *classes* of behaviors, not specific acts. Thus, if we hypothesize that a man unconsciously hates his father, we cannot be certain that he will have trouble with *all* persons in authority over him or any specific one, or that such trouble will take any particular form, but we can fairly confidently predict that he will behave in one or more ways that make up a describable *class of events* (e.g., "having trouble with authority figures"[2]). Or the analyst may similarly postdict a set of possible events that might have occurred in the patient's childhood to make him hate his father; and the analyst may verify the postdictions when and if the patient reports such events among his childhood memories. Every time such a prediction or postdiction is made and verified, the probability increases that the hypotheses giving rise to the prediction are credible. I would add, parenthetically, that the diagnostic tester proceeds in exactly the same way, forming particular clinical hypotheses by applying the clinical theory to items of test data and then attempting to confirm or disconfirm them on other such data [and that it is relatively easy to get large numbers of incidents or observations concerning a patient, making it possible to reach statistically secure conclusions about particular clinical hypotheses. But in order to *generalize* safely and legitimately, there is no substitute for large numbers of research subjects—patients.]

Ordinary clinical work is not sufficient, however: Predictions and postdictions must be regularly recorded, and then all relevant evidence recorded too, finally being judged blind, with control data, for relevance to the prediction (or postdiction). Needless to say, little such work has been published! Because so many thousands of us have successfully made predictions and postdictions about particular cases informally, however, the impression naturally arises that psychoanalytic theory has been thoroughly validated in clinical use. As we know, Freud said as much on several occasions.

Yet that is an illusion, based on an insufficient logical analysis of the process of clinical confirmation, which Rubinstein has now supplied. Note that if a particular clinical hypothesis yields correct predictions or postdictions, it does so via some *general* clinical hypotheses; hence the former may be said to be confirmed to a certain degree, "but *only* if the general clinical hypotheses involved in the confirmation are assumed to be true" (Rubinstein, 1976a, p. 257).[3]

The situation is even more disquieting, however. With an actual clinical case, Rubinstein shows how a set of confirmed predictions and postdictions produce data just as compatible with another particular hypothesis as with the one that had in fact occurred to him. "*The choice between the two hypotheses will be determined primarily by the nature of the general . . . hypotheses we decide . . . to adopt*" (Rubinstein, 1975, p. 43: italics in original). And that choice cannot be made on the grounds of clinical evidence.

Here is one of our central theoretical dilemmas. On the one hand, every confirmation of a specific hypothesis by a successful prediction or postdiction somewhat increases the probability that the more general hypotheses used to make the predictions are true also, though to a lesser and unspecifiable degree. As Rubinstein points out, that is "commonly accepted scientific procedure" (1975, p. 50). All too often, the full set of data used to confirm a particular clinical hypothesis (and which therefore partly confirm the special clinical hypotheses entailed in it) is equally compatible with *another* set of general hypotheses. For example, we are familiar with the fact that followers of non-Freudian schools of analysis or of nonpsychoanalytic clinical theories are ready with their own explanations of our cases. It is commonplace that most of these theories, with incompatible general hypotheses, are about equally capable of accommodating one another's data. All of them seem to be confirmed in clinical practice, but they cannot all be true.

The reason for this curious situation, Rubinstein says, lies in the general insistence of psychoanalysts on working exclusively with clinical data from the therapeutic encounter. With that restriction, it is impossible to test a great part of the general clinical hypotheses. Thus, they

> have the status of largely unproven *presuppositions*. A theory based on such presuppositions would be *strictly* clinical in the sense that no nonpsychological considerations would be able to affect it. For this reason such a theory may be regarded as essentially a *system of rules of interpretation*, a hermeneutic system . . . [which is] neither falsifiable or confirmable *as such*. (Rubinstein, 1975, p. 52; italics in original)

"I doubt," Rubinstein drily adds, "that analysts who advocate a strictly clinical theory are willing to accept this consequence of such a theory." There is an alternative, however: to treat all clinical hypotheses "as true scientific hypotheses, that is, as referring to at present unknown processes" (Rubinstein, 1975, p. 52). Notably, the hypothesis of unconscious processes can only refer to hypothetical processes in the brain [and possibly other parts of the body], probably similar in all respects except for one crucial (but unknown) one[4] to the brain processes accompanying conscious mental processes. So interpreted, the general hypotheses may ultimately be testable neurophysiologically. To be sure, at present that is only a program, but one that can "turn psychoanalysis from a system of rules of interpretation into a developing science" (p. 52). Notice that such a program entails expanding the clinical theory or supplementing it by what is in effect a metapsychology, old or new. And because we cannot yet develop a directly applicable neurophysiological theory of the general and special propositions of the clinical theory, we must be content with models that are, so far as we know, *structurally homologous* both to clinical theory and to neuroscience (Rubinstein, 1976b).

Rubinstein (1974, 1976b), Peterfreund (1971), Peterfreund and Franceschini (1973), Rosenblatt and Thickstun (1977), Reiser (1984), and a few others have begun work on such alternative extraclinical theories to replace metapsychology, but it is too early to say what will come of these efforts.

PSYCHOANALYSIS: HERMENEUTICS OR SCIENCE?

Surprisingly enough, there have appeared a number of analysts (e.g., Spence, 1982) who do seem willing to abandon any claim at historical truth, touting the virtues of merely establishing a satisfying, complete narrative or "hermeneutic circle" of meaning.

We have now arrived at the second major trend of the three with which I began. Ricoeur (1970) seems to have brought hermeneutics to the attention of psychoanalysts in a book where he argued that their theory was only partly if at all scientific, primarily belonging to another ancient group of intellectual disciplines that began with biblical exegesis. These hermeneutic disciplines, which deal with subjective meaning rather than external facts, were said to have their own methodology, distinct from but on a par with that of science. For the last 15 years, many a psychoanalyst has come under the influence of this misleading doctrine, (e.g., Klein, 1976; Spence, 1982; Schafer, 1976, 1978). Of late, an effective counterattack has begun.

I commend to you Blight's (1981) paper and Holzman's (1985), as well as Chapter 15 in Eagle's excellent book (1984) and the 94-page introduction to Grünbaum's (1984). Blight shows how the hermeneuts' entire position rests on their acceptance of an anachronistic and unnecessarily narrow conception of science. Caricature natural science as most advocates of hermeneutics do, and it is easy to accept the proposition that psychoanalysis should be something else—indeed, that there *is* some alternative, equally respectable and defensible way of attaining knowledge. Following Popper (1963), Blight undertakes to show that there *is no* such alternate methodology.

Grünbaum is not satisfied with Blight's argument, if only because it rests upon Popper's account. But Grünbaum (1984) has mounted his own withering attack on hermeneutics from within the citadel of philosophy. He takes on Habermas (1971) and his claim that psychoanalysis is not a natural science but a "critical discipline," and makes sausage meat out of it, as well as the position of those like Ricoeur (1970), Steele (1979), Schafer (1976), and Klein (1976), who argue on such grounds as the assumed difference between reasons and causes, and the special role they claim for *meanings* in psychoanalytic theory. Meticulously, he takes all of the arguments apart, examines them logically and empirically, and shows them to be either trivially true, false, or based on misunderstanding. *Inter alias*, he demonstrates that Habermas's argument is based on an idiosyncratic and partial reading of Freud, and on patently ill-informed misconceptions of the nature of natural science. By and large, the same is true of authors like Schafer, who say that psychoanalysis cannot be a natural science because they seriously misunderstand what science is and how scientists work.

RECENT THEORETICAL "DEVELOPMENTS"

The third major happening of recent years in psychoanalytic theory is the rise first of object relations theory and now of self psychology. Many of the same people who have been swept along by these trends have also been preoccupied with narcissism and so-called narcissistic disorders such as the borderline syndrome. As Eagle and Wolitzky (1989) point out, what all these topics have in common is a concern with preoedipal sources of psychopathology, which is in part a healthy reaction against the monotonous tendency of so many self-styled classical analysts to trace everything to the vagaries of the oedipal situation and its aftermath. One hears less talk about ego psychology these days; it is no longer modish.

The last comment betrays my basic reaction to the content of this third trend: that it is largely a matter of current fads. It is not, I think, a mere coincidence that these theories have arisen as metapsychology was declining, but neither one is a substitute for it. Indeed, despite certain attractive features of both object relations theory and self psychology, they fail to make any serious or searching critique of metapsychology, and—like ego psychology—they retain a good deal of it. As rebellions, they are much too limited to accomplish the needed radical (indeed, revolutionary) change. Surely it is closer to the truth to reject the primal hate of objects and to recognize the biological irreducibility of attachment, and if Bowlby (1969) is considered a member of the object relations school, the above remarks do not apply to his much more fundamental revisions. Fairbairn (1952), Guntrip (1969), and Winnicott (1958), however, all incorporate far too many of the defective parts of psychoanalytic theory to make their corrections much more than cosmetic, in my view (and in that of Grünbaum, 1984, pp. 246–247). Moreover, like Kohut (1971, 1977) and his followers, they show the same familiar obliviousness to the need for cogent evidence, the same willingness to accept unspecified "clinical experience" as a sufficient factual basis for confident assertions of fact as the traditional Freudians whom they claim to have transcended, but on scientifically unacceptable grounds.

THE CURRENT CRISIS

I would be surprised if some readers were not taken aback or even outraged by such a brief dismissal of most of what is interesting and controversial about current psychoanalytic theorizing. But I am trying to get across the depth and urgency of my feeling that when the foundations of our house are tottering, it makes no sense to argue about rival designs for new wallpaper. There are a few sound timbers under there, no doubt, but we have very little idea which ones they are; and we know that there is deep trouble in the philosophical footings themselves.

Perhaps I can clarify the reasons for my sense of crisis if I go back to the clinical theory and sum up its present status. Just as a theory, it shares many of the liabilities of metapsychology. It is a sprawling mess, without boundaries, without definitive formulation of its hypotheses or generally accepted definitions for its concepts, which are intermingled with metapsychological terms and some of disputed status (e.g., unconscious wish). The faults of reification and personification may be found here too. The philosophical foundations of the clinical theory are uncertain, no psychoanalyst having ever plainly specified them. The clinical theory is full of mutually contradictory hypotheses. Analysts keep making new observations, which clash with existing formulations. Instead of trying to figure out what sampling or situational parameters make the difference, the tradition has been merely to say, in effect, "No, *this* is how it is." And the resulting contradiction is never resolved.

So, at the least, the theory needs a tremendous amount of work, of a kind few psychoanalysts possess the qualifications for—notably, a good grounding in the philosophy of science. The unglamorous work of codifying, of defining concepts and formulating hypotheses, has been well begun by Rubinstein, but in the years since his groundbreaking pair of papers, there has been no perceptible rush to pick up the baton and hurry it forward. It would be gratifying if these words were to stimulate some theoretically inclined young analysts to become interested in the task and to start preparing themselves for it.

As to the validity of the theory, the picture is quite murky. Remember that probabilistic hypotheses cannot be either clearly confirmed or refuted by a single experiment or other empirical study—a point grasped by few experimenters. Of course, if repeated trials find *no* positive instances, such a hypothesis can be said simply to be false; but I very much doubt that a lot of weeding out will take place that way. More often, it is a question of the proportion between positive and negative outcomes. It is fair to say that virtually none of the needed work has been done—attaching a specific likelihood to every hypothesis in the theory, along with a statement of its parameters.

My own reaction after reading and reflecting on Rubinstein and Grünbaum was to do a sort of double take, and ask myself, "Can the situation really be *that* bad?" It is hard to admit how little *proof* there is for any psychoanalytic hypothesis after all these years of use, when the theory seems so clinically valuable and when such a large part of the intellectual world has adopted great hunks of the clinical theory and treats it not as a set of interesting hypotheses but as received knowledge. After all that, *must* we say, "Well, in fact we don't really know precisely what we mean when we talk about unconscious fantasies, or even whether they exist and have important effects"? Yes, we should! Actually, about all we can say on this particular issue is that it makes sense out of a great many otherwise puzzling observations to assume that such processes as unconscious fantasies are active and effective in people, and that alternative explanations lack the simplicity and power of the psychoanalytic hypothesis.

Further, we must admit that during the past three-quarters of a century, no one has been able to push this part of the theory forward appreciably.

We do not know how or when unconscious fantasies get started; we cannot reliably and confidently say about even a person in psychoanalytic treatment whether she or he has a given fantasy or not; how intense or active it is at any given moment when the person in question is not producing clearly recognizable derivatives;[5] or what determines whether it will be manifest in a dream, in conscious daydreaming, in some autoplastic symptom, in acting out, or in adaptive behavior. By "what determines whether . . . " I mean what situational circumstances other than subliminal activation of the kind Silverman (1982) used in his important researches, interacting with what aspects of personality in persons of various ages, sex, education, and so on, and from what culture and era. Such parameters are lacking for every one of the hypotheses making up the clinical theory, to the best of my knowledge.

When it has been possible to test parts of the clinical theory by use of *non*clinical data, it has often come off badly. Results of recent surveys of the attempts to test and verify the clinical theory (e.g., Fisher & Greenberg, 1977) are about as mixed and spotty as those of Sears's (1943) original review. The main reason is, as Rubinstein points out, that we must go to a nonbehavioral realm, such as neurophysiology, to test a great deal of the most distinctive parts of the clinical theory: Psychoanalysis is *not* autonomous, existing in self-sufficient isolation on an island remote from other sciences. No science can do that, and it was a great mistake for psychoanalysis to have cut its ties to the rest of the scientific world.

The role of whistle-blower does not particularly suit me. By nature I am a moderate, a compromiser who starts with the conviction that there is something valuable on each side of most controversies. But this time I feel I would be derelict if I did not seize every opportunity to say to psychoanalysts, "Hey, really, people—this is an emergency!" Things have gotten so bad that we have to start making radical changes. I believe that if psychoanalysts simply continue down their present path, making no effort at fundamental change, psychoanalysis will continue to shrink and wither, and will eventually collapse.

There is a kind of moral crisis in psychoanalysis about which very little is said, a clash between the values we profess and those we live out. In America, the mass media and the dominant corporations encourage an adjustive style of getting along and going along, but we profess an ideal of personal autonomy and integrity. Do we have the requisite guts really to live by those standards? We are surrounded by a culture of alarming mendacity and systematic disinformation, but we stand for and seek the truth. Yet some of us are happy to qualify that as "narrative truth"—not necessarily what really happened, but what makes a good story. In a mixed democratic and authoritarian society, we profess democratic values, but run our organizational affairs in a largely authoritarian way. Above all, Freud taught what Rieff (1959) called "an ethic of honesty," an unflinching readiness to forsake self-deception and to face the facts about oneself. In practice, however, Freud himself was no paragon of self-criticism. He was unusually intolerant of outside criticism, too; I cannot think of a single incident where he really listened to a critic who was not part of the inner circle and considered the critique on its merits. Yet he is our scientific model, and analysts have faithfully copied him in this respect.

American psychoanalysis has lived for so long within a snug cocoon of myth that it seems unable to go through the predictable pains of metamorphosis into a viably progressive discipline. The protective threads it has wound around itself include warding off all criticism as resistance, idolatry of Freud, and faithful internalization of all his faults as a scientist and writer. It has therefore failed to develop any *standards* for or means for *improving* (1) the accumulation of facts; (2) the formulation of hypotheses; (3) the testing of hypotheses, or other means to confront theory with fact; (4) the consolidation and collation of the huge theoretical literature; (5) the resolution of disputes, whether over facts or theories; or (6) the training of new generations of psychoanalytic scientists capable of doing anything better than their predecessors. Without self-criticism and a concerted effect to improve, there can be only stagnation.

I am sorry to have to add that though all of the above failings may be most egregiously true of many medical analysts from the Freudian mainstream, neither nonmedical psychoanalysts nor those of dissident schools have any reason to feel complacent. There are approximately as many medical as nonmedical analysts among the handful to whom one can point as sophisticated theorists or researchers in psychoanalysis.

SOME TENTATIVE PRESCRIPTIONS

Having gone this far in radical criticism, I feel an obligation to say at least something about what needs to be done.

For a good many years, I thought that the necessary reforms might be facilitated by bringing into psychoanalysis behavioral scientists who were already well trained and committed to scientific method and research. Briefly: We tried it and it didn't work. A sustained and fairly expensive attempt by the Foundations Fund for Research in Psychiatry did recruit and train a good many such scientists, but with a minimal impact upon organized psychoanalysis. Some became disillusioned and dropped out; some were totally co-opted and became analysts indistinguishable from any other. Most continued to do their original kinds of research alongside a psychoanalytic practice, maintaining an impermeable barrier between the two activities. So I believe that we know pretty well that that is not the way.

Few of the critiques of psychoanalysis have explicitly recognized the special problems of developing it beyond its present status as a sort of protoscience, or at least a science in an early phase of development. The fact is that it would be extraordinarily difficult to take the next steps to improve it. Those should include a theoretical phase and a research phase; ideally, they should proceed concurrently, one helping the other along.

The first step, then, must be to survey the theory, attempting to collect and separately consolidate its metapsychological and clinical-theoretical branches, purging them of obvious fallacies and errors—a job essentially completed as far as metapsychology goes. [That is, the operation was successful though the patient died.] The clinical theory, on the other hand, needs a great deal more work of the kind Rubinstein has so admirably begun. We must *restate the theory* in such a way as to make it as testable as possible, giving the relation between its theoretical and observational language a clear and unambiguous formulation.

Thirty years ago, at the Research Center for Mental Health, George Klein and I decided to make such an attempt. With the help of several younger colleagues, we tried to reformulate the psychoanalytic theory of thinking so that we could test it in our laboratory and more generally in empirical research. I focused on making the theory of the primary and secondary process operational in the form of a manual for scoring manifestations of primary-process thinking and its control in Rorschach responses (and, later, other kinds of data such as dreams, Thematic Apperception Test stories, and free associations). That gave rise to a good deal of research, and indirectly to some efforts to reconsider the theory in light of the findings. I was surprised, at first, by the fact that we never succeeded in finding any Freudian proposition about primary process that was directly testable. We did formulate and test a number of theoretical propositions, but they have not been much noticed by psychoanalysts—partly because I have not yet pulled it all together, asking what the theoretical yield has been.

Its theory of thinking is a relatively unrepresentative facet of psychoanalysis, however. What is distinctive about psychoanalysis as a psychology, what gives it a special claim to our attention aside from our personal involvement, is its concern with what is most important in human lives. Long before the birth of lifespan developmental psychology, Freud was virtually alone in attempting to make a theory about how human lives grow, how they are malformed and straightened out, and what determines their major features. Just because of this macroscopic approach—this orientation to the largest issues and the most perplexing dilemmas of human lives— psychoanalytic theory is especially interesting but extraordinarily difficult to test. The clinical psychoanalyst has an unrivaled opportunity to make observations of potentially broad importance, to formulate observed or intuited regularities, and to frame hypotheses. The treatment situation has many grave deficiencies as a setting in which to test and validate hypotheses, however; but how else are the necessary data to be obtained? The main trouble is that one has to expend enormous amounts of time, effort, and money to get such data on a single case, while the probabilistic nature of the theory demands statistical studies with *many* cases.

Too many analysts treat it as obvious that only the data of the psychoanalytic hour are relevant to answering questions about the clinical theory. Actually, a good deal can be done with the techniques of multiform personality assessment, particularly when applied in such longitudinal research as that of Jack and Jeanne H. Block (1980). Indeed, I am convinced that it is easy to exaggerate the comprehensiveness of psychoanalytic clinical data. Often enough, an analyst knows very little about several departments of a patient's life. Those can be probed by systematic inquiry of a kind the therapeutic enterprise does not need and in fact countermands. And such techniques can yield surprising amounts of confidential, highly personal, and conflict-ridden confessions to a skillful interviewer in a research setting (see, e.g., the work of Vaillant, 1977) and direct observations of familial interactions in place of one participant's reports (see, e.g., Hauser et al., 1984).

Therefore, systematic empirical research on the clinical theory must be done, using data other than those of the treatment. Let us have all of such research we can get; but do not expect to see much of it, especially not from the psychoanalytic institutes. It requires teams of highly trained clinical researchers; a favorable setting in which they can establish good rapport and gather data over long periods of time; and money—lots of it, providing secure support over long times. For many problems, that means decades. To some extent, such protracted work can be carried out with changing personnel if the attrition and replacement are gradual and if the main leadership remains constant.

Another needed and feasible kind of research that can feed back to the clinical theory uses tape recordings of complete psychoanalyses, or at least of multihour segments of them (e.g., the work of Gill & Hoffman, 1982; Luborsky, 1967, 1984; Silberschatz, 1978). Dahl has proposed and has begun assembling an eclectic library of such data, not limited to classical Freudian treatments; the data are available to any qualified researcher. Obviously, the value of each case grows as the recorded hours are accompanied by accessory data, and as various kinds of indexing, summarizing, compilation, and coding are performed and their results stored as a permanent addition to the library. Again, however, the work is very expensive; it requires many talents not likely to be found in single individuals; and virtually none of it can be done without the aid of psychoanalytically trained judges to perform various kinds of blind analysis of the raw data. This complex, demanding, expensive work has the great merit of solving the problems of public access (Wallerstein & Sampson, 1971).

It would be greatly helped along if training institutes would require all candidates to submit one recorded case of no less than 100 consecutive hours before graduation, along with their notes and a diagnostic workup.

Supervising analysts could be required to keep some kind of record of their observations also. If I may become even more fanciful, a condition of a senior psychoanalyst's attaining the status of training analyst could be the submission of the complete recording of a reasonably successful case. Those would be rather substantial contributions to research, which would cost something but not nearly as much as would be necessary otherwise to build up quickly enough a data base of substantial size.

If training institutes had active research branches where competent teams were working with the cooperative data base just described, it would contribute greatly to the training of future generations of more scientifically oriented psychoanalysts. The senior investigators could offer required courses in the institutes on the problems, rationale, and techniques of controlled clinical research. Candidates would naturally be drawn into the work, serving first as judges and learning at first hand what rigorous investigation is like. Obviously, only a minority would go on to take more important roles and to become investigators themselves, but the numbers would doubtless be considerably greater than at present, when the supply is alarmingly small.

In a thoughtful paper, Holzman (1985) attributes the neglect of research and the scientific stunting of psychoanalysis to its exclusive focus on therapy. He overlooks, however, the excellent economic reasons for this focus. The situation remains now as it has been since the beginning: The one way to make a secure living in psychoanalysis is private practice. No career lines exist for anyone who might have the fantasy of becoming a psychoanalytic scientist—no obvious job openings and no prospect that society will ever find enough of a need for such people to establish the necessary institutional base. We probably cannot expect working psychoanalysts literally to tithe in order to support research centers, though many are already voluntarily giving substantial amounts of their incomes to the American Psychoanalytic Association's Fund for Psychoanalytic Research, which has funded some much-needed work. Without a basic change in our crisis-ridden, absurdly expensive, and dilapidated system of providing medical care, I see no prospect that the necessary economic base can be provided for the heroic effort needed to reorganize, redirect, and reform psychoanalytic theory. Let's hope I am wrong! For it would be an enormous loss to psychology if the great insights of psychoanalysis faded away without ever having had a chance to be converted into a real science, and a huge loss to society if it were deprived of the unique contribution to human welfare that clinical psychoanalysis at its best can make.

PART VI

Toward the Future

CHAPTER 14

Freud and the Emergence of a New World Hypothesis

With Chapter 13, I have brought to an end my critique of metapsychology. In the process of writing this book, again and again philosophical issues came up. I became aware that Freud was, much more than I had imagined, the prisoner of his early assumptions—not only about methodological issues (which are ultimately epistemological), but about other metaphysical ones as well. As we saw in Chapter 9, his implicit theory of reality constituted a partial commitment to a materialist and mechanistic ontology. In several places, his stance on the mind-body problem turned out to have important consequences for his theories.

I have thus found myself brought up against the necessity to make these philosophical commitments explicit and to criticize them. That does not seem quite enough. At least, I should lay my own cards on the table. This chapter attempts, therefore, to discuss ways in which Freud helped to change the metaphysical scene onto which he was born, and to outline the systems metaphysics that appeals to me as a more adequate foundation for a future psychoanalytic theory than the pragmatism[1] that is so prevalent, especially among those who are drawn to hermeneutics.

Several times, in this book I have spoken about metaphysical systems, but now I want to change my terminology to conform to that of Stephen C. Pepper, and explain his concept, which appears in this chapter's title.

WORLD HYPOTHESES

A modest renewal of interest in the work of Pepper (1891-1972) is currently taking place, though his concept of "world hypothesis" does not yet have any wide currency. It is nevertheless highly suited to my purposes—a conception of basic philosophical assumptions that underlie, support, and subtly guide many aspects of our conscious thoughts and behavior, though we may not be focally aware of having adopted them.

Whether a person has ever given philosophy as much as a passing glance, he cannot help picking up and incorporating into his own outlook the prevailing definitions of reality (ontology), ideas about the place of humanity in the universe (cosmology),[2] and conceptions of knowledge and how we can know anything (epistemology). In short, we are all metaphysicians, implicitly if not explicitly, and we must take some stand on ethical principles as well. Pepper does not include a person's basic value positions in his conception of that thinker's world hypothesis, but I am impressed by the congruence of a school's handling of moral and ethical values with the rest of its world view.

Pepper's peculiar merit, in contrast to others who have surveyed and classified types of metaphysical positions, is that he searches for and finds a small number of independent, more or less equally comprehensive and adequate philosophical positions, each stemming from a distinctive *root metaphor*.

> A man desiring to understand the world looks about for a clue to its comprehension. He pitches upon some area of commonsense fact and tries if he cannot understand other areas in terms of this one. This original area becomes then his basic analogy or root metaphor. (Pepper, 1942, p. 91)

From this root grow categories, used as "basic concepts of explanation and description" and applied to all other areas of fact and speculation. The most fertile root metaphors generate the most adequate explanatory systems, or world hypotheses.

With remarkable neutrality, Pepper examines the range of metaphysical positions and settles upon four as "adequate"—formism (e.g., Plato), mechanism (e.g., Locke), contextualism (e.g., Dewey's pragmatism), and organicism (e.g., Hegel's idealism). He himself later added a fifth, which he called "selectivism." Though I have cited approximate examples, none of these world hypotheses is exactly identical with the philosophical system of any one man. Instead, it is an abstracted, internally coherent, implied position, a kind of ideal type toward which the "strain toward consistency" in human thought impels us.[3] At the same time, any given philosophical work is the outcome of various other influences, so that it is likely to be a compromise formation (in Freud's phrase) to some degree, even to the point of an attempt to hybridize fundamentally incompatible systems of ideas. Cartesian dualism, for example, is such a conjoining of two worlds— one of matter, one of spirit—each with its world hypothesis: mechanism and animism.

I hope to show (though more incidentally than through exposition) that, despite their somewhat shadowy and conceptual existence, world hypotheses have an important kind of reality in intellectual history.

FROM ANIMISM TO MECHANISM

The first major world hypothesis, which dominated European thought for many centuries, does not appear in Pepper's list of four, since he did not consider it adequate. He calls it *animism*, though in the form that is most familiar to us it is theology or religious supernaturalism. As Freud (1912–1913) noted, it is the oldest theory of the world; still vigorous in his time (and ours), it was the target of most of his polemical writing of a philosophical character (see also Freud, 1927c). Its perennial appeal despite its philosophical weakness, Pepper believes, arises from its being based on the most appealing of root metaphors: the human being. The spirits primitive people imagine in an effort to comprehend the events of nature are transparently projections of themselves, and no matter how profound, elevated, or sophisticated the theology, the concept of God can be traced back in an unbroken lineage to simple projective animism. That does not, of course, invalidate it. One secret of the staying power of this world hypothesis is its imperviousness to evidence. The principal inadequacy with which Pepper charges it, however, is its lack of precision. Since it begins by postulating a supernatural world beyond human ken except by revelation to persons who are able to persuade others that they have privileged access, it tends to be authoritarian and hostile to skeptics. The only limits on what can be asserted are set by the cognitive consciences and self-discipline of religious leaders and spokesmen.

Parenthetically, I should note that the first adequate world hypothesis, which Pepper calls *formism*, was developed by Plato and has long enjoyed the respect of many philosophers and educated people generally. Yet it has never, in modern times, been able to command the adherence of a large enough segment of the world of ideas (except perhaps in the classic era) for us to be able to call it the dominant theory.

Let me briefly sum up the major tenets of the animistic world hypothesis. Cosmologically, the ostensible center of everything is God, who created and oversees it, intervening at will. But it is also an anthropocentric universe: God made the world for man and set our habitation, the earth, in its literal center. However omnipotent and omniscient God may be, he is remarkably attentive to and solicitous of every mortal one of us. What is most real is the spiritual realm—our immortal souls, God, and the afterworld. The world of this life is a passing show of purely temporary importance, a brief prelude to an eternity in heaven or hell. Its only importance is that our behavior in this world may determine where we spend the infinite future. Man's knowledge is limited, but God is omniscient; the most important things we know by faith, not by observation or reasoning. If you would seek knowledge, go to the wise men or the sacred books, the traditionalistic sources of truth; it is impious folly to try to discover truth on your own. Religion can teach us the meaning of life: We are here for a purpose, because God put us here for ends of his own, and everything that happens is part of his (usually inscrutable) grand plan in a teleologically ordered universe. He has laid down moral rules for the guidance of our conduct, also; we must obey his commandments. Since we have immortal souls, not subject to the laws that govern brute matter, we are free to choose which path to follow and so are morally responsible for our acts.

As E. A. Burtt (1932) has brilliantly shown, the new physics of the 17th century brought with it a revolution in ways of conceiving of the entire world. The new formative image, the mechanical clock, was an important invention of the preceding medieval centuries. Machines were the main cultural artifacts usefully supplied by the new science, and the spring-driven clockwork made possible the construction of clever automata, mimicking the movements of living beings. The machine remains a principal guiding figure of our culture; witness the readiness with which it is invoked figuratively when we refer to the structure of anything from the galaxy to the atom, and particularly the human being and human institutions.

Even though such pioneers as Kepler and Newton were devoutly religious, they created a picture of the universe as a majestic clockwork requiring nothing more of God than that he create the machinery and serve as its prime mover. By the late-18th-century period of the Enlightenment, it became increasingly feasible to encompass all explanatory knowledge about the universe and man without needing to invoke God at all. He was read out of existence by such materialists as Baron d'Holbach (1770) and (in Freud's time) Büchner (1855), who were not afraid to be outright atheists. A complete and consistent world hypothesis of reductionistic mechanistic materialism emerged. It did not need to be adopted by scientists generally to have a profound influence upon them, however piously they might attend religious services and devoutly believe in God. It was no longer necessary to assume a spiritual reality behind the material (though one might if one liked). Simple location in time and place became the hallmark of the real, and the hard, tiny, grittily enduring atom was its very epitome.

In cosmology, a new grandeur of immensity, provoking a rather dismal sense of wonder, had to serve in place of religious reverence: The universe was far larger, emptier, lonelier, and more indifferent than before, and human beings seemed humble and trivial indeed, living on a minor planet of a modest, ordinary star without an easily specifiable place among billions of neighbors in a galaxy undistinguished among countless others. Our lives are the briefest flicker in a stony, insensate eternity of time, devoid of any special significance or claim to notice. It became meaningless to ask for the meaning of life; purpose had no more place in this austere and flavorless world, governed by abstract, quantitative laws, than did spiritual entities like souls, or secondary qualities like colors and feelings.

Alfred North Whitehead (1925) has shown how the new scientific world hypothesis required Locke's and Descartes's doctrine of primary and secondary qualities. If what was essential to science about an object was its quantifiable mass and its location in space and time, then by a procrustean logic all its other properties (color, sound, odor, etc.) were mere secondary qualities resulting from the operations of minds and not of interest to science. That is, the grand objective order of nature had been formulated without them, in terms of only the primary qualities, which soon were known merely as quantities. Such a drab and abstract nature would hardly interest anyone but a scientist, yet it is wonderfully useful to him. Precisely this impoverishment of their subject matter freed the scientists of that time to work with growing success, providing humankind with many concrete benefits.

Note how central was the role of analysis in this system. Newton succeeded so well because of his analytic ability to extract from apples and luminous heavenly spheres alike their elementary properties of mass and movement in space and time. Generations of scientists since have followed his methods, for Newton seemed to be saying: To succeed, simplify; assume an isolated system; find the basic elements; experiment to find their causal interrelations; seek the mathematical formula that will explain how they operate conjointly; and you have the answer—scientific law. The important new method of experimental control means taking pains to narrow one's field of vision to see more surely by looking at less; the subject matter is isolated from its natural setting by careful artifice. The thematic emphasis of atomism was highly congenial to the analytic scientific mind, though logically separate.

Despite what Freud (1917a) was to call the cosmological blow to man's narcissism delivered by Copernicus in destroying the geocentric world picture, science gave reason for pride and hope; for human knowledge, despite its fallibility, now becomes in principle indefinitely extensible if we only hew to the rules of the scientific method. We must receive all traditional wisdom with skepticism and demand to be shown evidence—that is, controlled observations. These are then organized by clear logic into testable laws. It was consistent with this world hypothesis to rely on the cool, lucid intellect to solve moral as well as empirical problems. But since all events are rigidily determined down to their tiniest details by gapless chains of cause and effect, freedom of choice is an illusion. By the late 19th century, morality had become a subject for dispassionate scientific examination, for no department of life or experience was exempt. Indeed, many tried to produce a new, scientifically based ethics, though without notable success.

Lewis Mumford (1970) has brilliantly argued the case that there has always been a close connection between materialistic, mechanistic science and political authoritarianism.[4] It is not just in the Reagan budget that by far the greatest expenditures for research and development are allocated to the war machine; the latter has always been science's most faithful patron. The hierarchical, machine-like structure of bureaucratic institutions requires of its human components that they perform as much like interchangeable mechanical parts as possible. The ultimate extension of this dreadful but powerful fantasy is what Mumford calls the "megamachine"—the entire society in a totalitarian organization, rolling along over everything in its path with one dictatorial despot in the driver's seat: Hitler conducting the Holocaust through his order-taking intermediaries.

Clearly, I do not mean to imply that everyone who is true to the ideals of 19th-century reductionistic science will end up doing the grisly "experiments" of the Nazi doctors. Human beings are not wholly consistent, and very few people have clearly espoused the entire mechanistic ethos. Yet the fact that all the elements of this ideological configuration exist and fit naturally together creates a subtle, implicit pressure to believe in most aspects of the whole system, or to act as if you did.

FREUD, RELATIVISM, AND PRAGMATISM

As soon as the mechanistic world picture began to unfold, it met opposition. The main new philosophical alternatives for a couple of centuries were idealisms, equally extreme attempts to reduce the material to the mental or spiritual instead of the reverse. In the hands of Hegel, a third and equally adequate world hypothesis took shape, which Pepper [somewhat misleadingly] calls *organicism*.[5] One can look on the romantic movement as another reaction against the austerity of the ethos of mechanistic science, and it is important to remember that most scientists were not handicapped as human beings because they were brought up in a culture where religious indoctrination began very early and the school system was pervaded by humanism.

It is obvious that in many ways, Freudian psychoanalysis was a natural outgrowth and expression of the mechanistic world hypothesis, especially so in its metapsychology. To be sure, Freud was just about as deeply committed to a contrasting set of ideas from the softer tradition of humanism, the central core of ideas and values conveyed by the humanities. His theories were always more or less successful struggles to synthesize the themes and outlook of humanism with those of mechanistic metaphysics. Humanism is not a consistent *Weltanschauung*, but a valuable partial set of themes opposed to and threatened by both the supernatural and the mechanistic world views. Any ideology broad and loose enough to attract the fealty of thinkers as diametrically opposed as Carl Rogers and B. F. Skinner can hardly be integrated or a workably consistent set of philosophical footings.

Fairly early in the 19th century, the mechanistic world hypothesis began to be challenged and stretched by some developments within the hard sciences themselves. In a growing variety of disciplines, notably crystallography and morphology, some concepts of structure and form began to be necessary. Ecology, in some ways the most typical scientific embodiment of an emerging emphasis on contexts and whole systems, had its beginnings in some of Humboldt's shrewd observations about landscapes as habitats, and in much that Darwin wrote, for example, about the evolutionary fitting of species to their environments. A number of facts began piling up in physics that were embarrassing to the Newtonian cosmology. All along, of course, advocates of the religious (supernatural) world view continued to thunder against scientific materialism, and we should keep in mind the fact that the great majority of humankind has always held a basically dualistic, supernatural set of metaphysical assumptions—to this very day, as the rise of fundamentalism and the challenge of creationism attest.

In many respects, the intellectual crisis of the 19th century that was precipitated by a reluctant Darwin only continued a task that had been begun by the Enlightenment and the romantic era—that of undermining settled, traditional, absolutist ways of thinking. As the intellectual bankruptcy of dogmatic doctrines became evident, one or another form of relativism took its place in the minds of literate people. A student of intellectual development in contemporary young people, W. G. Perry (1970), has regularly found the following sequence. Naive youngsters, so unquestioning of their basic beliefs that they may be called dogmatists, in secondary school or college first encounter multiplicity: a diversity of people, ideas, systems of values, ways of thinking, and so on. After several intermediate positions of attempting to come to terms with multiplicity, the student typically adopts the relativistic stance that "everyone is entitled to his own opinion."

Without too much oversimplification, the history of Western culture can be said to have followed a similar course during the past four centuries. In the era of great explorations, travelers brought back marvelous tales about the multiplicity of human beings and their cultures; eventually the pursuit of such exotic curiosities became anthropology. The particularistic romantic temper was especially fascinated by the diversity in the ethical systems by which the world's peoples have lived, and many people were at first shocked to discover that ideals which they had always taken as universal were ethnocentrically limited. If there were as many moral perspectives as cultures, the disquieting thought arose, perhaps all were equally valid. Thus cultural relativism in ethics was born.

But moral relativism also raised the possibility of what Piaget (Piaget & Inhelder, 1969) calls "decentering" (see below). That is, once we realize that there are various other cultures besides our own, with somewhat different moral views, we become aware of the possibility that what seems absolutely right and wrong to us may be so only because of our cultural conditioning. (We do not have to accept the premises that different cultures have fundamentally different moral views, or that our moral views would have been different if we had had different accidents of birth and rearing. The possibility alone is upsetting to orthodoxy and absolutism.) We can now envisage a new stance, previously invisible to us, outside of and perhaps above our culture, suspended in some hyperspace in which cultures are arrayed. From this new imaginary standpoint, it is possible to raise such questions as these: Are any of the moral systems or principles of any cultures absolutely right or wrong? Could another sentient and intelligent creature have quite a different moral sense or indeed none at all? Granted, there are no easy answers to these and similar questions, as D. H. Munro (1968) argues. Nevertheless, it was a striking intellectual achievement to have attained the decentered position, which alone permits questions of this type to be asked.

Consider also the relation between pragmatism and developments in mathematics. With the development of non-Euclidean geometries early in the 19th century, it became evident that a geometry was one of a number of possible formal systems, none of which had the absolute and eternal verity that had long been claimed for Euclid's. Likewise, language and mathematics generally are formal systems of this kind; their value is contingent upon the human purposes to which they were harnessed. C. S. Peirce could see that and put forward the first pragmatic theory of truth precisely because of his attainments in symbolic logic (Wiener, 1968).

This common theme of liberation from absolute, fixed dogmas swept through many fields of thought during the 19th century. Before the Darwinian revolution, the general conception of the biological universe was a fixed and stable one: The forms of life we know were created at one time and would persist unchanged until Judgment Day. Darwin not only upset the authoritarian dictates of the Christian churches about the "kingdom" of living things, but also substituted a view of ceaseless change with no logical goal or endpoint.

Freud did his best to apply this Darwinian view to human psychology. He did not conceive of a fixed and eternal human nature, but saw man as a continually evolving creature with different instincts and potentialities than his remote ancestors had had. In that respect, he was not very different from many of his contemporaries, for all ideational shores were wet by the rising Darwinian tide.

Freud did, however, make a more distinctive and personal contribution to the growth of relativism and the new possibilities of decentering, for what he (1917a) called the three "blows to man's narcissism" delivered by Copernicus, Darwin, and himself may also be pictured as three stages of decentering, each freeing us from an old dogmatism and introducing a type of relativism. When Copernicus dethroned the earth from its place at the center of the physical universe, he gave us a vaster vision: Long before space travel became a literal reality, people were freed to roam in imagination through a world of many worlds, a universe of universes, where before we had been confined within a single small and parochial one. When Darwin showed us that we were a species like any other, with a common ancestry and a future of continued modification, he greatly enlarged our self-knowledge, freeing and inspiring all the biological sciences. Our increased capacity to free ourselves from disease is only the most obvious benefit.

Freud likewise brought humankind unpalatable but nourishing truth. He correctly saw that many people would feel threatened by being told that they were not entirely masters of themselves, that they could not easily know even their own minds because of the veils of repression, and that most of us spend much of our lives endlessly enacting versions of simple but unconscious dramas from our early childhoods. In works such as *Totem and Taboo* he showed the imprint of impulse and defense, operating without the conscious will of the actor, on systems of religious and philosophical ideas as well as on neurotic symptoms. Here, then, was a psychological relativism growing up alongside the economic and sociological relativism of his contemporaries. The concept of rationalization—that we hold certain ideas not for their superficial and ostensible content, but because they satisfy the obscure imperatives of desire and fear—had a swift and enormous vogue if an unsettling effect. Who could be sure that one's beliefs were not clever fronts for wishful conclusions? One could not assume that everyone else shared the same psychic reality; what seems real for me is to you transparently determined by my unconscious wishes and defenses. The unremembered traces of infantile traumas and fixations leave a different coloring on everyone's personal spectacles.

In all the forms of relativism I have briefly sketched, the phenomenon of what Hofstadter (1979) calls the "strange loop" occurs: The relativist eventually discovers that he is sawing off the limb on which he himself is sitting. If each culture seems to have its own moral system, which anthropologists tell us fits it and seems necessary to it, perhaps all are equally valid or invalid—including the system of values within which I am making the present value judgment! If all ideological systems are ultimately determined by the economic system of producing and distributing wealth within which they grow up, then how could Marx himself claim to stand outside? Why are his own ideas—indeed, the very doctrine of economic determinism—not subject to the same caveat? If conscious ideas and arguments are often rationalizations for decisions made on the basis of unconscious wishes or fears, what guarantee is there that Freud's own theory—including the concept of rationalization itself—was not a vast rationalization? The problem of relativism, therefore, is that of the strange loop of self-referentiality, which produces so many of the familiar logical paradoxes. The oldest is that of Epimenides the Cretan, who baffled his listeners by declaring, "All Cretans are liars." Or, more baldly put, "This sentence is false." As a moment's reflection shows, it can be neither false nor true!

Relativism is hardly a comfortable position; it is inherently unstable. Perry (1970) finds that some college students lapse from it back into the values and outlooks with which they first entered the new milieu, while others move ahead to what he calls "commitment," the affirmation of an examined and personally integrated set of basic principles and goals. Nevertheless, near the end of the 19th century, a group of philosophers were able to transform relativism into a vigorous philosophical school, *pragmatism*, which ultimately constituted a new world hypothesis as adequate as any that had preceded it.

Pragmatism, according to P. P. Wiener (1968) has five major components:

(1) a *pluralistic* empiricism or method of investigating . . . ; (2) a *temporalistic* view of reality and knowledge as the upshot of an evolving stream of consciousness . . . or of *objects* of consciousness . . . ; (3) a *relativistic* or contextualistic conception of reality and values in which traditional eternal ideas of space, time, causation, axiomatic truth, intrinsic and eternal values are all viewed as relative to varying psychological, social, historical, or logical contexts . . . ; (4) a *probabilistic* view of physical and social hypotheses and laws in opposition to both mechanistic or dialectical determinism and historical necessity or inevitability . . . ; (5) a secular democratic individualism. (p. 553)

Pepper calls the world hypothesis of the pragmatists *contextualism*. The previous summary hints at some of its strengths and hospitality to a new temper that began developing in science around the turn of the 20th century. If an idea can be fully understood only in some context—for example, as someone's defense against anxiety, as an instrument of oppression, or as a gesture of rebellion against a social norm—any of these relativisms may be taken as a way of sensitizing us to the ways parts assume special meaning depending on the wholes in which they are embedded. Context thus can take on ontological significance; pattern gains a dignity and centrality it could never have in mechanism.

The very instability of relativism can be converted into a metaphysical principle. The root metaphor of contextualism, says Pepper, is the experienced event, which William James described as part of a stream of consciousness. One needs verbs, not nouns, to discuss the fundaments of reality. This is a philosophy of becoming rather than being, open to continual and basic change:

Change in this radical sense is denied by all other world theories. If such radical change is not a feature of the world, if there are unchangeable structures in nature like the forms of formism or the space–time structure of mechanism, then contextualism is false. (Pepper, 1942, p. 234)

Freud took little interest in pragmatism, showing much less openness to James's ideas than the American did to his. I don't know whether he would have been more amused or indignant if he had been told that part of his contribution to the history of ideas was to prepare the way for this philosophical development, this new world hypothesis to rival mechanism as a foundation for science.

Not that pragmatism (or contextualism) ever seriously threatened to displace mechanism in widespread appeal to scientists. Ironically, though in many respects the world hypothesis of mechanism is thoroughly out of date and far less congruent with modern physics, biology, computer science, and a good many other disciplines than contextualism, its metaphysical assumptions still silently suffuse many aspects of the contemporary ethos. In many universities, methodologists teach a conception of science that stresses analysis to elements as the primary method; reductionism as an ideal; an implicit conception of matter—especially in the form of its subatomic particles—as the ultimate reality; and the classical experiment as the model of investigative procedures, with values carefully segregated from facts and as far as possible excluded entirely from the realm of science. The computer, far more sophisticated than the old-fashioned clockwork but still a machine, seizes the imagination of our bright young people and bids fair to become the root metaphor of an updated new version of mechanism. Despite all the dazzling achievements of high technology, its underlying philosophical assumptions are rigid, cold, and authoritarian; moral values have no natural roots in them. These assumptions will not do as the foundations of a future world fit for ordinary organisms like human beings.

TOWARD A NEW, INTEGRATIVE WORLD HYPOTHESIS

Contextualistic metaphysics is evidently quite congruent with some versions of modern quantum theory, but not—despite the similarity of terminology—with relativity. Einstein never liked that term, which was introduced by Max Planck for what Einstein himself preferred to call *invariance theory* (Holton, 1979). His choice of terms indicates his commitment to finding just those "unchangeable structures in nature" that contextualism cannot tolerate. Far from implying merely that "everything is relative," Einstein's work made physics a simpler, more consistent, and universally applicable theory. Einstein did this through the very device of giving up Newton's absolute framework of a fixed reference system of space and time, though intuitively that feels more basic and necessary to many people than preserving a set of invariant equations for the laws of physics. We just have to keep our priorities straight: The most important thing is to know that the basic physical laws will always be the same, regardless of the circumstances under which observations are made.

How did Einstein reformulate the laws of nature in a form that is independent of any particular standpoint, freeing them from relativism? By developing sets of mathematical transformations that systematically take into account the circumstances under which observations are made and adjust them accordingly. If you are familiar with factor analysis, it may help to think of it this way: Represent space and time geometrically as a four-dimensional reference system, and the transformation equations become a way of rotating the axes of this coordinate system so as to achieve the same structure of relationships among your data unfailingly, no matter what form they originally had. It is strictly analogous to the successful effort of a factor analyst to attain a common, simple structure for sets of data based on various batteries of tests and different samples of subjects.

With this example, I want to suggest that Einstein's solution to the problem of relativism is extremely powerful and flexible, and applicable to many problems in psychology. Consider, for example, Piaget's work on children's perspective taking. In one of his classical experiments, children who lived around Lac Leman in Switzerland were shown a miniature construction or model of the lake and its surrounding mountains. "If you stand on the north shore of the lake," Piaget would tell a child, "this is how the mountains look; how do they look to a child standing over there, on the eastern shore?" The youngest children would say, in effect, "The same way they look to me, 'cause that's the way they are." When a major step of cognitive development takes place, the child becomes aware that how the mountains look depends on your point of view, and that different people can have different perspectives. Piaget saw, however, beyond the implied relativism to the fact that there is a single real structure to the lake and mountains, which *is* recoverable from the many reports if they are subjected to a set of transformations. Getting out of one's unquestioned position in the center of the universe, or decentering, takes a long time, for the process has to be repeated many times in increasingly abstract contexts.

In the experimental psychology of human perception, a similar story has been emerging, notably in the study of the perceptual constancies. Psychologists' curiosity was initially attracted by the observation of certain striking achievements of our senses in constructing a steady world. For example, white paper continues to look white in the moonlight, when it reflects to the eye far less light than the blackest paper does in direct sunlight. Even more astonishing was the realization that our eyes provide us with constantly moving scans of the surrounding world, which nevertheless seems to hold steady whether we stand still and stare fixedly or move eyes, head, and body in complex and jerky ways. It turns out that the brain computes a set of transformations of these fluctuating, relativistic inputs in order to emerge with the perceptual invariances that we experience as a stable external world (Hochberg, 1971).

Freud, too, went beyond psychological relativism in his discovery of transference and countertransference (Erikson, 1982). "Transference" is so called because the patient tends to transfer to a contemporary figure, notably the analyst, emotional reactions that properly belonged to another person in his own past.[6] The reaction is mediated by the *symbolic equivalence* of the two persons, an interesting generalization of Freud's original discovery of the way to interpret dreams: They must be subjected to a process of semantic (and figural) transformation, following the rules of primary-process thinking. In a more than trivial sense, I believe that there is a parallel between these transmutations of meanings and forms and Einstein's mathematical transformations;[7] both achieved invariant order out of bewildering particular or paradoxical data.

Freud went a crucial further step into relativism by recognizing that he himself was subject to the same process of assimilative distortion; he called it "countertransference." Here he moved decisively away from the naive absolutism of the assumedly objective expert; the psychoanalyst's perceptions and conceptions of the patient are likewise vulnerable to or are shaped by the unique life experiences that constitute his special perspective. Is that not a relativistic chaos, in which no one knows where the truth lies, if indeed one can now believe in the very possibility of valid human knowledge? It would have been, had Freud not seen a practical way out. The psychoanalyst must himself be subjected to successful analytic therapy. Such treatment does not claim to work by removing all conflicts or by lastingly opening the doors of the unconscious. Instead, the training analysis helps the neophyte learn his own characteristic ways of distorting reality, so that he can take appropriate distance from them and learn compensatory ways of correcting them. That comes close to being a set of transformations that yield an invariant lawfulness and the possibility of approaching true knowledge despite the facts of psychological relativism. It is an imperfect means of promoting decentering, but when it works well it illustrates the principle.

To return to philosophy for a moment, the process I have been describing can be called giving up naive realism for relativism and then replacing that by critical realism. It is often difficult for people to grasp the difference between the two kinds of belief in something solidly real and fixed in the universe. The naive form, which I have also called "absolutism," simply accepts things the way they appear to us from whatever standpoint we happen to inherit or find ourselves in and assumes that the resulting reality is absolutely trustworthy, because "seeing is believing." As we get older, we learn to be wary; as we discover that our eyes can deceive us, and that things do look different to different poeple, we gain a degree of sophistication or decentering. But it amounts to a further achievement in decentering to realize that, outside all the vantage points of all the individual observers, there is a constant and asymptotically approachable framework of reality. We cannot always—perhaps never—see it directly, but we can construct it. The qualitative operations of judgment used by the critical-realist philosopher are again analogous to the quantitative operations of the Lorentz transformations that Einstein rediscovered to save the laws of physics.

In an initial enthusiasm for Einstein's principle of finding invariant structures of laws by means of systems of transformations, I thought that this discovery might serve as the germinal cell for yet another world hypothesis. (It does not seem quite close enough to common-sense experience to be spoken of as a root metaphor.) But in reading over Burtt's (1943) appreciative critique of *World Hypotheses*, I was struck by an important weakness of the book's argument. Pepper argues that all eclecticism is confusing and that root metaphors must not be combined. That is, any attempt to combine in one system ideas that stem from different root metaphors will fail, he claims, because they will prove fatally incompatible. As Burtt notes, to have proved such a point Pepper would have had to have the metatheoretical advantage that only another world hypothesis could have provided, and Pepper was quick to deny that he had any such ambitions.[8]

The root metaphor hypothesis is indeed convincing, but as a bit of the psychology of ideas, not as a methodological principle. Such metaphors must be discovered by a creative—perhaps artistic—process of intuitive discerning, which has not been reduced to principles that can be reliably used by others. More to the point, no genetic analysis has probative value— it doesn't *prove* anything. We are left, then, with the ancient criterion of consistency. Surely it is desirable to strive for coherence and lack of contradiction. But the world is extraordinarily rich and various; why, then, should we not draw on more than one strand of experience or common sense in building a world hypothesis, as long as we do so carefully and with particular concern not to entail subtle forms of contradiction?

The ideals of simplicity and adequacy lead us in opposite directions. In a charming little prose poem Pepper tells us how much stronger, for him, was the emotional pull toward simplicity:

> . . . it occurs to me
> That when we find the truth
> It will be as simple as the blue sky of morning.
>
> (Quoted in Hahn, 1980, p. 75)

This appealing image in a way expresses the esthetic ideal that was so important to Einstein. Yet such a tranquil vision has no greater claim to be a sure guide to the truth than Darwin's "tangled bank"—itself a strong claimant to be the root metaphor of the ecological outlook (Hyman, 1962).

Pepper erred, I think, in failing to distinguish the feckless eclecticism of an intellectual pack rat from true synthesis, which is as demanding of disciplined thought as any single-rooted purity. If the four adequate world hypotheses have differing and somewhat complementary strengths, if they have endured so long despite their individual shortcomings, it would seem likely that a true synthesis could yield a more valuable and defensible set of metaphysical foundations for the work of the future than any pure system could hope to do. Repeatedly in the history of ideas, where competing but incompatible formulations have persisted, the outcome has not been the victory of one and rout of the other but a reorganization of the field, making it possible to transform and integrate what in untransformed guise had seemed irreconcilable. Einstein's invariance-finding principle (or algorithm) may thus help us to attain a true synthesis of world hypotheses.

In my more optimistic moments, I feel that progress is being made toward such a synthesis. The systems view of the world, as I understand and construe it, embraces much of humanism and mechanism.[9] It shares with contextualism an emphasis on the emergence of novel properties of wholes; with formism a regard for the importance of universals and formal systems; with naturalism a conception of enduring physical entities or material systems; and with organicism a respect for the reality of ideas, values, and subjective experience.[10] The religiously inclined can as easily add on to this world view, as they have done to any other, their faith in a supernatural creator and spiritual realm.

I know that such a statement is little more than a declaration of faith and hope. Not a metaphysician by training, I doubt that I am well suited to try the synthetic task in any more serious way. Yet I am firmly convinced that metaphysics does matter, that huge benefits will accrue if satisfactory philosophical foundations can be laid for a true concert of the disciplines— the arts and humane letters alongside all the sciences. Psychoanalysis will be an indispensable component, with many of Freud's ideas and discoveries finding a permanent place in any scheme to get all the resources of the human mind and heart to work together. So grounded, a new morality for human survival may take root and prosper, filling a gap that now seems to be dangerously widening.

CODA

In his moving funeral oration for Freud, Ernest Jones (1957, p. 247) said:

> At my first meeting with him so long ago three qualities in particular produced an impression on me that only deepened as the years passed. In the first place, his nobility of character, his *Erhabenheit*. It was impossible to imagine his ever doing a petty thing or thinking a petty thought. [Then he quoted a letter from Freud to Putnam in German, in which Freud declared, "Actually I have never done a mean thing."] How many of us, if we search our hearts, could truthfully say that? Those of us who have special knowledge concerning the imperfections of mankind are sometimes depressed when we consider ourselves and our

fellow men. In those moments we recall the rare spirits that transcend the smallness of life, give life its glory and show us the picture of true greatness. It is they who give life its full value. There are not many of those rare spirits and Freud was among the highest of them.

Here he confesses the reason for his need to deny Freud's occasional lapses from nobility (and from the two other ideal qualities the grieving disciple went on to attribute to him—unswerving devotion to truth and to justice). Jones apparently needed to believe that certain abstract ideals could in fact be concretely achieved, as if there was no point in trying to be truthful unless one could believe that absolute, total devotion to truth was attainable. That is a prepsychoanalytic idea, not one he got from Freud. Psychoanalysis teaches, rather, that every god has clay feet, but that we can nevertheless respect and admire anyone who succeeds relatively better than others in the never-ending struggle against evil or petty impulses. The facts of Freud's life show that he was not superhuman; he was, we know, occasionally mean, untruthful, and unjust. But his own reaction to evidence of such failings in others was not to collapse into cynicism; Freud himself had no such illusions about the perfection of others, and he tried to discourage his followers from idolizing him.

Perhaps, in that same spirit, we should not be too hard on Jones. When he wrote the words just quoted, he had just suffered a grievous loss, a blow that tends to bring up deeply infantile longings. We have enough distance, today, not to share his need to believe that Freud had somehow attained an impossible perfection. Life can have full value without the necessity of denying the existence of some imperfection in everyone.

Notes

Chapter 2. The Manifest and Latent Meanings of Metapsychology

1. In an attempt to make sure I have examined all his usages, I supplemented the index of the *Standard Edition* by use of the *Concordance* (Guttman, Jones, & Parrish, 1980). The former is erratic in its treatment of "metapsychology," faithfully noting every occurrence in some volumes and ignoring the term entirely in others where it does occur. On the whole, however, Freud used it a good deal less than many another technical term.

2. From the context, one might guess also that the term appears in Taine's book, but that is not the case. The work may have appealed to Freud because Taine's psychology made conspicuous use of unconscious ideas, characterized in dramatic imagery (e.g., "Outside a little luminous circle, lies a large ring of twilight, and beyond this an indefinite night . . ." [Taine, 1864, p. 181]). In the intellectual ancestry of his concepts Leibniz is more conspicuous than Herbart.

3. In this interpretation of "meta-" he seems to have been influenced by its common function in zoological and anatomical terminology to mean behind or hindmost, rather than by the original Greek sense "denoting chiefly sharing, joint action, pursuit, quest, and (esp.) change" (Onions, 1966, p. 572).

4. Mayr (1978) writes:

> Those who rejected natural selection on religious or philosophical grounds or simply because it seemed too random a process to explain evolution continued for many years to put forward alternative schemes with such names as orthogenesis, nomogenesis, aristo-genesis or the "omega principle" of Teilhard de Chardin, each scheme relying on some built-in tendency or drive toward perfection or progress. All these theories were finalistic: they postulated some form of cosmic teleology, of purpose or program. (p. 50)

5. Buckle (1871) was recommended to him by his close friend Heinrich Braun when he was an adolescent. The recommendation made enough of an impression that he recalled it 50 years later (see Freud, 1960, p. 379; Holt, 1988).

6. Sulloway added, in the discussion of this paper in San Juan, that "organic-sexual" was a shorthand expression for sexual biochemistry, in the Fliess correspondence; but even in this restricted sense, it was part of a thoroughly evolutionary biology.

7. He continued, "I became a therapist against my will . . ." How strikingly this foreshadows the passage of three decades later when he was describing how he came to be a physician:

> I became a doctor through being compelled to deviate from my original purpose; and the triumph of my life lies in my having, after a long and roundabout journey, found my way

back to my earliest path. . . . In my youth I felt an overpowering need to understand something of the riddles of the world in which we live and perhaps even to contribute something to their solution. (Freud, 1926e, p. 253)

8. And, it should be added, one that probably was not conscious except for a brief time. Never again did Freud link metapsychology and metaphysics; indeed, most of his subsequent references to philosophy are quite negative, indicating that he had consciously turned his back on it, abjuring his early longing to be a philosopher and contribute to the great intellectual issues that had plagued so many great minds. Yet we cannot fully understand the appeal of metapsychology to Freud if we do not hypothesize that the grandiose ambition expressed in the quoted passage from 1901 stayed with him as an important latent meaning.

9. See Burnham (1974) for the philological point that Freud's contemporaries and teachers used the same word (*Instinkt*) for the urges of animals and children.

10. In connection with this last point, it is pertinent to recall the context from which Freud drew the quoted words. Faust has rejected the more mundane and practical of Mephistopheles' two prescriptions for regaining his youth: to work hard with one's hands—like a peasant; so the latter turns to the witch as the only one who can brew the magic potion required to do it the miraculous way. My friend Benjamin Rubinstein (personal communication, May 31, 1981) points out the possibility that Freud was quite aware of these implications; metapsychology is called upon to perform a seemingly impossible task, and it is a dangerous tool, one that may purchase an immediate gratification at the risk of long-run perdition. The witch is not an entirely "split" (unambiguously bad) mother-image, then, but one who combines the allurements of instantaneous magical wish-fulfillment with castrative punitiveness—properties Freud may have attributed to his childhood nurse (or so I have concluded from a review of independent evidence; [see also Vitz, 1988]).

Chapter 3.   Freud's Cognitive Style

1. In *The Interpretation of Dreams*, Freud wrote:

As a young doctor I worked for a long time at the Chemical Institute without ever becoming proficient in the skills which that science demands; and for that reason in my waking life I have never liked thinking of this barren and indeed humiliating episode in my apprenticeship. On the other hand I have a regularly recurring dream of working in the laboratory, of carrying out analyses and of having various experiences there. These dreams are disagreeable in the same way as examination dreams and they are never very distinct. While I was interpreting one of them, my attention was eventually attracted by the word 'analysis,' which gave me a key to their understanding. Since those days I have become an 'analyst', and I now carry out analyses which are very highly spoken of . . . (1900a, p. 475)

2. In light of recent revelations about the extent and duration of Freud's use of cocaine (Swales, 1981), this hallucination was probably drug-induced and of little significance for his characterological style of imaging (Holt, 1972b).

3. Again, over two decades later, he wrote that psychoanalysis worked "by making an analytic dissection of both normal and abnormal phenomena" (1923b, p. 36).

4. It may be relevant that, in the realm of art, Freud strongly preferred the balance of classical antiquity; a 1930 letter to Romain Rolland speaks of his "Hellenic love of proportion" (1960, p. 392).

5. For further discussion of Freud's ambivalence concerning speculation, see Chapter 6. [Actually, Freud greatly exaggerated the empirical and observational aspect of his scientific work, except in the general life-historical sense that he developed psychoanalytic theories only after a good many years of clinical work. Undoubtedly, his techniques of psychotherapy did entail a great deal of listening, which is surely observational though not as systematic as, let us say, the naturalistic collecting of a Darwin on the *Beagle* voyage. But Freud probably succeeded in concealing from himself as well as from others the extent to which he always perceived the ramblings of his patients through the filters of extensive preconceptions, and the degree to which he drew on unacknowledged philosophical and scientific assumptions when he attempted to construct theories. "In fact," remarks Morris Eagle (personal communication, August 1988), "in important ways, his own psychoanalytic theory is closer to the philosophical approach he abjures than to an empirical discipline."]

6. Other examples of qualification by explicit self-contradiction may be found in the following works of Freud: 1905e, pp. 42–43; 1915e, p. 191; 1917d, pp. 224–225; 1920g, p. 39.

7. In fairness to Freud, he did occasionally take note of the dangers of such generalizing; for example: "A single case can never be capable of proving a theorem so general as this one" (1905e, p. 115).

In modern methodology, a consideration closely related to quantification is sampling. Today, when a conclusion is set forth, one wants to know not only the number of cases on which it is based but the method by which they were selected. K. H. Pribram (personal communication, 1961) points out the fact that neuroanatomy has always been and is even today surprisingly lax and undisciplined, by the standards of modern behavioral science. Very small samples have traditionally been used and the sample size not reported; nor in texts, where tracts are confidently described, is there usually any indication of the methods used to isolate them. Pribram believes that the concrete tangibility of the subject matter gives rise to unjustified confidence in the reliability of casual methods and samples of one or a few cases. Actually, even in this comfortingly concrete discipline, there are considerable individual variations in structure, even among normal brains, and neuroanatomy could profit by the application of more sophisticated methods.

8. Compare a similar image from *Inhibitions, Symptoms and Anxiety*: "An analogy with which we have long been familiar compared a symptom to a foreign body which was keeping up a constant succession of stimuli and reactions in the tissue in which it was embedded" (1926d, p. 98).

9. As a brief ecological aside, I would like to suggest that Freud might have been less of a fighter in his writing if he had worked from the protective security of an academic position. His precious professorship did not carry tenure or a salary; Freud operated always from the exposed and lonely situation of private practice [see pp. 61–63, below].

10. In the same paper, Linton adduces data showing that field-independent college students did in fact seem more hypochondriacal than the field-dependent

ones, reporting more bodily symptoms on the Minnesota Multiphasic Personality Inventory. One price of being able to hear signals from within oneself is more awareness of ordinary aches and pains.

Chapter 4. A Critical Examination of Freud's Concept of Bound versus Free Cathexis

1. I obviously have not been able to read all of Freud's works, as might have been an ideal procedure, searching for all possible usages. I have compromised, therefore, on a review of all his primarily theoretical works (specifically, those listed by Strachey, *Standard Edition*, Vol. 14, pp. 259–260). I have checked a large proportion of the passages that resulted from this search against the *Gesammelte Werke*, hoping that perhaps Freud was more consistent in his use of German than his translators have been with English, but that has not proved of great value. Not every usage seemed worth including here; *binden* is after all a rather common German verb, and it would have been unlike Freud to give up using it in its general literary sense of tying or restraining, just because he had decided to give it a technical meaning. Strachey tried to indicate the more technical usages, apparently, by the use of single quotation marks (which never appear in the German). In this respect, however, he was not entirely consistent. In the passages quoted, I have taken the liberty of making occasional slight alterations in the translations, usually in places where the English was unnecessarily ambiguous. I want to acknowledge the assistance in this revisionary endeavor of [my late friend] Dr. Ilse Bry, who helped with a number of passages.

[The recent availability of a concordance (Guttman et al., 1980) has enabled me to make the search for usages truly comprehensive. For further discussion, see the afterword to this chapter.]

2. [This concept of tonic excitation, named in analogy to muscular tonus, was a common neurophysiological assumption of the time (Amacher, 1965). One might think that Freud was using it in the following passage from Draft I, on migraine, written March 4, 1895, while he was still at work on his final chapter for the joint book: "The pain of neuralgia usually finds its discharge in tonic tension (or even in clonic spasms) (Freud, 1950 [1892–1899], p. 215). The context makes it evident that here Freud was speaking about the tonus of muscles, however, not nerves.]

3. [This is the only place in the *Standard Edition* where Freud used the phrase "tonically bound."]

4. [Something like it is implicit in the concept of nontransmitted excitation, however, and Breuer may have been aware of that implication—may even have discussed it with Freud. We have no way of knowing.]

5. I am indebted to Dr. M. M. Gill for bringing this point to my attention.

6. [It is also possible that he already had in mind the ideas he was to present in the last part of the Project, pp. 380ff. See below, pp. 80–81.]

7. This distinction is particularly clear on p. 301 [of the Project (Freud, 1950 [1895])]; I am grateful to Dr. Karl H. Pribram for pointing it out to me. Hereafter in this section, I have omitted the parenthetical indications of abbreviations—e.g., (Q)—since they add nothing to the present discussion.

8. [Knowing what we do today about the depth of Freud's ambivalence

toward Breuer at this time (Sulloway, 1979), I am inclined to believe that a defensive displacement was at work. Freud owed Breuer a great deal, not only in concrete financial terms but emotionally and intellectually, and was in no position to repay any of it. Therefore, he probably found it easier to credit his older friend handsomely for something he had not actually obtained from him than to begin to express the appropriate gratitude for his actual debts.]

9. So far as I know, this is the only passage in which Freud ever said that attention cathexis could be bound. He may have been using it in the same sense of "riveted" (a state he called *Fesselung*) in the following passage from a letter to Fliess written January 1, 1896. He was trying to explain some of the psychosomatic effects in which Fliess was interested. He remarked first that in the case of spastic movements, quantity was not "being *transferred* to the motor center but . . . being *liberated* there because the binding Q in the sensory center coupled with it may have diminished." Then he took up the case of "a continuous afflux" of quantity from organic sources into the ψ-system, lasting

> for a time. Certain [ω-perceptual] neurones then become *hyper*cathected, and produce a feeling of unpleasure, and they also cause attention to be riveted at that point. Thus 'neuralgic change' would have to be regarded as an afflux of quantity from some organ augmented beyond a certain limit, till summation is suspended, the [perceptual] neurones are hypercathected and free ψ-energy riveted. As you see, we have arrived at migraine. (1950 [1895], p. 390)

The riveting or binding of hypercathexis ("free ψ-energy") thus occurs only under the special conditions of the liberation of quantity in ψ, with its pathological consequences.

10. [It is difficult to be sure just what this brief, condensed passage hypothesizes. The basic premise of this "economic" thinking seems to be that action obviously expends more energy than thinking, so some must be held in reserve during thought for the larger expenditure that lies ahead. Binding accomplishes that holding-in-reserve while still allowing for the ready passage of the small quantities needed for what he was to call the experimental action of thought. It is possible that Freud had learned the concept of "bound charge" in physics, which has a roughly parallel meaning: "the portion of the electrical charge on a conductor that because of the inductive action of a neighboring charge will not escape to the earth when the conductor is grounded" (Gove, 1981, p. 260). Once the problem of what to do has been solved, the person starts to move toward his goal, expending large quantitites of energy. In the last pages of the Project, Freud seems to say that as soon as the current passes from the motor neurones into the musculature, there is an automatic undoing of the restraint (binding) of quantity within the ego neurones; the term "irresistibly" seems to imply an automatic, "wired-in" device of some kind. In the cybernetic spirit of the Project, one might assume that Freud had in mind a feedback circuit from the muscles to the ego, a signal from which would release much of the otherwise retained cathexis, which is then available for the assumedly large amounts needed for sustained action. Once again, however, the mechanical theory of neural functioning—which was all that Freud knew, or at least the only one he used—encounters difficulties in conceptualizing the opposite effects of different signals. If he had known of the existence of whole areas of the brain in which neural activity

has an inhibitory rather than excitatory effect, it would doubtless have been a great help. But perhaps this particular difficulty would have been obviated if Freud had known that the role of the nervous system in action is merely to give a signal to the muscles, which contain their own energy source. There is, accordingly, no need to assume any fundamental difference between nervous activity in thought and in action. (On this and similar matters, see McCarley & Hobson, 1977.)]

11. The conceptions of the Project [see especially pp. 368-369] are strongly echoed in this passage: The second system plays the role of the ego, inhibiting discharge by means of its lateral cathexes. The reference to raised potential recalls the assumption that a high potential of cathexis would enable the small currents involved in thought to flow freely.

12. [At the time of writing this paper, I was not yet aware of the subtle reifications and personifications implicit in these Freudian metaphors, which I uncritically adopted. The idea that energy "discharges" implicitly treats it in terms of the prevailing hydrological model of electricity as a fluid, which flows through channels, accumulates when damned up, and may be stored in or discharged from containers or reservoirs. And the notion of "pressing" assigns an attribute of the person to the energy itself—anthropomorphism, a mode of discourse that is appropriate for poetry but too primitive for any but the most sparing use in science, and then only in contexts where it is clearly employed for color or vividness (or cited as the nonrational source of a conjecture). See also Grossman and Simon, 1969, and Chapter 3, this volume.]

13. It is interesting that on pp. 615-617, Freud used the word *mobil* five times, referring to hypercathexis, though on p. 576 he referred to the "more mobile" state of attention just before waking as *beweglicher*. In the Project, the term he had used was *frei*. The latter two terms seem to have a connotation of unrestrainedness, while *mobil* connotes the property of being mobilizable—something that seems more appropriate to attention cathexis than to drive cathexis. It might have led to greater clarity if Freud had consistently called hypercathexis *mobil* (or, as he did in *The Ego and the Id, verschiebbar*), which he did not do, and had reserved the other terms (*frei, beweglich*) for the energies of the primary process, and if the translators had made a corresponding distinction. I am grateful to Dr. M. M. Gill for bringing to my attention the fact that the translators have rendered all of these terms as "mobile," regardless of the type of energy being discussed. I have inserted the German in square brackets occasionally, principally to clarify Freud's usage when he was referring to drive energy as opposed to hypercathexis. There is little problem about the translation of *binden* as "bind."

14. I am grateful to Dr. K. M. Colby for directing me to this passage. A number of similar usages occur after the quoted passage, but do not shed new light on the concept.

15. Freud even equated them by writing: "*primary process* (mobility of cathexes)" (1915e, p. 187).

16. I am grateful to Dr. David Rapaport for pointing out the similarity of this formulation to Freud's conceptualization of the pattern of jokes (1905c).

17. The principal passage of this kind is in "The Unconscious": "Anticathexis is the sole mechanism of primal repression; in the case of repression proper ('after-pressure') there is in addition withdrawal of the *Pcs.* cathexis. It is very possible that

it is precisely the [hyper]cathexis which is withdrawn from the idea that is used for *anticathexis*" (1915e, p. 181).

18. This is the process of the "taming of affects," to which Fenichel (1934) referred. [Notice that in the passage above, the primary and secondary processes themselves instead of their energies are now called "unbound" and "bound."]

19. [In the original paper, it seems that I quite overlooked this new idea, since 1914c, that the binding hypercathexis is narcissistic—an unelaborated specification of unknown significance. Presumably he meant that since an actual injury mobilizes a person's attention along with an attitude of self-concern, and since he had now decided that some libidinal energies were narcissistic, the latter type must be involved.]

20. [That is, "the original, erotogenic" masochism is or results from a 'taming' [*Bändigung*] of the death-instinct by the libido. . . . death instincts are . . . tamed in this way by being bound to admixtures of libido" (p. 164).]

21. [I did not notice the fact that this passage related the concept of bound energy and that of bound anxiety. For some years, Freud had been speaking about free and bound *anxiety* in passages such as this one. See the following note and the Afterword to this chapter.]

22. Speaking of the restrictions of the ego after a defense has become structuralized, Freud said that a new impulse, of the same kind as the defense had originally been directed against, may come along when the defense is no longer needed, but will be subject to the same "compulsion to repeat. . . . The fixating factor in repression, then, is the unconscious id's compulsion to repeat—a compulsion which in normal circumstances is done away with only by the freely mobile function of the ego" (p. 153). Likewise, the concept of "bound anxiety," which is so often encountered in psychoanalytic writing, appears here (p. 141: the ego tries "to save itself from anxiety . . . and to bind it by the formation of symptoms"). It is either to be interpreted in the sense of the passage above quoted from p. 144, or else does not refer to energies and so is not treated in the present paper. [See the Afterword.]

23. See also the discussion of the id: The energy of its "instinctual impulses is . . . far more mobile and capable of discharge" than elsewhere (1933a, p. 74).

24. Inhibition (*Hemmung*) is another term that Freud used in both a general and a specific sense. When he meant it nonspecifically, Freud used the concept to refer to defense and delay generally—the "restriction of a function . . . a simple lowering of function" (1926d, p. 87). But the term has also taken on the more specific connotation of one type of defense—the barricading of impulse by suppression, repression, or blocking, as opposed to a defense or sublimation that produces qualitative modification or transformation of the impulse. In this sentence, I am using it in the former, general sense, and wish to make a further specification about the other, clinical concept: The mere inhibition of an impulse does *not* result in the neutralization of its drive energy (which, indeed, may be of any degree of neutralization for other reasons), nor does the diversion of the impulse into pathological transformation. When, on the other hand, impulses are delayed in their plunge toward immediate gratification, and then are diverted into long-circuiting channels that ultimately allow some gratifying discharge—some adaptive work to be performed on the external reality—then neutralization does take place. [How certain I

was about matters about which I knew nothing directly, and about which no one else knew anything either!]

25. [I am pleased to acknowledge the assistance of my daughter, Dorothy Prickett, M.A., in this and other forays into German etymology.]

26. [Notice that even before writing the metapsychological papers, Freud was already assuming that there were other types of psychic energy besides the libidinal.]

Chapter 5. A Review of Some of Freud's Biological Assumptions and Their Influence on His Theories

1. I am grateful to Dr. M. P. Amacher for a helpful reading of this paper and several valuable corrections, and also for his permission to quote from his dissertation. My friend Dr. Benjamin B. Rubinstein also earned my gratitude by a critical reading and several suggestions.

2. [The list that follows obviously needs a great deal of supplementation. The most important corrective to the limited outlook of this chapter is the important book by Sulloway (1979); but see also the papers of Cranefield (1966, 1970) and Spehlmann (1953).]

3. [And from a variety of other sources, including doubtless his Gymnasium teachers, the works they assigned, and books Freud read on his own, among which Büchner (1855) is especially noteworthy (Holt, 1988).]

4. [A likely source of this notion is *Force and Matter* (Büchner, 1855), one of the books Freud and his friends read in 1871 or 1872 (Holt, 1988). Büchner devotes an entire chapter to "motion," using the word interchangeably with "energy." It "is the very essence of force itself. . . . molecular vibration as heat or as electrical or magnetic action" (p. 75). Later, he declares that "thinking . . . is . . . an activity or motion of the substances and material compounds [of] the brain" (p. 304). Again, ". . . psychical activity is nothing more than a motion going on between the cells of the grey matter, caused by an external impression" (p. 305).]

5. He had already formulated the principle of constancy in an 1893 lecture in these words: "If a person experiences a psychical impression, something in his nervous system which we will for the moment call the sum of excitation is increased. Now in every individual there exists a tendency to diminish this sum of excitation once more, in order to preserve his health" (1893h, p. 36). In another paper of the same year, he wrote: "Every event, every psychical impression is provided with a certain quota of affect (*Affektbetrag*) of which the ego divests itself either by means of a motor reaction or by associative psychical activity" (1893c, pp. 171–172). Incidentally, it is only fair to Breuer to point out that the latter did not share the view that the only energies in the nervous system are introduced from the outside: "Spontaneous awakening, which . . . can take place in complete darkness and quiet without any external stimulus, proves that the development of energy is based on the vital process of the cerebral elements themselves. A muscle remains unstimulated, quiescent, however long it has been in a state of rest . . . This is not so with the cerebral elements" (Breuer & Freud, 1895, p. 196). Nevertheless, he included without ques-

tion "the fact that there exists in the organism a 'tendency to keep intracerebral excitation constant' (Freud)." (Emphasis is Breuer's, p. 197; he cites no specific work of Freud's.)

[Cranefield (personal communication, September 29, 1975) emphasizes how widely neurophysiologists of the early to mid-19th century believed that the nervous system is perpetually active. He concedes, however:

> One could, I suppose, argue that there is behind all of this a model in which the nervous system is a "passive instrument in a state of rest until stimulated" but 19th-century neurophysiologists were, I believe, well aware that the nervous system is in fact never in a state of rest since it is never free from rather extensive sensory input.]

6. [Büchner (1855, p. 83) quoted some very similar words from Baron d'Holbach's (1770) *Système de la Nature*: "the world is nothing more than matter and motion. . . ." Note, incidentally, that in 1895 this was already an anachronistic concept of physical reality. Field theory had been implicit in Newton's laws of motion and had been made quite explicit by Maxwell in 1864; it was by no means universally believed any more that all energy consisted of "masses in motion." Note also the overwhelming role of energy in this concept of reality: Nothing whatever is said about the static structure of the environment, the configurations of nonvibrating masses. Here is a harbinger of Freud's later persistent neglect of structural considerations and his steady preference for dynamic and economic explanations; cf. also Brücke's remark about forces as the only causes.

7. Despite the clarity of the text, many psychoanalysts nevertheless interpret "quantity" as referring to psychic rather than to physical energy (see Modell, 1963). This interpretation is attributable to the historical accident that the Project was published only in 1950, after many analysts had studied and taught the 20th-century versions of psychoanalytic theory for many years. In those familiar works, "cathexis" does refer to psychic energy, and so it is natural to read in the later meaning when one encounters the same words, even though written at a time when Freud had a strong emotional identification with physicalistic physiology, one of the central tenets of which was the rejection of vitalistic notions like psychic energy (Holt, 1963 and Chapter 4, this volume).

8. To be sure, they spoke about "instinct," to make the point that it was a superfluous concept for human physiology; but they used the term *Instinkt*, not *Trieb*. No confusion would be entailed if it were not for the unfortunate British insistence on rendering *Trieb* as "instinct," despite the fact that both German words have unambiguous cognates in English. Exner, in his theory of emotions, came closest to what could pass today as a theory of drives; Amacher points out a number of resemblances between his account and Freud's in the *Three Essays on the Theory of Sexuality* (1905d). In a personal communication (1961), Amacher adds: "Meynert was critically concerned with drives as they determined the reaction of the *Ich*. Exner's whole book leads up to his chapter on the instincts, which involved excitation from endogenous nerve endings." [See also Chapter 4, this volume.]

9. An even clearer statement of the male sexual drive as originating in a somatic tension that pours drive stimuli into the psychic apparatus until removed by appropriate action may be found (Freud, 1895b [1894], pp. 108–109).

10. In a panel discussion on psychic energy (Modell, 1963), I found myself very much in the minority in the position I argue here.

11. Boring (1963) has written:

> In the last couple of decades the model has been brought out to replace the theory, which has fallen into disrepute because it has claimed to state truth without assimilating its contradictions. Truth is all-or-none. There are would-be truths but no half truths. The model does not claim truth-value. It is an aspiration for a generalization. It may be employed for a limited universe. You see how well you can get your data to fit, perhaps adjusting the model to make the fit better. If the fit is good, you have a good summary of these data and then you may use the model to predict other data and test it empirically. If the prediction is borne out, the model gains in dignity and importance.

For a discussion paralleling and supporting that in the text paragraph, see Black (1962). [And for my present position on this matter, see Chapter 12, this volume.]

12. Another possible explanation for Freud's overemphasis on the dynamic besides the influence of Brücke et al. may be the following: He was committed to a belief in exceptionless determinism; but he also had a fundamental concept of reality as random. Environmental influences he persistently called "accidental factors" (e.g., 1905d, *passim*); he only dimly and occasionally admitted that there was a sociocultural patterning of the individual's surround, a nonpsychological structure that persisted without the mediation of individual heredity (instead, he tried to account for social regularity and the transmission of social forms by the genetic inheritance of acquired characteristics!). Therefore, to maintain a lawful and deterministic view, he *had* to look predominantly to internal motivation. Overdetermination usually means that there are several *motives* (some of them unconscious), rather than the sort of thing Waelder (1936) had in mind with the principle of multiple function, or Rapaport and Gill's (1959) metapsychological approach, which takes it for granted that every event has structural, sociocultural, and external-environmental causes as well as dynamic–economic ones.

13. For example, in 1905 he wrote:

> The concepts of 'psychical energy' and 'discharge' and the treatment of psychical energy as a quantity have become habitual in my thoughts since I began to arrange the acts of psychopathology philosophically. . . . It is only when I speak of the 'cathexis of psychical paths' that I seem to depart from the analogies commonly used by Lipps. . . . To avoid misunderstanding, I must add that I am making no attempt to proclaim that the cells and nerve fibres, or the systems of neurones which are taking their place today, are these psychical paths, even though it would have to be possible in some manner which cannot yet be indicated to represent such paths by organic elements of the nervous system. (1905c, pp. 147–148)

In 1920:

> the system *Pcpt.-Cs.* . . . must lie on the borderline between outside and inside; it must be turned towards the external world and must envelop the other psychical systems. It will be seen that there is nothing daringly new in these assumptions; we have merely adopted the views on localization held by cerebral anatomy, which locates the 'seat' of consciousness in the cerebral cortex—the outermost, enveloping layer of the central organ. (1920g, p. 24)

At the end of the same work:

> The deficiencies in our description [of the relations between drives] would probably vanish if we were already in a position to replace the psychological terms by physiological or chemical ones. . . . Biology is truly a land of unlimited possibilities. We may expect it to give us the most surprising information and we cannot guess what answers it will return in a few dozen years to the questions we have put to it. They may be a kind which will blow away the whole of our artificial structure of hypotheses. (1920g, p. 60)

In 1923: "We have said that consciousness is the *surface* of the mental apparatus; that is, we have ascribed it as a function to a system which is spatially the first one reached from the external world—and spatially not only in the functional sense but, on this occasion, also in the sense of anatomical dissection" (1923b, p. 19). A few pages on (p. 25): "we learn from cerebral anatomy" that "the ego wears a 'cap of hearing'"—a region marked "acoust," on the accompanying diagram—"on one side only." In 1924: "We are without any physiological understanding of the ways and means by which this taming of the death-instinct by the libido may be effected" (1924c, p. 164), in reference to fusion, indicating that he was still considering the psychic energies of drives potentially describable in physiological terms. In 1940: "The phenomena with which we have to deal [in psychoanalysis] do not belong only to psychology; they have also an organic and biological aspect" (1940a, pp. 103–104); a page or so later, "We have adopted the hypothesis of a psychical apparatus, extended in space, appropriately constructed, developed by the exigencies of life, which gives rise to the phenomena of consciousness only at one particular point and under certain conditions. This hypothesis has put us in a position to establish psychology upon foundations similar to those of any other science, such as physics" (p. 105). To the end, Freud was reluctant to give up physicalism and unwilling to create a "pure psychology" without some attempt at coordination with anatomy and physiology.

14. [Cranefield (personal communication, September 29, 1975) disagrees:

> It is, I think, very difficult to ascertain what Freud knew or believed about these facts, but rather less difficult to ascertain whether or not most of them "have become familiar to us only since his death." I believe, on the contrary, that most of them were familiar to physiologists at the time of Freud's student days.

His specific comments about the five points are given in notes 15–18.]

15. [Cranefield comments with a helpful corrective: "Visual and auditory stimuli certainly *initiate* activity; they do not merely encode existing activity."]

16. [Again Cranefield disagrees:

> The concept of the nerve impulse as propagated is rather old. . . . The core-conductor or cable theory which provides the correct physical analogy (to a telegraph cable rather than to a wire carrying a flow of current) was well established (by Ludiman Hermann) in the late 1870s and early 1880s.]

17. ["As far as I know," says Cranefield, "all neurophysiological theories as far back as Descartes and Willis took this view. . . . I am not aware of any serious doubt

cast on the idea that an end organ is a 'transducer' at any time during the 19th century (or now)."]

18. ["This was known, indeed . . . the most sensitive detectors of electrical energy known in their time . . . were used to detect the tiny electrical changes associated with the nerve impulse," states Cranefield. I stand corrected. Nevertheless, the works of Brücke, Meynert, and Exner may be read as Amacher and I understood them, and I remain confident that Freud did *not* know these five points even though some of his peers did.]

19. [For a later, and fuller, discussion of the psychoanalytic theory of motivation, see Chapter 7, this volume.]

20. For the preceding facts in this paragraph, I am grateful to Dr. M. P. Amacher (personal communication).

Chapter 6.   Beyond Vitalism and Mechanism: Freud's Concept of Psychic Energy

1. [For a slightly more expanded account of the rise of the mechanistic world view, see Chapter 14, this volume.]

2. It is interesting to note that Descartes is probably the father of the "hydrodynamic" metaphors of metapsychological energy theory, since he conceived of the nerves as tubes filled with a special fluid and operating essentially like a modern hydraulic brake system.

3. It became so in the work of his followers; Newton himself remained a devout Christian to the end. See also Koryé (1956), as paraphrased later in this chapter. In connection with Freud's treatment of quantity and quality in the Project (see later text), it is interesting to read Bergson's (1911) remarks about the impact of Newtonian physics on philosophy:

> The first result of the new science was to cut the real into two halves, quantity and quality, the former being credited to the account of *bodies* and the latter to the account of *souls*. The ancients had raised no such barriers either between quantity and quality or between soul and body. (p. 349)

4. [Lamarck is particularly interesting in this context, for in his own time he was considered a materialist rather than a vitalist, probably because he attempted to reduce life to motion, denounced the personification of Nature, and made various programmatic statements of a mechanistic kind. Yet he spoke of nature as a creative "intermediary between God and the various parts of the physical universe for the fulfilling of the Divine Will" (from his *Philosophie Zoologique*; quoted by Nordenskiöld, 1928, p. 328). He managed to be as teleological as any avowed vitalist and to postulate hypothetical tensions that, despite their materialistic pretentions, have all the properties of a vital force or entelechy.]

5. A century later, Bergson (1911, pp. 34–35) was repeating essentially the same argument: "Science has reconstructed hitherto nothing but waste products of vital activity; the peculiarly active plastic substances obstinately defy synthesis." Also favoring Müller's position was the fact that the substance Wöhler had begun his synthesis with, ammonium cyanate, was not for some years to be synthesizable from inorganic elemental sources.

6. Compare the parallel statement by du Bois-Reymond (1884):

We can imagine the knowledge of nature arrived at a point where the universal process of the world might be represented by a single mathematical formula, by one immense system of simultaneous differential equations, from which could be deduced, for each moment, the position, direction, and velocity of every atom of the world.

Einstein and Infeld (1938) comment on the quotation from Helmholtz: "This view appears dull and naïve to a twentieth-century physicist. It would frighten him to think that the great adventure of research could be so soon finished, and an unexciting if infallible picture of the universe established for all time" (p. 58). For an even more devastating critique of this position, as stated by Laplace, see Polanyi (1962, pp. 137–142).

7. The parallel between Cope's concepts and Freud's life and death instincts (1920g) is particularly striking.

8. [Cranefield (1966) has corrected a number Bernfeld's (1944) historical errors. The University of Vienna was hardly a hotbed of extreme materialistic mechanism; indeed, most of Freud's teachers were humanistic graduates of the classical Gymnasium system who in their lives and works sought to integrate their hard scientific ideas with the softer components of their general culture.]

9. Galdston (1956) has pointed out the ways in which Fliess's grandiose speculations show how he, too, had been influenced by nature-philosophical ways of thinking. [See also Sulloway (1979).]

10. Compare Democritus on quality, almost 23 centuries earlier:

By convention sweet is sweet, by convention bitter is bitter, by convention hot is hot, by convention cold is cold, by convention color is color. But in reality there are atoms and the void. That is, the objects of sense are supposed to be real and it is cutomary to regard them as such, but in truth they are not. Only the atoms and the void are real. (Quoted in Einstein & Infeld, 1938, p. 56)

11. As Lashley put it:

Neural activity has been sufficiently well explored to rule out such broad assumptions as of the energy of the libido or of the id. Summation, potentiation, irradiation, and inhibition are fairly well, though not completely, understood. The energy of the nervous system is that of transmitted excitations, with its implied limitations and specificities. Energy dissociated from this, as postulated by field theories, is ruled out by definite experimental evidence. In particular, the derivation of psychic energy from one or a few "instincts" finds no support in the nature of neural activity. . . . Where instinctive activities have been analyzed experimentally, as in our studies of hunger, mating and maternal behavior, there is nothing that suggests free or transferable energy . . . behavior can be explained without assumption of any energy other than the interaction of specific neural elements. (Lashley & Colby, 1957, p. 234)

12. Freud never explicitly said, so far as I know, that psychic energy does not operate in space. To be sure, the issue does not come up in a pure psychology any more than in mathematics: The theoretical terms are simply not interpreted existentially (as referring to anything real). Some of the time (1900a), Freud took this stance; at others (1915c), he wrote as if the nervous system were virtually identical with the psychic apparatus. Often, however, he either indicated that at some point in

the body (physical) neural energy is converted into psychic energy (1895b [1894]), or else he simply implied an interactionism. This last doctrine must entail an existential interpretation of psychic energy, but since there is no room in the head for a psychic appartus in addition to the brain, the former must not exist in the same spatial world. Freud does not seem to have been as loath to make such an assumption as his early radical materialism and many explicit rejections of mysticism and the supernatural would imply. Perhaps one reason why Freud did not explicitly embrace vitalism was the fact that its adherents so often have been religious mystics. Yet he did believe in telepathy and other "psychical phenomena." Just as vitalism opens the door to such concepts as extrasensory perception (Driesch was once president of the Society for Psychical Research in England), so too does a teleological, nonspatial, anthropomorphic psychic energy. If a mentalistic entity can affect the body operating from outside of three-dimensional physical space, why cannot the psychic energy from one person directly affect the mind and behavior of another, unhindered by the intervening gap in physical space? None of these implications proves that there is anything intrinsically invalid about psychic energy, and in the minds of some they may constitute arguments for it. My intention is not to try to induce any theoretical "guilt by association" either, but simply to note that scientists usually choose not to use concepts having these properties once they are pointed out. As long as the facts do not positively require the assumption of real but nonspatial entities, it is more parsimonious to try to get along with the realities we are accustomed to.

13. My impression is that doctrines resembling vitalism as much as Freud's have been advanced by a number of prominent figures in psychology in recent years. McDougall, who violently rejected psychoanalysis as a whole, nevertheless had his own properly named dynamic (or hormic—i.e., purposive) psychology, an instinct theory complete with a doctrine of energies. On the mind–body problem he was an avowed interactionist; like many vitalists, he was a believer in the spontaneity of life, in human free will, and in Lamarckian inheritance of acquired characteristics; and by making purpose the central fact of behavior he links up with a major theme of vitalism. But he is long dead and without heirs. The author of the following is still quite influential, however [though he died recently]:

> Whether one calls it a growth tendency, a drive toward self-actualization, or a forward-moving *directional* tendency, it is the mainspring of life. . . . It is the urge which is evident in *all organic and human life*—to expand, extend, become autonomous, develop, mature—the tendency to express and activate all the capacities of the organism. (Rogers, 1961, p. 35; emphasis added)

Similar words are being written by a good many other contemporary psychotherapists who have been influenced by existentialism.

14. [I have found, however, in a book (Büchner, 1855) Freud read as an adolescent, an extensive account of vitalism in the guise of an attack on it by a reputedly extreme materialist who nevertheless inadvertently adopted a good many vitalistic concepts and ways of thinking (Holt, 1988). What more insidious way of picking up ideas could there be than by reading a purported devastation of them!]

15. [Lloyd Silverman told me (in a personal communications, 1982) that in a number of his early experiments on the effects on conscious cognition of sublimi-

nally presented pictures with aggressive content, the closed-system economics of psychic energy suggested some of the hypotheses he tested, and in his discussions he tried to conceptualize the findings in economic terms. He came to realize that his experiments in no way tested the theory, which was in fact quite expendable. For about the last decade of his tragically foreshortened life, therefore, he no longer found the concept of psychic energy useful, and abandoned it.]

16. One could hardly find a clearer example of Platonic essentialism than the following statement by Driesch (1929, p. 6): "It is the final object of all biology to tell us what it ultimately means to say that a body is 'living,' and it what sorts of relation body and life stand one to the other."

17, In the first draft of this paper, presented in a panel discussion on psychic energy (Modell, 1963), I made statements to the effect that the concept had clinical usefulness, and I have been so quoted (Apfelbaum, 1965). I still believe that Freud may have been aided in a number of ways by his economic concepts, which probably helped him make certain types of observations, and I was impressed by the claim of a number of psychoanalytic clinicians that they found the concept useful in their work. On further reflection, however, I have become more fully aware of the numerous ways in which emphasis on economic considerations may be clinically deleterious: It fits certain kinds of facts better than others and so creates a bias to consider observations that fit as more basic, important, or valid. Elsewhere (Holt, 1968; see also Chapters 5 and 8, this volume), I have cited a number of examples, and Apfelbaum (1965) contributes several others. It would be difficult to strike a balance and say whether the economic point of view has been more helpful clinically or more misleading. [Rubinstein (1975) presents a modern version of the clinical theory, free from fallacies and anachronistic concepts like psychic energy.]

18. "All life, animal and vegetable, seems in its essence like an effort to accumulate energy and then to let it flow into flexible channels, changeable in shape, at the end of which it will accomplish infinitely varied kinds of work" (Bergson, 1911, pp. 253–254). He contrasts this to the world of inorganic nature, in which the second law of thermodynamics holds sway.

19. Culbertson (1963) writes:

> In this [cybernetic] analysis afferent impulses are not in any way regarded as "messages" to the brain. Only in a far-fetched and misleading sense could we call them messages, or regard them as such. This term, and its equivalents, would presumably imply a "receiver" of these messages. The basic perception problem would then begin over again, at the alleged boundaries of this "receiver."

20. Apfelbaum (1965) has shown the fallacies of the assumption that such clinical phenomena as fatigue demand an explanation in terms of psychic energy. He goes too far, however, in rejecting all use of quantitative concepts. My own belief is that psychoanalysis needs much more quantification, but that there is little point in measurement for its own sake. We need to develop quantitative concepts, not simply to try to measure whatever we have. In this sense, then, I do not mean to argue against an economic point of view in any blanket fashion, nor do I deny that in a protoneurophysiological model there will be a place for measurements of physical energy. I am persuaded that the neural impulse is on the whole more usefully considered from the standpoint of information engineering than from that of power

engineering, but it would be rashly premature indeed to assert that quantities of neural energy can be of no interest to psychoanalysis.

Chapter 7. Drive or Wish?: A Reconsideration of the Psychoanalytic Theory of Motivation

1. Even here, Freud characteristically went off in several directions, following up various lines of thought as they arose, even when they made him begin implicitly to postulate another basic theory. He was usually confident that synthesis would take care of itself in the long run—truth would prevail—whereas too much concern for consistency could hamper creativity. His was no little mind to be frightened by Emerson's hobgoblin! [See Chapter 3, this volume.]

2. For more detailed treatments of the following points, with references, see Chapters 5 and 9, this volume.

3. His way of trying to handle meanings was to treat them as "drive derivatives," a concept that enabled him to go ahead and consider the clinical facts of motivation in more or less their own terms. Some critics of this chapter have complained that I have not given adequate stress to this fact. I did not highlight it in the text because it seems to be a theoretically unsatisfactory way of trying to patch up a major deficiency in metapsychology. Meanings still have no recognized place in metapsychology; "drive derivative" and equivalent expressions are merely a back door by which they are smuggled in, despite their lack of proper scientific credentials. For the odd paradox of metapsychology is that despite its apparent reliance on "psychical" concepts, these are modeled after the concepts of physics (energy, force, structure) and physiology (excitation, pathway), and the mere addition of "derivative" does not convert them into units or dimensions of semantic, phenomenal, or other meaningful realms.

4. I deal here with only the basic definition, not the full theory as Rapaport presented it, because it does not seem to me that he made fundamental changes in Freud's conception. True, Rapaport's version of psychic energy does not have some of the confusions of Freud's, but he leans on it and also on the concept—equally dubious, methodologically—of psychic structure as central explanatory constructs, though both concepts are still subject to most of the objections I have cited above.

5. For a critique of the concept of tension, see Chapter 5, this volume.

6. I hope my position is clear: I do not mean to deny the obvious importance of the biological (anatomical, physiological, biochemical, etc.) determinants of sexual behavior, but only the drive concept itself. Even though the concept of instinct or drive is becoming an anachronism, we are so used to it that my attempt to replace it can easily give the false impression that I refuse to face either of two realities: the facts of biology, or the facts of psychoanalytic observation.

7. That is, the original explicit model. Implicitly, I believe that the model was probably urination, the one activity that clearly does have the alleged course (a buildup of fluid generating an increase of unpleasant internal sensation, followed by a literal discharge and a subjective sense of pleasure through relief). Note that hydrodynamics is even relevant here—literally, not metaphorically—and there *is* a set of the "interconnecting pipes," to which Freud was wont to allude, in the male urinogenital apparatus.

8. There are some obvious similarities between my reformulation of Klein's theory and the conception of motivation advanced by McClelland as long ago as 1951 (see also McClelland, Atkinson, Clark, & Lowell, 1953). I cannot undertake here to explain in detail why I do not find the McClelland theory entirely satisfactory; but in general I agree with the critique of Cofer and Appley (1964, pp. 382–386). Helson's (1959) concept of adaptation level is plainly useful, perhaps necessary, but I believe that the problem of value is far too complex to be reduced to degrees of deviation from adaptation level. For some further parallels to contemporary theories, see my footnotes on p. 91 of Klein (1967). [After the original version of this chapter was in press, I found that many of its ideas had been anticipated in two more highly developed theories, which also embody the cybernetic and systems approach: Rubinstein (1974) and Powers (1973).]

9. [In retrospect, it is evident that two important and interrelated issues were silently ignored in this chapter: how motives are learned, and how the aggressive motive works. Recent research on the role of neuropeptides in motivation and emotion (see, e.g., Pert, 1988) offers some exciting prospects of breakthroughs on some of these problems.]

10. The human being is designed and functions so as to process and produce meanings. That being the case, so long as the person is alive and well, he cannot help but deal with meanings and make meaningful sense out of experience. To say that we have a *need* to find meaning is thus no more accurate than, and is as misleading as, to say that an automatic knitting machine has a need to knit or that a seed has a need to germinate. Those activities are simply what they do, each in its own fashion, carrying out the function its structure makes more or less inevitable. I believe that the structure of the human nervous system, in its organismic setting, makes the generation of meanings as natural as the generation of sweat from sweat glands. In a certain sense it is true that we do need to sweat, but that sense is simply that sweating is useful, adaptive, even necessary to the maintenance of a steady temperature within the body, just as we need to have something solid to walk upon without our necessarily wishing for it more than occasionally.

11. This unpsychoanalytic-sounding proposition needs some amplification. I think it is safe to say that all *extended* behavior sequences are determined by wishes, usually by a number of them with varying degrees of consciousness. But viewed more microscopically, behavior is at times automatized, in Hartmann's (1964) sense of the term, or habitual; as Rapaport (1960b) put it, to consider that *all* behavior is in all components motivationally determined is to return to the old and fallacious "seething cauldron" conception of Freud's early writings.

Chapter 8.   The Past and Future of Ego Psychology

1. Let us take note here of the fact that the body image is a relatively unambiguous, operational (i.e., concrete) concept, and that Freud never clarified in what way it was related to the other components of his complex concept of ego—the functions, the abstract structural concept, the identifications, the ego energies, and so on. The organ of synthesis itself was left in an unsynthesized state.

2. I quite agree with Royce (1973) that the terms "person" and "self" need not imply dualism, but I am not persuaded by his argument that the concept of the soul,

as used in Catholic Thomist psychology following Aristotle, does not imply dualism and in fact represents an alternative to both dualism and monism. He extends the argument quite far back in time, claiming that

> the ancient Sumerians and Egyptians . . . held a unified view of the nature of man. . . . and that the Hebrew Old Testament tradition was not dualistic in any Platonic or Cartesian sense, and the biblical expressions "I said to my soul" or "to lose one's soul" would be better translated as "I said to myself" or "to lose one's self." (p. 883)

This gloss on the rendition of the Bible's Hebrew I find interesting, though I cannot evaluate it, and I remain unconvinced that the ancient religions he cites were free of implicitly dualistic animism.

3. [As noted in previous chapters (see also Clark, 1980, pp. 33–34), Freud did read a good deal of philosophy in his adolescence and during his university years, when he even considered philosophy as a career. The present text may give the false impression that he was the complete empiricist he presented himself as being, whereas there is a great deal of evidence that his underlying (preconscious?) preconceptions, assumptions, and ways of framing issues were deeply influenced by the philosophers he read during his second decade.]

4. It is worth noting that the modifications of classical technique that have made it possible to treat psychotics have not been of the kind that would be necessary to study the characteristic psychotic defects in perception, memory, conceptual thinking, motor coordination, and the like; hence it should not be surprising that no great advances in ego psychology have come from analysts who have learned ways of treating schizophrenics.

Chapter 9.   Ego Autonomy and the Problem of Human Freedom

1. [As in earlier chapters, I have made no effort to change the implicitly sexist language of my original paper, but let it stand with this brief apology.]

2. In this review, I am much indebted to Rapaport's unpublished seminars on ego psychology and some of his papers (particularly 1958a and 1959). I have deliberately kept it as narrow as possible, not from a lack of appreciation for the work of many analysts within and without the Freudian mainstream who have contributed to the contemporary picture of the ego as at least potentially strong and autonomous, but for the sake of brevity.

3. Rapaport cites facts and makes formulations on the basis of which it is extremely easy to take the step of postulating a positive correlation of the autonomies. For example (1958a, p. 731): "Both autonomies require external and/or drive stimulation of a specific intensity and quality for maintenance and effectiveness." He was clear that the same structures were involved in both types of autonomy:

> Cognitive organization, ego interests, values, ideals, ego identity and superego influences—all of which are relatively autonomous from the drives—also play a causal role in the persistence of many behavior forms [that are countermanded by the environment— the kind of persistence he was just discussing]. However, since the autonomy of these is secondary, they may be regarded as only *proximal guarantees* of the ego's autonomy from the environment. (p. 726)

He overlooked the fact that the structures of primary autonomy also were involved in both autonomy from the id and from the environment, and perhaps was too much charmed by the dialectical paradox he glimpsed of a reciprocal relation, ultimately, between the two great classes of determinants.

It was characteristic of Rapaport to work on a number of theoretical issues more or less simultaneously, letting them interact in his mind and enrich one another. During the years between his two autonomy papers, he was working on many such issues; the problem of adaptation as a metapsychological point of view and the problem of activity and passivity were prominent among them. In his 1953 paper on activity and passivity (Rapaport, 1967), which he was never content to publish, he introduced a number of subtle new considerations that required a rethinking of many autonomy issues. He wrote to me on October 25, 1958: "The main reason I did not publish this paper as yet is that the adaptive problem, i.e., the relation to the external environment and the passivity–activity implications of that, prevented me from publishing. I had to digest those first." Likewise, he wrote on November 19, 1958, speaking about the second autonomy paper:

> I gave at the end of that paper a tentative solution of the relationship [between activity-passivity and autonomy]. But I have not convinced myself about the nature of this relationship in a final way. It is, however, quite certain that activity–passivity has implications which reach far beyond autonomy.

I cite these passages to indicate that Rapaport was far from content with the way he left his discussions of either activity and passivity or autonomy in these two papers, and that he was aware of many problems that remained to be worked out in the relations between them, particularly with respect to relations to reality.

Miller (1962) gives a misleading impression of some controversy or conflict between Rapaport and his students on these matters. But as Dr. Gill has confirmed in a letter to me (of May 20, 1962) about the hypnosis book, "he read over Chapter V in several different versions . . . and to the best of my knowledge agreed with it as a more acceptable formulation than his in so far as they differed."

Similarly, Rapaport was fully aware of David Shapiro's development of a rationale of the color response in the Rorschach test on the basis of his own paper on activity and passivity (see Shapiro, 1956, 1960), implying a correlation between the two autonomies, and he knew and approved my paper (Holt, 1960) in which I made this implication quite explicit in summarizing Shapiro's ideas. By these examples, I merely mean to point out the fact that it was a matter of indifference to Rapaport whether his ideas were developed explicitly by himself or by his students. He had little pride of authorship, was generous to a fault (e.g., often urging others to accept joint authorship with him when they had only commented on a manuscript of his), and in general considered it nothing regrettable when an advance in theory was made that contradicted an earlier published statement of his.

4. Rapaport was well aware of this point. He acknowledged that he was neglecting "freedom to," but deferred for the future what he described as "the crucial task . . . the study of the autonomous ego motivations, the ego's methods of setting its goals and the ego's capability to give free rein to and to execute derivative id motivations" (1958a, p. 731 n.). [In a personal communication, L. W. Brandt has pointed out to me that the distinction between "freedom from" ("*Frei wovon?*") and

"freedom to" ("*frei wozu?*") is at least as old as *Also Sprach Zarathustra* (Nietzsche, 1896).]

5. [To be sure, we can and do make useful gross judgments about the accuracy of perception every day, as when two people differ in their hearing of a third party's words and one's interpretation is validated by the speaker, or when there is a consensus about an aspect of reality but one person's percepts are so deviant that they are judged to be hallucinatory. The fact that consensual percepts sometimes prove to be physically impossible—like the "rising" or "setting" of the sun—is only one indication that it is difficult to generalize simply from successful everyday judgments of perceptual veridicality or accuracy.]

6. Perhaps Rapaport was thinking about the skilled piano playing of psychotic or near-psychotic patients he had known, in which case a criterion is readily available. [In general, it may justly be protested that we can and do make useful judgments of a gross kind. As Morris Eagle has pointed out (in a personal communication of August 1988),

> we can and do evaluate, without much difficulty, whether or not motor functioning is efficient. . . . [as in these] examples: walking vs. stumbling; coordinated vs. uncoordinated; a smooth, experienced, and talented athlete, say, fielding an infield grounder vs. an untalented novice doing the same thing.

My point is that once we go beyond such obvious extremes, it gets quite difficult to make quantitative judgments, except in the case of quite specific and circumscribed acts, such as the acrobatic routines judged in athletic competitions.]

7. Compare the role of the closely related concept of freedom (or liberty) in democratic ideology. [In both instances, we show our ethnocentrism if we leave these values unexamined and even unrecognized as such.]

8. [I originally wrote "memory-trace structures," a term I now avoid using; see Paul (1967) and my notes accompanying it.]

9. [As Rubinstein (1967b) points out, however, most skills depend a great deal on practice, which could be called "structure-specific nutriment." In the short run, skills and memories alike seem to be more disrupted by disarranged, inappropriate inputs than by deprivation; clearly, however, with very prolonged disuse (as in strabismus), a perceptual function may be irreversibly lost.]

10. [It is embarrassing to see the anthropomorphism with which I endowed "the apparatus" with homuncular properties of searching, trying, and fouling up. It is so much easier to criticize such lapses in others than to avoid them oneself!]

11. [One must not be confused by Freud's making a sharp antithesis between "internal psychical reality" and "the reality of the external world," for the latter is equally likely to be a meaning. In the passage just cited (1939a [1937–1939], p. 76), he is talking about the same kind of incompatibility between delusion and social fact in psychosis as he had been in 1894.]

12. [In this section, the unbracketed material is an excerpt, with minor alterations, from my rejoinder (Holt, 1967a) to critics of the autonomy paper (Holt, 1965b).]

13. [After I had written the text, I discovered that this solution to the problem of free will is a familiar one to philosophers. Bertrand Russell (1929, p. 239), for example, wrote: "Freedom, in short, in any valuable sense, demands only that our

volitions shall be, as they are, the result of our own desires, not of an outside force compelling us to will what we would rather not will." On the lack of conscious feelings of intent or purpose on the part of impulsive people, whose whims are demonstrably the acting out of unconscious wishes, see Shapiro (1965).]

Chapter 10. The Development of the Primary Process: A Structural View

1. For example: "The principal feature of the primary process is a tendency to the complete discharge of mental energies without delay"; "the assumption that there are two types of mental functioning [the primary and secondary processes] . . . has to do essentially with mental energies" (Arlow & Brenner, 1964, pp. 15, 84); "The terms primary and secondary process as described by Freud in *The Interpretation of Dreams* refer only to modes of discharge of psychic energy" (Beres, 1965a, p. 19).

2. This is the correlation between the percentage of Rorschach responses containing content indications of primary process (drive-dominated imagery) and the percentage containing manifest evidences of such formal indications as condensations, autistic logic, symbolism, tolerated contradiction, and so on. The correlation between the raw numbers of responses containing these two types of material is higher (.71), the difference reflecting the extraneous factor of total number of responses. They are based on a sample of 305 mixed cases, including 121 college students and other relatively normal persons, 81 schizophrenics (mostly in VA hospitals), the remainder being diagnosed in a variety of neurotic and character-disordered categories. The correlations in the normal and schizophrenic subsamples are virtually the same as the ones cited. [In 1967], I would justify the use of drive domination as a criterion of primary process not in terms of any presumed lack of neutralization, but in terms of the pleasure principle as central to the definition of primary process (see Gill, 1967, and Wolff, 1967). Likewise, its formal features can be conceptualized without reference to free versus bound cathexis (see below).

3. "[I]deas and affect-charge already presuppose 'psychic structure,' and cannot be derived alone from the cathectic dynamics" (Rapaport, 1951a, p. 691). Though at least lip service is generally given to the applicability of the structural point of view to the primary process, it often amounts to little more than referring the primary process to the id. Gill (1967) provides a brief treatment of the primary process from all five metapsychological points of view. That is one reason I have concentrated exclusively on structural considerations in this chapter; another is the lack of a detailed discussion of the primary process from the standpoint of structure. The concept of structure is general enough to include at least the following three meanings: the largest divisions of the psychic apparatus (ego, superego, id), at the most general; the organization of particular mental contents (e.g., the structure of a percept or of a fantasy), at the most specific; and an intermediate level in which I am most interested—the operative elements of a theory that will explain how thought and behavior come about. In this context, such an expression as "primary-process structure" does not refer to the architectonics of dream imagery; below I make limited use of the organization of dreams only as a kind of datum to suggest the need for the postulation of further structures in the model of an organism that can produce such dreams. On the general relevance of the structural point of view to the primary process, see also Wolff (1967).

4. A psychic structure, Rapaport said, is a process characterized by a slow rate of change. It is difficult to quarrel with this assertion, since all empirical structures of whatever kind do undergo change and therefore can be looked upon as processes. But as a definition, it fails to specify the very features that distinguish some slow processes from others. Consider, for example, a glacier, a proverbial instance of slow change. Because it is a sluggishly moving mass of ice, it appeals to us as more structural than an ordinary river of water. But consider an even slower process: the melting of the polar icecaps, including glaciers, which is uncovering Viking ships that have been frozen in Greenland for a millennium. Because this process is of a slower rate of change than a glacier, is it even more structural? On the contrary; I doubt that anyone would call this melting "a structure." The processes that shape the landscape are in themselves less structural than a soap bubble, which may come into being and perish in a fraction of a second. The central defining feature of structure, as I see it, is its organization: It is an arrangement of parts in a pattern, which does not necessarily have to have any simple kind of ordering and does not necessarily endure for long, though we are usually most interested in structures that persist for a matter of months or years. Logically, if the psychoanalytic model includes psychic energy, structures must have the property of conducting or insulating against it, as well as subserving all hypothesized functions and setting limits on them.

The great difficulty in defining psychic structure is its ontological unclarity, with the twin dangers of mentalism and reductionism always hovering in the background. As Beres (1965b) has pointed out, the danger of reifying the structural concepts of metapsychology is also a besetting one, though it seems odd that he singles out this particular aspect of the theory as prone to such danger, which is quite general. I cannot undertake here to demonstrate why I disagree with Beres's rejection of structural concepts, despite the fact that he makes a number of cogent critical points.

It should be obvious from the above discussion that the traditional definition of "structures" as "groups of functions," adopted by Beres and by Arlow and Brenner (1964), seems to me as unsatisfactory as Rapaport's, and on similar grounds. That is, I agree with Rubinstein (1967a) that ego, superego, and id are best thought of as groups of functions, but this last phrase does not therefore constitute an acceptable definition of structures generally. There is an ambiguity in the term "structure," in that it is used in various contexts to refer to three rather different kinds of hypothetical entities: (a) In the traditional sense of the "structural hypothesis," ego, superego, and id are structures; the corresponding great subdivisions of the topographic model might also be called structures in this sense, and I have adopted that usage in referring to the two systems Freud associated with the primary and secondary processes in 1900. (b) The smaller component elements of the theory are called structures, particularly by Rapaport; for example, defenses, thresholds, cognitive styles, anticipations. (c) Specific mental contents—thoughts or percepts—are organized and satisfy the definition I have just advanced; these are the structures with which gestalt psychology has been especially concerned. In the passage quoted above from p. 610 of The Interpretation of Dreams, the "particular mental grouping" might be a structure in this restricted sense, but that is not relevant to my point. Throughout this chapter, except in the passage noted where I briefly adopted sense (a), I use the term in sense (b).

5. Rapaport made this point in passing: "Objections might be raised against discussing these primary-process mechanisms as structures, but I cannot attempt to justify this here" (1959, p. 128 n.).

6. Peter Wolff (personal communication, 1966) points out the fact that "*all* meaning implies structure, since any connection of meaning must be cast in structural–functional terms." That is to say, meaning necessarily entails persisting linkages between ideas, between symbols and their referents, and so on, which constitute an organization satisfying the criteria for structure contained in note 4, above.

7. [Difficult, that is, within the purview of the mechanistic world hypothesis (Pepper, 1942). From the standpoint of the theory of living systems and the world hypothesis or metaphysical system in which it is grounded, however, what seems an impossibility is recognized as a everyday reality. See Weiss (1969) for several telling examples of regular order maintained in a living system without mechanical means. That much said, I believe that the argument still has some merit. Even though organisms lack the precise micromechanical control presumed in mechanistic theories, there are and must be some structures setting the recorded parameters of the dynamic system play.]

8. [In this chapter, I have let stand a terminology I no longer use. What Freud called "mechanisms of defense" are ways of defining (one's sense of security, of safety, of self-esteem, etc.) against various threats. One of the revelations of my own personal analysis was the realization that I had (have) recurrent strategies of defending myself that did not fit any of the standard lists of "*the* defense mechanisms." That made me realize that I had been implicitly visualizing such a mechanism as a kind of complex mechanical gadget, a component of a larger "apparatus"; in addition, I had been assuming that repression, projection, reaction formation, and so forth were the names of standard interchangeable parts, pretty much the same from one person's psychic apparatus to the next. The root metaphor of the machine is all too evident in such thinking, once one becomes aware of it.]

9. Rapaport (1960a) spoke about "structuralized primary-process mechanisms," though he conceived of them in a somewhat narrower way than Gill (1963, 1967) and I do:

> The primary-process mechanisms (displacement, condensation, substitution) are basically means of immediate drive discharge. In this role they have a structural characteristic, since the discharge attained through them is slower than a discharge which can take place without them. Nevertheless, they are at best *ad hoc*, short-lived structures. When they appear in a form which is integrated into the secondary process, their lifetime is increased: they have become further structuralized. (p. 844 n.)

10. Cf. Gill (1963, p. 13): "In a recurrent dream, a pattern of functioning has been formed which repeats the pattern of the *ad hoc* primary-process event. In short, a structure has developed."

11. [I would no longer choose this example, which presupposes acceptance of the dual-drive theory of aggression. For a much more tenable conceptualization of bullying, see Olweus (1986).]

12. The other half of his reluctance seems to have been his experience that patients could not decipher symbols by the process of association, and resisted his symbolic interpretations when he offered them. A simpler explanation of this obser-

vation than the postulation of a mysterious "racial memory" would start from ordinary resistance, and [his assumption] that the great majority of symbols refer to sexual organs and activities. In any event, other analysts today do *not* find that, uniformly, "nothing occurs to a person under analysis in response to" symbols (Freud, 1916-1917, p. 149). For another and perhaps more likely interpretation of the relation between symbolism and displacement, see Gill (1967).

13. G. S. Klein's astute warnings are relevant here:

> Psychical organization is assumed to be a hierarchic arrangement of structures recognizable by their function. Such functions as perceiving, remembering, anticipating, intending, are assumed to have a structural basis. Not necessarily a single structure for a single function, for a function can be represented by relationships among many activated structures. (Klein, 1962, p. 182)

One should therefore be "wary of assuming that thought products that appear to be formally identical are the products of the same structures and mechanisms" (1962, p. 189).

14. [Here I originally wrote "model," as I did also above, where I have substituted the words "theoretical conception of a human being," because in 1967 I was uncertain what "model" meant (in contradistinction to "theory"; see Chapter 12). I still have not found a good word to denote what Freud called "the psychic apparatus"—the linked set of theoretical abstractions conceptualizing the human person and his or her functioning. The term "apparatus" implies the mechanistic outlook; my adoption of Waters's term "mechanomorphism" shows a vague awareness that something was wrong with this mechanical terminology, but at the time I had not yet realized that the underlying problem was a clash of metaphysical systems (Holt, 1984a, 1984b). The remainder of this paragraph is a trifle glib, ignoring the difficult problem of specifying just what subsystem has the functions of knowing, willing, and initiating action. Even at the time of this revision, however, I do not feel ready to set forth a complete theory of the self, much less a comprehensive rewriting of the clinical theory of psychoanalysis, in spite of the fine spadework that has been done by Rubinstein (1975).]

15. Suzette H. Annin points out (in a personal communication, 1966) a generally overlooked implication of the undifferentiated-phase conception: that the primary and secondary processes should develop simultaneously, not sequentially. Moreover, she notes, if the primary process is as closely linked to the drive organization of memories and the secondary process to the conceptual organization as Rapaport (1951a) maintained, these two organizations of memories also would have to develop simultaneously; all of which seems quite discrepant with the usual understanding. The difficulty is only apparent, however. It is quite possible for the two systems of thought to make their *beginnings* more or less simultaneously—or even for the line of development that most clearly eventuates in the secondary process to begin a little earlier—and for the sequence that Freud described to be still grossly correct. As I shall argue below, the primary process is probably synthesized into what could be called a system of thought at a time when the organization of realistc, logical thinking is still quite crude and primitive; and it seems likely that the primary process *completes* its development before the secondary, too. Both of these "processes" are actually quite complex, and the various structures subserving them

(including the organizations of memory) undergo gradual rather than saltatory development and at varying, partly independent rates. [All such rumination becomes unnecessary once we abandon the assumption, which is warranted primarily by tradition, that we must postulate an ego and an id. Without that requirement, the need for an undifferentiated phase vanishes.]

16. On this process, see Werner (1948) and Werner and Kaplan (1963) [and see also Hochberg, 1971].

17. This picture of the perceptual world of the infant, in stressing fluidity, may seem inconsistent with the work of such investigators as Fantz (1958, 1964), Hershenson, Munsinger, and Kessen (1965), and other students of attention in the neonate (e.g., Kagan, Wolff; [see also Stern, 1985]). The recent discoveries of this group of investigators have resulted from advances in method, a central aspect of which is careful control over the visual displays presented to the baby. The infant's "task" is often to look at one of two pictures, which are presented in constant illumination and position, in such a way that there is a minimum of distracting or interacting stimuli from other senses or from other parts of the visual field, and with the child lying quietly on its back, tested during the brief periods of alert inactivity. The experimental conditions thus ingeniously but artificially make unnecessary the as-yet-undeveloped perceptual constancies: Most of what must be slowly learned, as the baby extracts invariances from fluctuating stimulus fields, is supplied for him. In these circumstances, the infant shows that there are various innate "categories" (to use Wolff's [1967] term) operating to direct attention selectively, which is an important finding. It should not blind us, however, to the likelihood that the average expectable environment of the neonate, during most of the time he is awake and [hungry], lacks the properties that can provide perceptual stability. It may well be that the important early advances in cognitive growth take place under conditions of quiet but gently varying stimuli, which mothers intuitively seek for their infants. Work such as that of Riesen (1961) has shown the profoundly disruptive effects on development of keeping animals in environments with minimal sensory variation; it may well be that too much variation would have equally deleterious effects by straining the capacity of the developing organism to find invariances and construct a stable world of recurrent objects.

18. I do not mean to imply that the neonate is "confused," or experiences the world as a chaos, in anything like the adult sense. As I read him, James implied that the infant's world was *not yet* structured, rather than *dis*ordered. Suzette H. Annin comments (in a personal communication, 1966) that in this paragraph the description of the primitive mental state seems to have "an overtone of the terrifying" (which is not intended), and that though Freud did characterize the id as "a chaos" as a synonym for the primitive state of drives, he seems not to have postulated chaotic infantile *cognition*. Terror is, however, a form of anticipation (Freud, 1926d), a relatively advanced type of cognitive function which presupposes the capacity to imagine what is not perceptually present. [So do many motives, even those Freud considered infantile instinctual drives. Hence the paradoxical observations about ability to wait: Younger infants sometimes tolerate delay better than older children. It is easy to wait if you can expect nothing, however; an infant who has not yet learned to think of an absent and wanted object, for example, is not aware of waiting for it.] One of the greatest difficulties in the way of our imagining what the

consciousness of the neonate must be like is our inability to conceive an entirely passive and diffuse awareness of a succession of wholly unfamiliar presentations, with an inability to reflect on them in any way. As Schachtel (1954) has suggested, it is probably a consciousness without focal attention.

19. The general consensus is that subprimates do not give evidence of capacity for thought of any kind, in the sense of manipulating images or symbols, having very meager capacity for "conserving an object" that is not perceptually present. Skinner's intention was not to attribute magical thought to the pigeon, but to try to explain it away in the human being as just a type of conditioning. But though newborn infants (and even fetuses) are capable of being conditioned (Mann, 1946), what Piaget described may not be a simple conditioned response. My objection to the term "magical phenomenalism" is that the adjective implies a kind of primary-process thinking in the baby, even if it is used only descriptively and without such an intent. It can mislead the reader, as it apparently misled Wolff; see below.

20. In a personal communication (1966), Wolff agrees with the above critique of this part of his 1960 work, and says that he slipped into "adultomorphism"; we cannot say that at the third stage of sensorimotor development the infant's schemes do function according to the primary process, only that his actions give us the impression that they do.

21. I find it difficult to follow Rapaport here. He precedes the quotation above by noting that a model's

> fate depends on its usefulness . . . dreams . . . [and] Observations reported by persons who have been on the brink of death by starvation or dehydration, as well as observations on toxic hallucinoses (Meynert's amentia), schizophrenic hallucinations, illusions of normals, daydreams, and so on, further demonstrate that such hallucination phenomena do occur. (1951c, p. 411)

He implies that they occur "when drive discharge is delayed." My reading of the evidence does not agree; hallucinations do arise in circumstances of stress when integrative functioning has been weakened, in such situations as shipwrecks or maroonings. Many motives are frustrated in disasters of these kinds, to be sure, but a great deal else that is abnormal is going on, too. I have seen no evidence that the specific frustration of drives plays a special role. (See Goldberger & Holt, 1958; Holt, 1964 and Chapter 9, this volume). Moreover, it is dangerous to apply a model based mainly on observations from adulthood to earliest infancy.

22. Suzette H. Annin (in a personal communication, 1966) suggests a further argument against this classic assumption about the origins of the secondary process: "Suppose the infant does hallucinate the breast when he gets hungry; the mother always does come and feed him. Why shouldn't he keep on hallucinating until food does come?" Hallucinated gratification is ultimately unsatisfactory only if the mother never comes; but the nursling is hardly capable of foraging for himself even if he were to "decide" to turn toward reality. Annin's main point, however, is that we exaggerate the unsatisfactoriness of the assumed hallucination: If it occurs, it is adaptive in that it helps the baby wait for the gratification that must eventually come. If one accepted the common psychoanalytic assumption about infantile omnipotence of thought, it would be reasonable to suppose that such sequences

teach the child that he makes the mother come by hallucinating her—and the secondary process would *never* develop!

23. It is easy to slip into hypostasis when using a concept as "the synthetic function of the ego." My intention is to avoid this fallacy even at the cost of having to ask the reader to accept usages to which he may not be accustomed. Such discussions as Rapaport's, just quoted, urge that many kinds of uniting, organizing, integrating, and gestalt formation occur in the human being, even at a single level of development. To assume, as Nunberg (1931) did, that all processes having any of these synthesizing or binding-together properties are at bottom one and can be attributed to a single ego function, is consistent with some of Freud's theoretical idiosyncrasies but has little to recommend it; the unity may be merely in the metaphorical language we use to describe these processes. Even within the realm of testable abilities, there is no general factor for all tests of synthesizing and organizing; positive evidence for the identity of all integrative functions has never been offered.

24. In this connection, see Schafer (1967) on the magical quality of early ideals and ideal objects. Most of the anthropological literature on relevant topics with which I am familiar deals with the question of the *universality* of mythic themes and ways of thought. Kluckhohn (1959) has summarized a good deal of this literature, the main purport of which is that impressive regularities of theme and content occur in the myths—especially the hero stories—of all culture areas. Kluckhohn (1959, p. 48) notes: "There are two ways of reasoning that bulk prominently in all mythological systems. These are what Sir James Frazer called the 'laws' of sympathetic magic (like causes like) and holophrastic magic (the part stands for the whole)." (Note the implication of displacement in the first of these laws and condensation in the second.) Similarly, Freud (1912-1913), Werner (1948), Lévy-Bruhl (1922), and numerous others emphasize the *similarities* in the (primary-process) modes of thought among primitive peoples generally. When diversity or cultural uniqueness of myth is stressed, the emphasis is put upon idiosyncrasies of content.

25. Dahl (1965) has produced a persuasively argued case that certain data from Helen Keller's (1908) recollections are so well conceptualized by the primitive model of cognition as to constitute evidence of its utility. The critical passage he cites is as follows: Miss Keller is speaking about her life before the advent of her teacher, Annie Sullivan:

> When I wanted anything I liked,—ice cream, for instance, of which I was very fond,—I had a delicious taste on my tongue (which, by the way, I never have now), and in my hand I felt the turning of the freezer. I made the sign, and my mother knew I wanted ice cream. I 'thought' and desired in my fingers. (Keller, 1908, pp. 115-116)

This, Dahl argues, is a report of the primitive model actually in operation: "*She hallucinated the previous experience of satisfaction*—the 'delicious taste' of the ice cream" (p. 537). Did she? Possibly so, depending in large measure on just how you want to define "hallucination." My preference is for a narrower, stricter definition that would exclude this example on the grounds that the child did not have any failure of reality testing: She did not accept the taste on her tongue as a real gratification, as we do in dreams, but proceeded to give "the sign," which Dahl tells us was "her hand turning the freezer handle."

This example seems to me much better conceptualized in Piaget's theory than in Freud's. Note the emphasis on enactive representation, the fact that the subjective part of the experience was not separate from but an integral part of a total sensorimotor functioning. It was not just the memory trace of an earlier experience of gratification that was activated, but a sensorimotor scheme. It is indeed interesting that the wish *was* the condensed (and possibly reversed) sequence of turning the freezer handle and tasting the ice cream, and that the taste image had in effect an eidetic quality, being experienced *at* the receptor. Perhaps the relative sensory deafferentiation produced by little Helen's illness made it possible for her to experience the iconic aspect of the sensorimotor totality with such quasi-hallucinatory vividness; see the discussion of infantile dreaming, below.

26. See Paul (1967) and Wolff (1967) for the relevant evidence and arguments.

27. A few weeks later, I was able to observe, during a briefer REM period, that the vicissitudes of my son's penile erections seemed meaningfully related to other observable behavior: A smile occurred after a period of tumescence to maximum erection, and detumescence accompanied frowning and larger, aversive-looking movements followed by awakening (see Fisher, 1965).

[Over 30 years] ago, Aserinsky and Kleitman (1955) reported that neonates spend more than half of their sleeping time in an active phase marked by bodily movements, both fine and gross, with rapid eye movements [REMs] and fluttering of the eyelids. Roffwarg, Dement, and Fisher (1964) confirmed these observations, noting that the eye movements closely resemble those of adults, and adding:

> In the active phase, there are almost continuous fine twitches, grimaces, smiles, and tremors with frequent, but intermittent large athetoid excursions of the limbs and stretching of the torso. Occasionally, vocalization occurs. Bursts of muscle movement and irregular respirations generally appear concurrently with the REM bursts. (p. 62)

These observations were of babies 15 days of age and younger; the next group they observed were from 14 to 20 weeks old. The authors comment on the present topic only: "Body movement is very prominent during the REM periods and hence the phrase, 'active phase,' may still be applied to this portion of the sleep cycle. However, the body movement is not nearly as frequent as in the neonate" (p. 63). They add that muscular movements gradually diminish up to young adulthood, and that Jouvet has reported a similar developmental sequence in the cat.

Roffwarg et al. (1964) raise the question whether these facts mean that dreaming is present at birth, and comment:

> If by dreaming is meant the occurrence of hallucinatory visual imagery which is correlated with the specific spatial patterns of the REM's, as in adults, then the possibility . . . must be negated. . . . REM's in neonates . . . seem to be an attribute of a unique physiological sleep state which later becomes associated with patterned dreaming. . . . It is likely that what goes on in the infant's mind during the REM period of sleep is fairly closely related to what goes on in his mind while awake . . . it is possible that as perception and memory functions develop in the growing infant, dreaming develops in a parallel fashion and takes place as a more or less obligatory concomitant of the quasi-awake neurophysiology of the REM period. . . . The occurrence of REM's in newborns, therefore, may be analogous to their presence in decorticates. That is, in both instances, the phenomenon of REM periods is most likely a *pure* brain-stem function. Prior to the

acquisition of visual perception and visual memory, it seems possible that dreaming may be expressed in other modalities (olfactory, gustatory, tactile, kinesthetic, etc.). (pp. 68–69)

The authors do not relate the decline of muscular activity with age to the development of sensorimotor intelligence; their only hypothesis about it is as follows:

> It may be that in infants, whose waking life is limited in time and scope and offers little occasion for activity, the REM period allows for a substantial discharge of activity during sleep. Perhaps as waking activity increases, the need for its discharge during sleep decreases. (p. 70)

This rather forced effort to invoke a tension reduction theory is not very convincing, since it does not fit other data.

My observations on a single infant have only suggestive value, of course, but besides confirming the report just cited, they point to the need for further studies to test a new hypothesis: that the activity seen in the neonate during activated sleep is largely random and unpatterned, and shows a developmental course during the first weeks, the elements becoming linked together into affectively meaningful, quasi-thematic units. I was fortunate in the accidental circumstance that my son developed a distinct position habit during his second month, a preferred direction of gaze to the right, which was so strong as to interfere with his nursing from the right breast. Once the preference had begun, it was reinforced by the fact that his environment accommodated to it, so that he always found his favorite toys placed to his right. In order to interpret observational data of the kind I suggest, investigators may need to know the life circumstances of their subjects equally well, and in any event research of the kind I am advocating will have to be studies of individual cases over a period of time, not cross-sectional surveys of groups of successive age levels.

Chapter 11. The Present Status of Freud's Theory of the Primary Process

1. As I shall demonstrate below, some of the time he did treat them as observables.

2. I do not try here to approach the question of origins in the manner of a historian of science, who would undoubtedly have begun by discussing Meynert's strikingly similar concept of a primary and a secondary ego, as well as other historical antecedents.

3. I mean "mysterious" here only in the sense that the ways in which emotions are evoked are concealed, not obvious.

4. He says so rather explicitly earlier in the same work: "It must be allowed that the great bulk of the thoughts which are revealed in analysis were already active during the process of forming the dream" (Freud, 1900a, p. 280).

5. In this connection, see Schimek's (1975, pp. 177–178) thoughtful discussion of these issues, in which he points out a fact I overlooked when I was writing my scoring manual, to be discussed below: "Symbolism, although now often listed as one of the characteristics of primary process ideation, is not on a par with the concept of displacement and condensation (it was never included in the theoretical formulations of the seventh chapter of 'The Interpretation of Dreams')."

6. See, however, Schimek (1975), who independently comes to the same conclusion about Freud's theory of perception.

7. How strikingly similar is the following paragraph from Freud's last work, the *Outline*:

Conscious processes on the periphery of the ego and everything else in the ego unconscious—such would be the simplest state of affairs that we might picture. And such may in fact be the state that prevails in animals. But in men there is an added complication through which internal process in the ego may also acquire the quality of consciousness. This is the work of the function of speech, which brings material in the ego into a firm connection with mnemic residues of visual, but more particularly of auditory, perceptions. Thenceforward the perceptual periphery of the cortical layer can be excited to a much greater extent from inside as well, internal events such as passages of ideas and thought-processes can become conscious, and a special device is called for in order to distinguish between the two possibilities—a device known as *reality-testing*. The equation "perception = reality (external world)" no longer holds. Errors, which can now easily arise and do so regularly in dreams, are called *hallucinations*. (1940a, p. 162)

8. Romanes, whose "book on animal intelligence is the first comparative psychology that was ever written" (Boring, 1929, p. 473), concluded in his third and final book, published in 1888, "that 'simple ideas,' like sensory impressions, perceptions and the memories of perceptions, are common to all animals and man" (Boring, 1929, p. 474).

9. In a personal communication, Merton Gill points out the fact that Pötzl's (1917) well-known experiment, to which Freud alluded approvingly (1900a, pp. 181–182, in a footnote added in 1919), and others that have been stimulated by it (summarized by Fisher, 1960b), "seem to represent the demonstration of a veridical input changed by primary processes." Some of these experiments do strongly suggest that there is a virtually photographic registration of pictures too briefly exposed for the observer to become conscious of more than small fragments of them, while his subsequent dreams and mental images contain what look like derivatives of the unreported registrations modified by condensation and displacement. Yet the data do not coerce this interpretation; like most experimental findings, they are disconcertingly amenable to other interpretations, which do not assume separate processes of accurate registration and distorting transformation. We are up against the indeterminacy inherent in the fact that we have no way of learning about any perception other than our own except through verbal, graphic, or other responses by the perceiver, all of which require postperceptual processing. I want also to note that Schimek (1975) has come to the same conception of the primary process as that which distorts an originally correct or veridical thought or percept.

10. Never, that is, in any published work; but his very first mention of the concept of the primary process, in the unpublished "Project," occurred in a discussion of how the ego is endangered by cathecting the memory of the need-satisfying object or situation of gratification so intensely as to give rise to an "indication of reality" from the ω (perceptual) system. Thus, his first definition of the primary process is "Wishful cathexis to the point of hallucination (1950 [1895], pp. 325, 326).

Chapter 12. The Death and Transfiguration of Metapsychology

1. For further details of the history of this late-romantic methodological movement and an attempt at a detailed refutation of its major arguments, see Holt, 1978a, Vol. 1, Chapter 1.

2. He is not alone in being properly critical of metapsychology as a language for the psychoanalytic domain; Rado (1956, 1962) and Sullivan (1953a, 1953b, 1956) devoted many pages to their sustained attempts to create an alternative and more satisfactory language, free of the old connotations of ambiguous terms.

3. There is a great deal that I might say about Schafer's contributions to the present topic in his two books (1976, 1978), both positive and negative. I have enormous respect for the psychoanalytic content of Schafer's writings, but disagree with a large part of the philosophy of science and metaphysics in them. See Spiro (1979) for a detailed critique of the latter, and also Holt (1979).

4. These laws were so strikingly similar that this model has been turned round, and electrical analog computers have been built to model the behavior of large and expensive hydraulic systems to discover the optimal configuration of a small and cheap system of wires before the expensive system of pipes and pumps is built (Hempel, 1965).

5, Perhaps precisely *because* we are still in the grip of materialistic prejudice, to which relationships are never as real as things. (See Whitehead, 1925.)

6. Bertalanffy (1964) proposed a somewhat similar idea.

Chapter 13. The Current Status of Psychoanalytic Theory

1. Most attempts to specify the clinical theory have concentrated on the special hypotheses, omitting the *general* clinical hypotheses, which obscures the critical role this part of the clinical theory plays in clinical inference.

2. To be convincing, a test of the prediction would have to use uncontaminated judges, applying the rules and definitions to unlabeled case data from the critical patient and from another, judged by the investigator not to hate his father unconsciously. A statistical test of the resulting data would be necessary to confirm the prediction.

3. I omit here the complicating circumstances that, strictly speaking, any scientific hypothesis can be tested only with the aid of a considerable apparatus of auxiliary assumptions, stipulations about conditions of measurement, and so on. If the prediction fails, some part of this scaffolding may logically be responsible, so the matter is never simple.

4. The hypothesis that the involvement of the reticular activating system makes the critical difference is plausible but not verified.

5. Which we cannot even confidently call derivatives until they have been reliably detected as such by independent and uncontaminated judges.

Chapter 14. Freud and the Emergence of a New World Hypothesis

1. [I mean "pragmatism" here in the metaphysical sense, as a school of relativistic contextualism. Thus, one may be a pragmatist—in my meaning—and reject the pragmatic (practical, no-nonsense, dollars-and-cents) outlook, as many people do who are attracted to hermeneutics.]

2. ["Cosmology" is an unfortunately ambiguous term, used in two somewhat overlapping senses. In science, it is used to refer to the endeavors of astrophysicists, astronomers, and other theorists to develop theories of the origin and development

of the physical universe. In philosophy, however, the same term has the sense intended here—as a branch of metaphysics concerned with the cosmos, all of reality, its origins, and our place in it.]

3. The coherence of a world hypothesis is not that of a formal system and should not be taken to mean the rigid lucidity of deductive interconnectedness.

4. [In a personal communication (August 1988), Morris Eagle argues that science—"including materialistic and mechanistic science"—has had "an *anti-authoritarian* historical role and influence. . . . The centrality of empirical evidence and the skepticism of science seem to me *inherently* antiauthoritarian." He is undoubtedly correct, I believe: Respect for truth and fidelity to the most objective methods of attaining it are surely antithetical to the authoritarian ethos. It is, however, difficult to know how to cast the balance, and to determine whether these considerations or the influence of mechanism had the greater influence at any given period of history.]

5. ["Organicism" is the term Pepper uses to refer to a philosophical position more usually called "idealism"—confusingly, to me, because I associate the former term with the organismic outlook, which is part of systems philosophy (see below). During the 19th century, idealism captured a larger sector of the popular imagination, especially in America, than formism or contextualism (Kuklick, 1980). Nevertheless, I give it short shrift here because it had relatively little impact upon science; indeed, it seems poorly suited indeed to be the philosophical infrastructure for the scientific enterprise. As a simple absolutism, it has a good deal in common with the mechanism it so fiercely opposed: Neither is synthetic, and each attempts to dismiss the entire reality of the other reductionistically.]

6. It is instructive if saddening to notice how often transference is construed— even by psychoanalysts themselves—as meaning simply falling in love with your analyst. Here Freud's own sexual reductionism joined forces with the regressive temptation to which thought is always vulnerable. That tendency itself, incidentally, is another manifestation of the same thought pattern as transference, which Piaget called "assimilation."

7. More precisely, those of Lorenz and Minkowski.

8. Later (Pepper, 1967), he did attempt to state his own adequate world hypothesis.

9. See, for example, Ackoff (1974), Laszlo (1972), Weiss (1969), and Chapters 6 and 9, this volume.

10. Near the end of his life, Pepper (1972a, p. 151) hailed Laszlo's (1971) systems philosophy as "a breath of fresh air" toward which he felt "extremely sympathetic." He believed that it closely resembled "(and certainly includes) my own presently favored paradigm of 'selective system' for a world theory" (1972a, p. 151). Its root metaphor, the dynamic self-regulating system, he considered "possibly the most fruitful or even the correct one for a detailed synthetic comprehension of the structure of the universe" (1972b, p. 548). Perhaps Pepper was right in seeing it as having a single root metaphor rather than as I have presented it, as itself a synthesis of valid elements from preceding world hypotheses.

References

In a couple of ways, the following list of references and the system of citation in the text differ from the standard of the American Psychological Association's *Publication Manual* (3rd ed.), which I have otherwise followed.

First, because most of the present inquiry is of a historical nature, I have thought it best to cite republished works by their original date of publication, giving dates of editions actually consulted in the list of references. Thus, a reader who wishes to consult the context of a quotation will do best to look not in the original source (when more than one place of publication is given), but in the later, usually more convenient one. For example, in the case of papers by David Rapaport, all page references in the text are to the collection edited by Merton Gill.

Second, in the following listing I have referred to *The Standard Edition of the Complete Psychological Works of Sigmund Freud* as merely *Standard Edition*, also omitting reference to the general editorship of James Strachey in collaboration with Anna Freud, Alix Strachey, and Alan Tyson, and to the translators (generally James Strachey). I have also adopted the designation of specific works used in the *Standard Edition*, under which (for example) "Analysis Terminable and Interminable" is 1937c though it is the only work of that date that is cited. For other authors, lettered suffixes after dates always begin with "a" when there is more than one from the same year.

Numbers in parentheses at the end of each entry list the pages in the text on which the work is cited.

Ackoff, R. L. (1974). *Redesigning the future: A systems approach to societal problems*. New York: Wiley. (229, 394)

Amacher, M. P. (1962). *The influence of the neuroanatomy, neurophysiology and psychiatry of Freud's teachers on his psychoanalytic theories*. Unpublished doctoral dissertation, University of Washington. (115, 116)

Amacher, P. (1965). Freud's neurological education and its influence on psychoanalytic theory. *Psychological Issues, 4* (Monograph No. 16). (77, 78, 114, 117, 174, 366)

Angyal, A. (1941). *Foundations for a science of personality*. New York: Commonwealth Fund. (244)

Apfelbaum, B. (1965). Ego psychology, psychic energy, and the hazards of quantitative explanation in psycho-analytic theory. *International Journal of Psycho-Analysis, 46*, 168–182. (377)

Apfelbaum, B. (1966). On ego psychology: A critique of the structural approach to psychoanalytic theory. *International Journal of Psycho-Analysis, 47*, 451–475. (210)

Applegarth, A. (1971). Comments on aspects of psychic energy. *Journal of the American Psychoanaltyic Association, 19*, 379–416. (324)

Arieti, S. (1955). *Interpretation of schizophrenia*. New York: Robert Brunner. (273)

Arlow, J. A. (1975). The structural hypothesis: Theoretical considerations. *Psychoanalytic Quarterly, 44*, 509–525. (199, 207, 209, 211, 212, 213)

Arlow, J. A., & Brenner, C. (1964). *Psychoanalytic concepts and the structural theory*. New York: International Universities Press. (199, 209, 264, 383, 384)

Aserinsky, E., & Kleitman, N. (1955). A motility cycle in sleeping infants as manifested by ocular and gross body activity. *Journal of Applied Physiology, 8*, 11–18. (390)

395

Bach, S. (1960). *Symbolic associations to stimulus words in subliminal, supraliminal, and incidental presentation.* Unpublished doctoral dissertation, New York University. (104)

Bahm, A. J. (1977). *Comparative philosophy: Western, Indian, and Chinese philosophies compared.* Albuquerque, NM: World Books. (243)

Bahm, A. J. (1988). Comparing civilizations as systems. *Systems Research, 5,* 35–47. (243)

Bailey, P., & Davis, E. W. (1942). The syndrome of obstinate progression in the cat. *Proceedings of the Society for Experimental Biology, 51,* 307. (180)

Bakan, D. (1966). *The duality of human existence.* Chicago: Rand McNally. (244)

Barr, H. L., Langs, R. J., Holt, R. R., Goldberger, L., & Klein, G. S. (1972). *LSD: Personality and experience.* New York: Wiley-Interscience. (61)

Barratt, B. B. (1976). Freud's psychology as interpretation. *Psychoanalysis and Contemporary Science, 5,* 443–478. (311)

Basch, M. F. (1973). Psychoanalysis and theory formation. *Annual of Psychoanalysis, 1,* 39–52. (324)

Beach, F. (1956). Characteristics of masculine sex drive. In M. R. Jones (Ed.), *Nebraska Symposium on Motivation* (Vol. 4, pp. 1–32). Lincoln: University of Nebraska Press. (182, 183)

Bellah, R. N. (1985). *Habits of the heart: Individualism and commitment in American life.* Berkeley: University of California Press. (244)

Beres, D. (1965a). Symbol and object. *Bulletin of the Menninger Clinic, 29,* 3–23. (263, 383)

Beres, D. (1965b). Structure and function in psycho-analysis. *International Journal of Psycho-Analysis, 46,* 53–63. (264, 384)

Bergson, H. (1911). *Creative evolution* (A. Mitchell, Trans.). New York: Holt. (152, 155–157, 242, 374, 377)

Berlinski, D. (1976). *On systems analysis: An essay concerning the limitations of some mathematical methods in the social, political, and biological sciences.* Cambridge, MA: MIT Press. (320)

Bernfeld, S. (1944). Freud's earliest theories and the school of Helmholtz. *Psychoanalytic Quarterly, 13,* 341–362. (114–116, 149, 152, 254, 375)

Bernfeld, S. (1951). Sigmund Freud, M.D., 1882–1885. *International Journal of Psycho-Analysis, 32,* 204–217. (59, 115, 116, 152)

Bertalanffy, L. von. (1950). The theory of open systems in physics and psychology. *Science, 111,* 23–29. (134, 164)

Bertalanffy, L. von. (1964). The mind–body problem: A new view. *Psychosomatic Medicine, 26,* 29–45. (393)

Bettelheim, B. (1983). *Freud and man's soul.* New York: Knopf. (108)

Bexton, W. H., Heron, W., & Scott, T. H. (1954). Effects of decreased variation in the sensory environment. *Candian Journal of Psychology, 8,* 70–76. (131)

Bishop, M. P., Elder, S. T., & Heath, R. G. (1963). Intracranial self-stimulation in man. *Science, 140,* 394. (132)

Black, M. (1962). *Models and metaphors: Studies in language and philosophy.* Ithaca, NY: Cornell University Press. (372)

Blight, J. (1981). Must psychoanalysis retreat to hermeneutics? Psychoanalytic theory in the light of Popper's evolutionary epistemology. *Psychoanalysis and Contemporary Thought, 4,* 147–206. (337)

Block, J. H., & Block, J. (1980). The role of ego-control and ego-resiliency in the organization of behavior. In W. A. Collins (Ed.), *Development of cognition, affect, and social relations: The Minnesota Symposia on Child Psychology* (Vol. 13, pp. 39–101). Hillsdale, NJ: Erlbaum. (343)

Boring, E. G. (1929). *A history of experimental psychology* (3rd. ed.). New York: Appleton-Century-Crofts, 1957. (24, 148, 290, 392)

Boring, E. G. (1963). Science keeps on becoming [Review of *The structure of scientific revolutions,* by T. S. Kuhn]. *Contemporary Psychology, 8,* 180–182. (372)

Bowen, M. (1978). *Family therapy in clinical practice.* New York: Jason Aronson. (239)

Bowlby, J. (1969). *Attachment and loss: Vol. 1. Attachment.* London: Hogarth Press. (244)

Bowlby, J. (1973). *Attachment and loss: Vol. 2. Separation.* New York: Basic Books. (244)

Breger, L. (1967). Function of dreams. *Journal of Abnormal Psychology, 72*(5, Pt. 2), 1-28. (112)

Breuer, J., & Freud, S. (1895). Studies on hysteria. *Standard Edition, 2*, 1-305. London: Hogarth Press, 1955. (73, 102, 116, 186, 221, 230, 242, 261, 287, 370)

Bronowski, J. (1965). *Science and human values* (rev. ed.). New York: Harper. (61, 62)

Brücke, E. (1876). *Vorlesungen über Physiologie* (Vol. 2). Vienna: W. Braumüller. (117)

Bruner, J. S. (1961). The cognitive consequences of early sensory deprivation. In P. Solomon, P. E. Kubansky, P. H. Leiderman, J. H. Mendelson, R. Trumbull, & D. Wexler (Eds.), *Sensory deprivation* (pp. 195-207). Cambridge, MA: Harvard University Press. (237)

Bruner, J. S. (1964). The course of cognitive growth. *American Psychologist, 19*, 1-5. (269)

Büchner, L. (1855). *Force and matter, or, principles of the natural order of the universe. With a system of morality based thereon* (Trans. from 15th German ed. of *Kraft und Stoff*; 4th English ed.). London: Asher, 1884. (32, 215, 240, 241, 350, 370, 371)

Buckle, H. T. (1871). *History of civilization in England.* New York: Appleton-Century-Crofts, 1934. (21, 32, 363)

Burnham, J. C. (1974). The medical origins and cultural use of Freud's instinctual drive theory. *Psychoanalytic Quarterly, 43*, 193-217. (364)

Burtt, E. A. (1932). *The metaphysical foundations of modern physical science* (2nd ed.). London: Routledge & Kegan Paul. (350)

Burtt, E. A. (1943). The status of world hypotheses. *Philosophical Review, 52*, 590-601. (360)

Butler, R. A., & Harlow, H. F. (1957). Discrimination learning and learning sets to visual exploration incentives. *Journal of General Psychology, 57*, 257-264. (131)

Cannon, W. B. (1929). *Bodily changes in pain, hunger, fear, and rage.* New York: Appleton. (184)

Cantril, H. (1941). *The psychology of social movements.* New York: Wiley. (4)

Carmichael, L. (Ed.). (1946). *Manual of child psychology.* New York: Wiley. (290)

Chein, I. (1962). The image of man. *Journal of Social Issues, 18*, 1-35. (219, 251)

Chein, I. (1972). *The science of behavior and the image of man.* New York: Basic Books. (203)

Clark, R. W. (1980). *Freud: The man and the cause.* New York: Random House. (24, 380)

Cofer, C. N. (1959). Motivation. *Annual Review of Psychology, 10*, 173-202. (130)

Cofer, C. N., & Appley, M. H. (1964). *Motivation: Theory and research.* New York: Wiley. (181, 245, 379)

Colby, K. M. (1963). Computer simulation of a neurotic process. In S. S. Tomkins & S. Messick (Eds.), *Computer simulation of personality* (pp. 165-179). New York: Wiley. (264)

The compact edition of the Oxford English dictionary (2 vols.). (1971). Oxford: Oxford University Press. (109)

Cope, E. D. (1896). *The primary factors of evolution.* Chicago: Open Court. (152)

Cranefield, P. F. (1958). Josef Breuer's evaluation of his contribution to psycho-analysis. *International Journal of Psycho-Analysis, 39*, 319-322. (51)

Cranefield, P. F. (1966). Freud and the "school of Helmholtz." *Gesnerus, 23*, 35-39. (114, 370)

Cranefield, P. F. (1970). Some problems in writing the history of psychoanalysis. In G. Mora & J. L. Brand (Eds.), *Psychiatry and its history* (pp. 41-55). Springfield, IL: Charles C Thomas. (114, 370, 375)

Creager, J. A. (1967). Freedom–determinism controversies: Some whys and wherefores. *American Psychologist, 22*, 235-236. (249)

Cronbach, L. J. (1957). The two disciplines of scientific psychology. *American Psychologist, 7*, 173-196. (71)

Culbertson, J. T. (1963). *The minds of robots.* Urbana: University of Illinois Press. (145, 263, 377)

Dahl, H. (1965). Observations on a "natural experiment": Helen Keller. *Journal of the American Psychoanalytic Association, 13*, 533-550. (389)

Dahl, H. (1968). Psychoanalytic theory of the instinctual drives in relation to recent developments. *Journal of the American Psychoanalytic Association, 16*, 613-637. (185)

Dahl, H. (1972). A quantitative study of a psychoanalysis. *Psychoanalysis and Contemporary Science, 1,* 237-257. (331)

Dahl, H. (1979). The appetite hypothesis of emotions: A new psychoanalytic model of motivation. In C. E. Izard (Ed.), *Emotions and personality in psychopathology* (pp. 201-225). New York: Plenum. (322)

Darwin, C. (1859). *On the origin of species.* Cambridge, MA: Harvard University Press, 1964. (151)

d'Holbach, Baron [P. H. Thiry]. (1770). *The system of nature.* New York: Garland Press, 1984. (350, 371)

Dorer, M. (1932). *Historische Grundlagen der Psychoanalyse.* Leipzig: Felix Meiner. (32)

Driesch, H. A. E. (1914). *The history and theory of vitalism* (O. K. Ogden, Trans.). London: Macmillan. (143)

Driesch, H. (1929). *The science and philosophy of the organism* (2nd ed.). London: Black. (143, 155-157, 377)

du Bois-Reymond, E. (1884). *Über die Grenzen des Naturerkennens.* Leipzig: Veit, 1892. (375)

Duffy, E. (1957). The psychological significance of the concept of "arousal" or "activation." *Psychological Review, 64,* 265-275. (131)

Eagle, C. J. (1964). *An investigation of individual consistencies in the manifestations of primary processes.* Unpublished doctoral dissertation, New York University. (274)

Eagle, M. N. (1983). A critical examination of motivational explanation in psychoanalysis. In L. Laudan (Ed.), *Mind and medicine: Problems of explanation and evaluation in psychiatry and the biomedical sciences* (pp. 311-353). Berkeley, CA: University of California Press. (313)

Eagle, M. (1984). *Recent developments in psychoanalysis.* New York: McGraw-Hill. (324, 326, 337)

Eagle, M., & Wolitzky, D. (1989). The idea of progress in psychoanalysis. *Psychoanalysis and Contemporary Thought, 12,* 27-72. (338)

Einstein, A., & Infeld, L. (1938). *The evolution of physics.* New York: Simon & Schuster. (150, 375)

Ellenberger, H. F. (1956). Fechner and Freud. *Bulletin of the Menninger Clinic, 20,* 201-214. (32)

Ellenberger, H. F. (1970). *The discovery of the unconscious: The history and evolution of dynamic psychiatry.* New York: Basic Books. (66, 174, 203, 204)

Erikson, E. H. (1939). Observations on Sioux education. *Journal of Psychology, 7,* 101-156. (274)

Erikson, E. H. (1950). *Childhood and society* (rev. ed.). New York: Norton, 1963. (212, 229, 274)

Erikson, E. H. (1954). The dream specimen of psychoanalysis. *Journal of the American Psychoanalytic Association, 2,* 5-56. (274)

Erikson, E. H. (1956). The first psychoanalyst: Crisis and discovery. *Yale Review, 46,* 40-62. Also in E. H. Erikson, *Insight and responsibility.* New York: Norton, 1964. (121)

Erikson, E. H. (1958). *Young man Luther: A study in psychoanalysis and history.* New York: Norton. (212)

Erikson, E. H. (1964). *Insight and responsibility: Lectures on the ethical implications of psychoanalytic insight.* New York: Norton. (214, 277)

Erikson, E. H. (1968). *Identity: Youth and crisis.* New York: Norton. (214)

Erikson, E. H. (1969). *Gandhi's truth: On the origins of militant nonviolence.* New York: Norton. (214)

Erikson, E. H. (1982). Psychoanalytic reflections on Einstein's centenary. In G. Holton & Y. Elkana (Eds.), *Albert Einstein: Historical and cultural perspectives* (pp. 151-173). Princeton, NJ: Princeton University Press. (358)

Exner, S. (1894). *Entwurf zu einer physiologischen Erklärung der psychischen Erscheinungen.* Vienna: Deutike. (73, 78, 118, 205)

Eysenck, H. J. (1954). The science of personality: Nomothetic! *Psychological Review, 61,* 339-342. (311)

Fairbairn, W. R. D. (1952). *Psycho-analytic studies of the personality.* London: Routledge & Kegan Paul. (338)

Fantz, R. L. (1958). Pattern vision in young infants. *Psychological Reports, 8,* 43–47. (387)

Fantz, R. L. (1964). Visual experience in infants: Decreased attention to familiar patterns relative to novel ones. *Science, 146,* 668–670. (277, 387)

Fechner, G. T. (1873). *Einige Ideen zur Schopfungs- und Entwicklungsgeschichte der Organismen.* Leipzig: Breitkopf & Haertel. (124)

Fenichel, O. (1934). On the psychology of boredom. *Imago, 20,* 270–281. Also in H. Fenichel & D. Rapaport (Eds.), *The collected papers of Otto Fenichel* (Vol. 1, pp. 292–302). New York: Norton, 1953. (101, 369)

Fenichel, O. (1938). The drive to amass wealth. *Psychoanalytic Quarterly, 7,* 69–95. Also in H. Fenichel & D. Rapaport (Eds.), *The collected papers of Otto Fenichel* (Vol. 2, pp. 89–108). New York: Norton, 1954. (22)

Fisher, C. (1954). Dreams and perceptions. *Journal of the American Psychoanalytic Association, 2,* 389–445. (292)

Fisher, C. (1956, May). *The concept of the primary process.* Paper presented at the Annual Meeting of the American Psychoanalytic Association. (Summarized in Panel Report, The psychoanalytic theory of thinking. *Journal of the American Psychoanalytic Association,* 1958, *6,* 143–153.) (253)

Fisher, C. (1957). A study of preliminary stages of construction of dreams and images. *Journal of the American Psychoanalytic Association, 5,* 5–60. (292)

Fisher, C. (1960a). Subliminal and supraliminal influences on dreams. *American Journal of Psychiatry, 116,* 1009–1017. (104, 292)

Fisher, C. (1960b). Introduction to "Preconscious stimulation in dreams, associations, and images." *Psychological Issues, 2* (Monograph No. 7), 1–40. (392)

Fisher, C. (1965, March 15). *Relationships between dream content and nocturnal REMP erection.* Paper presented at opening ceremonies, Research Center for Mental Health, New York University. (390)

Fisher, C. (1966). Dreaming and sexuality. In R. M. Loewenstein, L. M. Newman, M. Schur, & A. J. Solnit (Eds.), *Psychoanalysis: A general psychology* (pp. 537–569). New York: International Universities Press. (183)

Fisher, C., Gross, J., & Zuch, J. (1965). Cycle of penile erection synchronous with dreaming (REM) sleep. *Archives of General Psychiatry, 12,* 29–45. (274)

Fisher, C., & Paul, I. H. (1959). The effect of subliminal visual stimulation on images and dreams: A validation study. *Journal of the American Psychoanalytic Association, 7,* 35–83. (105)

Fisher, R. A. (1945). *The design of experiments* (4th ed.). London: Oliver & Boyd. (68)

Fisher, S., & Greenberg, R. P. (1977). *The scientific credibility of Freud's theories and therapy.* New York: Basic Books. (340)

Fodor, N., & Gaynor, F. (Eds.). (1950). *Freud: Dictionary of psychoanalysis.* New York: Philosophical Library. (68)

Frank, P. (1955). Foundations of physics. In O. Neurath, R. Carnap, & C. Morris (Eds.), *International encyclopedia of unified science* (Vol. 1, Part 2). Chicago: University of Chicago Press. (160)

Freedman, S. J. (1961). Perceptual changes in sensory deprivation: Suggestions for a conative theory. *Journal of Nervous and Mental Disease, 132,* 17–21. (235)

Freedman, S. J., & Greenblatt, M. (1959, September). *Studies in human isolation* (USAF Wright ADC Technical Report No. 59-266). Wright–Patterson Air Force Base, OH: Aerospace Medical Laboratory, Aeronautical Systems Division. (234, 235)

Freud, A. (1937). *The ego and the mechanisms of defence.* New York: International Universities Press, 1946. (212, 213)

Freud, S. (1891b). *On aphasia.* New York: International Universities Press, 1953. (178)

Freud, S. (1892-1893). A case of successful treatment by hypnotism. *Standard Edition*, 1, 117-128. London: Hogarth Press, 1964. (204)

Freud, S. (1893c). Some points for a comparative study of organic and hysterical motor paralyses. *Standard Edition*, 1, 160-172. London: Hogarth Press, 1966. (370)

Freud, S. (1893h). On the psychical mechanism of hysterical phenomena: A lecture. *Standard Edition*, 3, 27-39. London: Hogarth Press, 1962. (370)

Freud, S. (1894a). The neuro-psychoses of defence. *Standard Edition*, 3, 45-61. London: Hogarth Press, 1962. (102, 135, 221, 241)

Freud, S. (1895b [1894]). On the grounds for detaching a particular syndrome from neurasthenia under the description "anxiety neurosis." *Standard Edition*, 3, 90-115. London: Hogarth Press, 1962. (135, 154, 181, 212, 241, 242, 371)

Freud, S. (1895f). A reply to criticisms of my paper on anxiety neurosis. *Standard Edition*, 3, 123-139. London: Hogarth Press, 1962. (43)

Freud, S. (1896). Letter 52 to Wilhelm Fliess (December 6). *Standard Edition*, 1, 233-239. London: Hogarth Press, 1966. (288, 289)

Freud, S. (1896c). The aetiology of hysteria. *Standard Edition*, 3, 191-221. London: Hogarth Press, 1962. (242)

Freud, S. (1900a). The interpretation of dreams. *Standard Edition*, 4, 1-338; 5, 339-627. London: Hogarth Press, 1953. (9, 10, 25, 26, 40-42, 44, 47, 51-53, 58, 73, 78, 84-87, 96, 101-103, 121-123, 128, 153, 157, 184, 186, 202, 206, 208, 209, 212, 215, 221, 240, 242, 254, 257-260, 262, 263, 271, 283, 285, 288, 293, 294, 317, 364, 375, 384, 391, 392)

Freud, S. (1901a). On dreams. *Standard Edition*, 5, 633-686. London: Hogarth Press, 1953. (283, 285)

Freud, S. (1901b). The psychopathology of everyday life. *Standard Edition*, 6, 1-310. London: Hogarth Press, 1960. (25, 37, 38, 45, 47, 53, 65, 208, 247)

Freud, S. (1905c). Jokes and their relation to the unconscious. *Standard Edition*, 8, 1-243. London: Hogarth Press, 1960. (87, 208, 212, 262, 284, 372)

Freud, S. (1905d). Three essays on the theory of sexuality. *Standard Edition*, 7, 125-245. London: Hogarth Press, 1953. (30, 132, 174, 177, 181, 371, 372)

Freud, S. (1905e [1901]). Fragment of an analysis of a case of hysteria. *Standard Edition*, 7, 15-122. London: Hogarth Press, 1953. (29, 186, 190, 205, 206, 365)

Freud, S. (1906a). My views on the part played by sexuality in the aetiology of the neuroses. *Standard Edition*, 7, 271-279. London: Hogarth Press, 1953. (48, 52)

Freud, S. (1910a [1909]). Five lectures on psycho-analysis. *Standard Edition*, 11, 9-55. London: Hogarth Press, 1957. (208)

Freud, S. (1910e). The antithetical meaning of primal words. *Standard Edition*, 11, 155-161. London: Hogarth Press, 1957. (25)

Freud, S. (1910i). The psycho-analytic view of psychogenic disturbance of vision. *Standard Edition*, 11, 211-218. London: Hogarth Press, 1957. (286)

Freud, S. (1910k). 'Wild' psychoanalysis. *Standard Edition*, 11, 221-227. London: Hogarth Press, 1957. (135)

Freud, S. (1911b). Formulations on the two principles of mental functioning. *Standard Edition*, 12, 218-226. London: Hogarth Press, 1958. (52, 88, 102, 103, 177, 298)

Freud, S. (1911c). Psycho-analytic notes on an autobiographical account of a case of paranoia (dementia paranoides). *Standard Edition*, 12, 9-82. London: Hogarth Press, 1958. (102)

Freud, S. (1912f). Contribution to a discussion of masturbation. *Standard Edition*, 12, 243-254. London: Hogarth Press, 1958. (47)

Freud, S. (1912-1913). Totem and taboo. *Standard Edition*, 16, 1-161. London: Hogarth Press, 1955. (24, 29, 240, 272, 349, 389)

Freud, S. (1914c). On narcissism: An introduction. *Standard Edition*, 14, 73-102. London: Hogarth Press, 1957. (48, 49, 103, 125, 139, 140, 164, 210, 222, 265, 280)

Freud, S. (1915c). Instincts and their vicissitudes. *Standard Edition, 14*, 117–140. London: Hogarth Press, 1957. (42, 48, 56, 110, 124–126, 137, 138, 174–177, 179, 242, 265, 290, 316)

Freud, S. (1915d). Repression. *Standard Edition, 14*, 146–158. London: Hogarth Press, 1957. (49)

Freud, S. (1915e). The unconscious. *Standard Edition, 14*, 166–215. London: Hogarth Press, 1957. (17, 26, 37, 49, 73, 74, 88, 89, 101, 103, 139, 140, 171, 184, 210, 212, 242, 254, 256, 365, 368, 369)

Freud, S. (1916–1917). Introductory lectures on psycho-analysis. *Standard Edition, 15*, 1–240; *16*, 241–496. London: Hogarth Press, 1963. (37, 43, 58, 110, 111, 128, 212, 263, 386)

Freud, S. (1917a). A difficulty in the path of psycho-analysis. *Standard Edition, 17*, 137–144. London: Hogarth Press, 1955. (110, 350, 354)

Freud, S. (1917d [1915]). A metapsychological supplement to the theory of dreams. *Standard Edition, 14*, 222–235. London: Hogarth Press, 1957. (25–27, 78, 102, 118, 208, 210, 365)

Freud, S. (1917e [1915]). Mourning and melancholia. *Standard Edition, 14*, 243–258. London: Hogarth Press, 1957. (55, 89, 92)

Freud, S. (1918b). From the history of an infantile neurosis. *Standard Edition, 17*, 7–122. London: Hogarth Press, 1955. (111)

Freud, S. (1919g). Preface to Reik's *Ritual: Psychoanalytic Studies. Standard Edition, 17*, 259–263. London: Hogarth Press, 1955. (103)

Freud, S. (1920g). Beyond the pleasure principle. *Standard Edition, 18*, 7–64. London: Hogarth Press, 1955. (26, 27, 39–41, 44, 46, 52, 55–57, 73, 79, 89–95, 102, 103, 111, 119, 124–126, 132, 136, 365, 372, 373, 375)

Freud, S. (1921c). Group psychology and the analysis of the ego. *Standard Edition, 18*, 69–143. London: Hogarth Press, 1955. (27, 48, 52, 138, 240)

Freud, S. (1922a). Dreams and telepathy. *Standard Edition, 18*, 197–220. London: Hogarth Press, 1955. (45, 241)

Freud, S. (1923a). Two encyclopedia articles. *Standard Edition, 18*, 235–259. London: Hogarth Press, 1955. (135, 286)

Freud, S. (1923b). The ego and the id. *Standard Edition, 18*, 12–66. London: Hogarth Press, 1961. (6, 37, 40–43, 48, 49, 96, 98, 103, 125, 199, 200, 207–212, 216, 373)

Freud, S. (1923e). The infantile genital organization: An interpolation into the theory of sexuality. *Standard Edition, 19*, 141–145. London: Hogarth Press, 1961. (286)

Freud, S. (1924b). Neurosis and psychosis. *Standard Edition, 19*, 149–153. London: Hogarth Press, 1961. (286)

Freud, S. (1924c). The economic problem of masochism. *Standard Edition, 19*, 159–170. London: Hogarth Press, 1960. (97, 103, 125, 133, 373)

Freud, S. (1924e). The loss of reality in neurosis and psychosis. *Standard Edition, 19*, 183–187. London: Hogarth Press, 1961. (286)

Freud, S. (1925a). A note upon the "Mystic Writing-Pad." *Standard Edition, 19*, 227–232. London: Hogarth Press, 1961. (79, 102)

Freud, S. (1925d). An autobiographical study. *Standard Edition, 20*, 7–70. London: Hogarth Press, 1959. (26, 27, 47, 49, 60, 135, 152, 204, 266, 329)

Freud, S. (1925e). The resistances to psycho-analysis. *Standard Edition, 19*, 213–224. London: Hogarth Press, 1961. (63)

Freud, S. (1925h). Negation. *Standard Edition, 19*, 235–239. London: Hogarth Press, 1961. (128)

Freud, S. (1925i). Some additional notes on dream-interpretation as a whole. *Standard Edition, 19*, 127–138. London: Hogarth Press, 1961. (45, 241)

Freud, S. (1925j). Some psychical consequences of the anatomical distinction between the sexes. *Standard Edition, 19*, 248–258. London: Hogarth Press, 1961. (286)

Freud, S. (1926d). Inhibitions, symptoms and anxiety. *Standard Edition, 20*, 87–174. London: Hogarth Press, 1959. (26, 40, 97, 98, 102, 103, 112, 212, 365, 369, 387)

Freud, S. (1926e). The question of lay analysis. *Standard Edition, 20*, 183–258. London: Hogarth Press, 1959. (58, 364)

Freud, S. (1927c). The future of an illusion. *Standard Edition, 21*, 5–56. London: Hogarth Press, 1961. (44, 52, 207, 247, 349)

Freud, S. (1927d). Humor. *Standard Edition, 21*, 161–166. London: Hogarth Press, 1961. (27)

Freud, S. (1927e). Fetishism. *Standard Edition, 21*, 152–157. London: Hogarth Press, 1961. (287)

Freud, S. (1928b). Dostoevsky and parricide. *Standard Edition, 21*, 177–194. London: Hogarth Press, 1961. (30)

Freud, S. (1930a). Civilization and its discontents. *Standard Edition, 21*, 64–145. London: Hogarth Press, 1961. (39, 40)

Freud, S. (1933a). New introductory lectures on psycho-analysis. *Standard Edition, 22*, 5–182. London: Hogarth Press, 1964. (44, 45, 49, 58, 65, 98, 102, 103, 125, 128, 136, 264, 265, 279, 288, 369)

Freud, S. (1937c). Analysis terminable and interminable. *Standard Edition, 23*, 216–253. London: Hogarth Press, 1964. (27, 98, 103, 110, 111, 222)

Freud, S. (1939a [1937–1939]). Moses and monotheism. *Standard Edition, 23*, 7–137. London: Hogarth Press, 1964. (201, 265, 382)

Freud, S. (1940a). An outline of psycho-analysis. *Standard Edition, 23*, 144–207. London: Hogarth Press, 1964. (50, 99, 103, 104, 110, 128, 265, 287, 373, 392)

Freud, S. (1940e). Splitting of the ego in the process of defence. *Standard Edition, 23*, 275–278. London: Hogarth Press, 1964. (287)

Freud, S. (1941d [1921]). Psychoanalysis and telepathy. *Standard Edition, 18*, 177–193. London: Hogarth Press, 1955. (45, 241)

Freud, S. (1941f [1938]). Findings, ideas, problems. *Standard Edition, 23*, 299–300. London: Hogarth Press, 1964. (265)

Freud, S. (1950 [1895]). Project for a scientific psychology. *Standard Edition, 1*, 295–391. London: Hogarth Press, 1966. (19, 20, 23, 76–84, 102, 103, 119, 124, 138, 153, 175, 184, 205, 215, 241, 261, 287, 289, 366, 392)

Freud, S. (1950 [1892–1899]). Extracts from the Fliess papers. *Standard Edition, 1*, 177–280. London: Hogarth Press, 1966. (28, 76, 366)

Freud, S. (1960). *Letters of Sigmund Freud* (E. L. Freud, Ed.; T. & J. Stern, Trans.). New York: Basic Books. (41, 47, 363)

Freud, S. (1985 [1887–1904]). *The complete letters of Sigmund Freud to Wilhelm Fliess, 1887–1904* (J. M. Masson, Ed. & Trans.). Cambridge, MA: Harvard University Press. (16, 18–20, 28, 53, 55, 122, 241, 284)

Freud, S., & Abraham, K. (1965). *A psycho-analytic dialogue: The letters of Sigmund Freud and Karl Abraham 1907–1926* (H. C. Abraham & E. L. Freud, Eds.). New York: Basic Books. (27)

Freud, S., & Jung, C. G. (1974). *The Freud/Jung letters: The correspondence between Sigmund Freud and C. G. Jung* (W. McGuire, Ed.; R. Mannheim & R. F. C. Hull, Trans.). Princeton, NJ: Princeton University Press. (41, 48, 53, 60)

Freud, S., & Oppenheim, D. E. (1957 [1911]). Dreams in folklore. *Standard Edition, 12*, 180–203. London: Hogarth Press, 1958. (263)

Freud, S., & Pfister, O. (1963). *Psychoanalysis and faith: The letters of Sigmund Freud and Oskar Pfister* (E. L. Freud & H. Meng, Eds.; E. Mosbacher, Trans.). London: Hogarth Press. (35, 61)

Fromm, E. (1939). Selfishness and self-love. *Psychiatry, 2*, 507–524. (139)

Fromm, E. (1959). *Sigmund Freud's mission: An analysis of his personality and influence.* New York: Grove Press, 1963. (63)

Galatzer-Levy, R. M. (1976). Psychic energy: A historical perspective. *Annual of Psychoanalysis, 4*, 41–61. (324)

Galdston, I. (1956). Freud and romantic medicine. *Bulletin of the History of Medicine, 30*, 489–507. (375)

Gardner, R. W., Holzman, P. S., Klein, G. S., Linton, H. B., & Spence, D. P. (1959). Cognitive control: A study of individual consistencies in cognitive behavior. *Psychological Issues, 1* (Monograph No. 4). (63, 65, 66, 214)

Gay, P. (1988). *Freud: A life for our time.* New York: Norton. (63)

Gedo, J. E., & Pollock, G. H. (1975). Freud: The fusion of science and humanism. *Psychological Issues, 9* (Monograph No. 34/35). (307)

Genung, J. F. (1900). *The working principles of rhetoric.* Boston: Ginn. (55)

Gesell, A., & Ilg, F. G. (1943). *Infant and child in the culture of today.* New York: Harper & Bros. (202)

Ghent, E. (1962, September 26). *Governing principle in man's functioning.* Paper presented to the Postdoctoral Colloquium, New York University. (139)

Gill, M. M. (1959). The present state of psychoanalytic theory. *Journal of Abnormal and Social Psychology, 58,* 1-8. (127, 254)

Gill, M. M. (1963). Topography and systems in psychoanalytic theory. *Psychological Issues, 3* (Monograph No. 10). (101, 199, 209, 210, 253, 255, 261, 265, 266, 297, 385)

Gill, M. M. (1967). The primary process. In R. R. Holt (Ed.), Motives and thought: Psychoanalytic essays in honor of David Rapaport. *Psychological Issues, 5* (Monograph No. 18/19), 260-298. (253, 254, 257, 260, 264, 284, 293, 297, 299, 383, 385, 386)

Gill, M. M. (1976). Metapsychology is not psychology. In M. M. Gill & P. S. Holzman (Eds.), Psychology versus metapsychology: Psychoanalytic essays in memory of George S. Klein. *Psychological Issues, 9* (Monograph No. 36), 71-105. (16, 18, 19, 307, 324)

Gill, M. M. (1977). Psychic energy reconsidered: Discussion. *Journal of the American Psychoanalytic Association, 25,* 581-597. (307)

Gill, M. M. (1978). Metapsychology is irrelevant to psychoanalysis. In S. Smith (Ed.), *The human mind revisited: Essays in honor of Karl A. Menninger* (pp. 349-368). New York: International Universities Press. (29)

Gill, M. M. (1982). *Analysis of transference: Vol. 1. Theory and technique (Psychological Issues,* Monograph No. 53). New York: International Universities Press. (331)

Gill, M. M., & Brenman, M. (1959). *Hypnosis and related states.* New York: International Universities Press. (225, 230)

Gill, M. M., & Hoffman, I. Z. (1982). *Analysis of transference: Vol. 2. Studies of nine audio-recorded psychoanalytic sessions (Psychological Issues,* Monograph No. 54). New York: International Universities Press. (331, 343)

Gill, M. M., & Klein, G. S. (1964). The structuring of drive and reality: David Rapaport's contributions to psycho-analysis and psychology. *International Journal of Psycho-Analysis, 45,* 483-498. (256)

Gillispie, C. C. (1958). Lamarck and Darwin in the history of science. *American Scientist, 46,* 388-409. (148)

Goldberger, L. (1961). Reactions to perceptual isolation and Rorschach manifestations of the primary process. *Journal of Projective Techniques, 25,* 287-302. (300)

Goldberger, L., & Holt, R. R. (1958). Experimental interference with reality contact (perceptual isolation): I. Method and group results. *Journal of Nervous and Mental Disease, 127,* 99-112. (231, 301, 388)

Goldberger, L., & Holt, R. R. (1961). *Studies on the effects of perceptual alteration* (USAF ASD Technical Report No. 61-416). Wright-Patterson Air Force Base, OH: Aerospace Medical Laboratory, Aeronautical Systems Division. (61)

Goodwin, L. (1965). Using the feedback theory of action to reshape the freedom-determinism controversy. *American Psychologist, 20,* 234-235. (249)

Gould, S. J. (1977a). *Ever since Darwin: Reflections in natural history.* New York: Norton. (21)

Gould, S. J. (1977b). *Ontogeny and phylogeny.* Cambridge, MA: Harvard Press. (20)

Gove, P. B. (Ed.). (1981). *Webster's third new international dictionary of the English language, unabridged.* Springfield, MA: Merriam-Webster. (317, 367)

Graham, E. (1955). Inner-directed and other-directed attitudes. Unpublished doctoral dissertation, Yale University. (65)

Greenfield, N. S., & Lewis, W. C. (Eds.). (1965). Psychoanalysis and current biological thought. Madison: University of Wisconsin Press. (114)

Grossman, M. I., & Stein, L. F., Jr. (1948). Vagotomy and the hunger-producing action of insulin in man. Journal of Applied Physiology, 1, 263-269. (185)

Grossman, W. I., & Simon, B. (1969). Anthropomorphism: Motive, meaning and causality in psychoanalytic theory. Psychoanalytic Study of the Child, 24, 78-111. (324, 368)

Grünbaum, A. (1976). Is falsifiability the touchstone of scientific rationality? Karl Popper versus inductivism. In R. S. Cohen, P. K. Feyerabend, & M. W. Wartofsky (Eds.), Boston studies in the philosophy of science: Vol. 38. Essays in memory of Imre Lakatos (pp. 213-252). Dordrecht, The Netherlands: Reidel. (327, 328)

Grünbaum, A. (1977). How scientific is psychoanalysis? In R. Stern, L. Horowitz, & J. Lynes (Eds.), Science and psychotherapy (pp. 219-254). New York: Haven Publications. (327, 328)

Grünbaum, A. (1979). Is Freudian psychoanalytic theory pseudoscientific by Karl Popper's criterion of demarcation? American Philosophical Quarterly, 16, 131-141. (327, 328)

Grünbaum, A. (1980a). The role of psychological explanations of the rejection or acceptance of scientific theories. Transactions of the New York Academy of Sciences, 39, 75-90. (327)

Grünbaum, A. (1980b). Epistemological liabilities of the clinical appraisal of psychoanalytic theory. Nous, 14, 307-385. (327, 328)

Grünbaum, A. (1981). The placebo concept. Behaviour Research and Therapy, 19, 157-167. (327)

Grünbaum, A. (1983a). The foundations of psychoanalysis. In L. Laudan (Ed.), Mind and medicine: Problems of explanation and evaluation in psychiatry and the biomedical sciences (pp. 143-309). Berkeley: University of California Press. (327)

Grünbaum, A. (1983b). Freud's theory: The perspective of a philosopher of science (1982 Presidential Address to the American Philosophical Association, Eastern Division). Proceedings and Addresses of the American Philosophical Association, 57, 5-31. (327, 329)

Grünbaum, A. (1984). The foundations of psychoanalysis: A philosophical critique. Berkeley: University of California Press. (316, 327-329, 337, 338)

Grünbaum, A. (1985). Explication and implications of the placebo concept. In L. White, B. Tursky, & G. F. Schwartz (Eds.), Placebo: Clinical phenomena and new insights (pp. 9-36). New York: Guilford Press. (327, 328)

Guilford, J. P. (1967). The nature of human intelligence. New York: McGraw-Hill. (38)

Guntrip, J. (1967). The concept of psychodynamic science. International Journal of Psycho-Analysis, 48, 32-43. (311)

Guntrip, J. (1969). Schizoid phenomena, object relations and the self. New York: International Universities Press. (338)

Guthrie, E. R., & Horton, G. P. (1946). Cats in a puzzle box. New York: Rinehart. (269)

Guttman, S. A., Jones, R. L., & Parrish, S. M. (Eds.). (1980). Concordance to the standard edition of the complete psychological works of Sigmund Freud. Boston: G. K. Hall. (72, 363, 366)

Habermas, J. (1971). Knowledge and human interests (J. J. Shapiro, Trans.). London: Heinemann. (337)

Hahn, L. E. (1980). The Stephen C. Pepper papers, 1903-1972. Paunch, 75, 53-54. (360)

Haley, J. (1963). Strategies of psychotherapy. New York: Grune & Stratton. (239)

Harlow, H. F. (1953). Mice, monkeys, man, and motives. Psychological Review, 60, 23-32. (130, 131)

Harlow, H. F. (1958). The nature of love. American Psychologist, 13, 673-685. (131)

Hartmann, E. (1966). The psychophysiology of free will: An example of vertical research. In R. M. Loewenstein, L. M. Newman, M. Schur, & A. J. Solnit (Eds.), Psychoanalysis—A *general psychology* (pp. 521–536). New York: International Universities Press. (246, 247, 252)

Hartmann, H. (1939). *Ego psychology and the problem of adaptation.* New York: International Universities Press, 1958. (205, 212, 223, 266, 269, 289)

Hartmann, H. (1950). Comments on the psychoanalytic theory of the ego. *Psychoanalytic Study of the Child, 5,* 74–96. (93, 101, 255)

Hartmann, H. (1964). *Essays on ego psychology: Selected problems in psychoanalytic theory.* New York: International Universities Press. (15, 293, 307, 379)

Hartmann, H., Kris, E., & Loewenstein, R. M. (1946). Comments on the formation of psychic structure. In Papers on psychoanalytic psychology. *Psychological Issues, 4* (Monograph No. 14), 27–55. (50, 266)

Hauser, S. T., Powers, S. I., Noam, G. G., Jacobson, A. M., Weiss, B., & Follansbee, D. J. (1984). Familial contexts of adolescent ego development. *Child Development, 55,* 195–213. (343)

Heath, D. H. (1965). *Explorations of maturity.* New York: Appleton-Century-Crofts. (295)

Hebb, D. O. (1955). Drives and the C.N.S. (conceptual nervous system). *Psychological Review, 62,* 243–254. (74, 128, 130, 131)

Hebb, D. O., & Thomspon, W. R. (1954). The social significance of animal studies. In G. Lindzey (Ed.), *Handbook of social psychology* (pp. 532–561). Cambridge, MA: Addison-Wesley. (200)

Held, R. (1961). Exposure-history as a factor in maintaining stability of perception and coordination. *Journal of Nervous and Mental Disease, 132,* 26–32. (235)

Held, R., & White, B. (1959). Sensory deprivation and visual speed: An analysis. *Science, 130,* 860–861. (234)

Helson, H. (1959). Adaptation level theory. In S. Koch (Ed.), *Psychology: A study of a science. Vol. 1. Sensory, perceptual and physiological formulations* (pp. 565–621). New York: McGraw-Hill. (379)

Hempel, C. G. (1965). *Aspects of scientific explanation, and other essays in the philosophy of science.* New York: Free Press. (317, 318, 393)

Heron, W., Doane, B. K., & Scott, T. H. (1956). Visual disturbance after prolonged perceptual isolation. *Canadian Journal of Psychology, 10,* 13–18. (235)

Hershenson, M., Munsinger, H., & Kessen, W. (1965). Preference for shapes of intermediate variability in the newborn human. *Science, 147,* 630–631. (277, 387)

Hilgard, E. R. (1962). The scientific status of psychoanalysis. In E. Nagel, P. Suppes, & A. Tarski (Eds.), *Logic, methodology, and philosophy of science* (pp. 375–390). Stanford, CA: Stanford University Press. (16)

Hochberg, J. (1971). Perception. In J. W. Kling & L. A. Riggs (Eds.), *Woodworth & Schlosberg's experimental psychology* (3rd ed., pp. 395–550). New York: Holt, Rinehart & Winston. (358, 387)

Hofstadter, D. R. (1979) *Gödel, Escher, Bach: An eternal golden braid.* New York: Basic Books. (355)

Holt [Howe], L. P. (1948). *Psychoanalysis and the social process.* Unpublished doctoral dissertation, Harvard University. (8)

Holt, R. R. (1960). Recent developments in psychoanalytic ego psychology and their implications for diagnostic testing. *Journal of Projective Techniques, 24,* 254–266. (381)

Holt, R. R. (1961). Clinical judgment as a disciplined inquiry. *Journal of Nervous and Mental Disease, 133,* 369–382. (312)

Holt, R. R. (1962). A critical examination of Freud's concept of bound versus free cathexis. *Journal of the American Psychoanalytic Association, 10,* 475–525. (324)

Holt, R. R. (1963). Two influences on Freud's scientific thought: A fragment of intellectual biography. In R. W. White (Ed.), *The study of lives: Essays on personality in honor of Henry A. Murray* (pp. 364–387). New York: Atherton Press. (114, 127, 254, 371)

Holt, R. R. (1964). Imagery: The return of the ostracized. *American Psychologist, 19*, 254-264. (388)

Holt, R. R. (1965a). A review of some of Freud's biological assumptions and their influence on his theories. In N. S. Greenfield & W. C. Lewis (Eds.), *Psychoanalysis and current biological thought* (pp. 93-124). Madison: University of Wisconsin Press. (114, 324)

Holt, R. R. (1965b). Ego autonomy re-evaluated. *International Journal of Psycho-Analysis, 46*, 151-167. (Reprinted with critical evaluations by S. C. Miller, A. Namnum, B. B. Rubinstein, J. Sandler & W. G. Joffe, R. Schafer, & H. Weiner. *International Journal of Psychiatry*, 1967, 3, 481-523.) (218, 324, 382)

Holt, R. R. (1966). Measuring libidinal and aggressive motives and their controls by means of the Rorschach test. In D. Levine (Ed.), *Nebraska Symposium on Motivation (Vol. 14*, pp. 1-47). Lincoln: University of Nebraska Press. (295)

Holt, R. R. (1967a). On freedom, autonomy, and the redirection of psychoanalytic theory: A rejoinder. *International Journal of Psychiatry, 3*, 524-536. (218, 229, 324, 382)

Holt, R. R. (1967b). The development of the primary process: A structural view. In R. R. Holt (Ed.), Motives and thought: Psychoanalytic essays in honor of David Rapaport. *Psychological Issues, 5* (Monograph No. 18/19), 345-383. (324)

Holt, R. R. (1967c). Beyond vitalism and mechanism: Freud's concept of psychic energy. In J. H. Masserman (Ed.), *Science and psychoanalysis: Vol. 11. Concepts of ego* (pp. 1-41). New York: Grune & Stratton. Also in B. Wolman (Ed.), *Historical roots of contemporary psychology* (pp. 192-226). New York: Harper & Row, 1968. (141, 324)

Holt, R. R. (Ed.). (1967d). Motives and thought: Psychoanalytic essays in honor of David Rapaport. *Psychological Issues, 5* (Monograph No. 18/19). (10, 253, 298)

Holt, R. R. (1968). Freud, Sigmund. In D. Sills (Ed.), *International encyclopedia of the social sciences* (Vol. 6, pp. 1-12). New York: Macmillan. (324, 377)

Holt, R. R. (1969). (with collaboration and assistance of J. Havel, L. Goldberger, A. Philip, & R. Safrin). *Manual for the scoring of primary-process manifestations in Rorschach responses* (10th ed.). New York: Research Center for Mental Health, New York University. (295)

Holt, R. R. (1970). Artistic creativity and Rorschach measures of adaptive regression. In B. Klopfer, M. M. Meyer, & F. B. Brawer (Eds.) *Developments in the Rorschach technique* (Vol. 3, pp. 263-320). New York: Harcourt Brace Jovanovich. (296)

Holt, R. R. (1972a). Freud's mechanistic and humanistic images of man. *Psychoanalysis and Contemporary Science, 1*, 3-24. (64, 324)

Holt, R. R. (1972b). On the nature and generality of mental imagery. In P. W. Sheehan (Ed.), *The function and nature of imagery* (pp. 3-33). New York: Academic Press. (364)

Holt, R. R. (1974). On reading Freud. Introduction to C. L. Rothgeb (Ed.), *Abstracts of the standard edition of the complete psychological works of Sigmund Freud* (pp. 3-79). New York: Jason Aronson. (324)

Holt, R. R. (1975). The past and future of ego psychology. *Psychoanalytic Quarterly, 44*, 550-576. (324)

Holt, R. R. (1976a). Drive or wish?: A reconsideration of the psychoanalytic theory of motivation. In M. M. Gill & P. S. Holzman (Eds.), Psychology versus metapsychology: Psychoanalytic essays in memory of George S. Klein. *Psychological Issues, 9* (Monograph No. 36), 158-197. (324)

Holt, R. R. (1976b). Freud's theory of the primary process—present status. *Psychoanalysis and Contemporary Science, 5*, 61-99. (324)

Holt, R. R. (1978a). *Methods in clinical psychology: Assessment, prediction and research* (2 vols.). New York: Plenum. (392)

Holt, R. R. (1978b). Ideological and thematic conflicts in the structure of Freud's thought. In S. Smith (Ed.), *The human mind revisited: Essays in honor of Karl A. Menninger* (pp. 51-98). New York: International Universities Press. (306, 324)

Holt, R. R. (1979). Review of *Language and insight* by Roy Schafer. *Psychoanalytic Quarterly,* 48, 496–500. (393)

Holt, R. R. (1981). The death and transfiguration of metapsychology. *International Review of Psycho-Analysis,* 8, 129–143. (324)

Holt, R. R. (1982). The manifest and latent meanings of metapsychology. *Annual of Psychoanalysis,* 10, 233–255. (324)

Holt, R. R. (1984a). Freud's impact upon modern morality and our world view. In A. L. Kaplan & B. Jennings (Eds.), *Darwin, Marx, and Freud: Their influence on moral theory* (pp. 147–200). New York: Plenum. (386)

Holt, R. R. (1984b). Freud, the free will controversy, and prediction in personology. In R. A. Zucker, J. Aronoff, & A. I. Rabin (Eds.) *Personality and the prediction of behavior* (pp. 179–208). New York: Academic Press. (218, 386)

Holt, R. R. (1985). The current status of psychoanalytic theory. *Psychoanalytic Psychology, 2,* 289–315. (324)

Holt, R. R. (1988). Freud's adolescent reading: Some possible effects on his work. In P. E. Stepansky (Ed.), *Contributions to Freud Studies: Vol. 3. Freud: Appraisals and reappraisals* (pp. 167–192). Hillsdale, NJ: Erlbaum. (32, 240, 363, 370, 376)

Holt, R. R., & Havel, J. (1960). A method for assessing primary and secondary process in the Rorschach. In M. A. Rickers-Ovsiankina (Ed.), *Rorschach psychology* (pp. 263–315). New York: Wiley. (255, 297)

Holt, R. R., & Luborsky, L. (1958). *Personality patterns of psychiatrists* (2 vols.). New York: Basic Books. (10, 114)

Holton, G. (1973). *Thematic origins of scientific thought: Kepler to Einstein.* Cambridge, MA: Harvard University Press. (242, 312)

Holton, G. (1979). Einstein's task as a universe builder: His early years. *Bulletin of the American Academy of Arts and Sciences, 33,* 12–28. (357)

Holzman, P. S. (1976). The future of psychoanalysis and its institutes. *Psychoanalytic Quarterly, 65,* 250–273. (324)

Holzman, P. S. (1985). Psychoanalysis: Is the therapy destroying the science? *Journal of the American Psychoanalytic Association, 33,* 725–770. (324, 344)

Home, H. J. (1966). The concept of mind. *International Journal of Psycho-Analysis, 47,* 42–49. (307, 311)

Hyman, S. E. (1962). *The tangled bank.* New York: Atheneum. (360)

Immergluck, L. (1964). Determinism–freedom in contemporary psychology: An ancient problem revisited. *American Psychologist, 19,* 270–281. (246)

James, W. (1890). *The principles of psychology.* New York: Dover, 1950. (13, 166, 180, 204, 234, 242)

James, W. (1892). *Textbook of psychology: Briefer course.* New York: Holt. (268)

Jahoda, M. (1977). *Freud and the dilemmas of psychology.* New York: Basic Books. (15)

Jones, E. (1953). *The life and work of Sigmund Freud: Vol. 1. The formative years and the great discoveries, 1856–1900.* New York: Basic Books. (35, 36, 46, 60, 71, 117, 241)

Jones, E. (1955). *The life and work of Sigmund Freud: Vol. 2. Years of maturity, 1901–1919.* New York: Basic Books. (15, 35, 36, 38, 44, 54)

Jones, E. (1957). *The life and work of Sigmund Freud: Vol. 3. The last phase, 1919–1939.* New York: Basic Books. (95, 361)

Jones, T. (Ed.). (1963). *Harrap's standard German–English dictionary.* London: G. E. Harrap & Sons. (109)

Joseph, E. D. (1975). Clinical formulations and research. *Psychoanalytic Quarterly, 44,* 526–533. (212, 213)

Jouvet, M. (1961). Telencephalic and rhombencephalic sleep in the cat. In G. E. W. Wolstenholme & M. O'Connor (Eds.), *The nature of sleep* (pp. 188–206). Boston: Little, Brown. (276)

Jouvet, M. (1962). Recherches sur les structures nerveuses et les mécanismes responsable des différentes phases du sommeil physiologique. *Archivos Italianos Biologicos, 100*, 125–206. (276)

Kafka, H. (1963). *The use of color in projective tests and dreams in relation to the theory of ego autonomy.* Unpublished doctoral dissertation, New York University. (229, 274)

Kagan, J. (1955). Differential reward value of incomplete and complete sexual behavior. *Journal of Comparative and Physiological Psychology, 48*, 59–65. (183)

Kahn, M. W. (1965). A factor-analytic study of personality, intelligence, and history characteristics of murderers. In *Proceedings of the 73rd Annual Convention of the American Psychological Association, 1*, 227–228. (295)

Kaplan, A. (1964). *The conduct of inquiry.* San Francisco: Chandler. (66, 160)

Kardiner, A., Karush, A., & Ovesey, L. (1959). A methodological study of Freudian theory: I. Basic concepts; II. The libido theory. *Journal of Nervous and Mental Disease, 129*, 11–19, 133–143. (160)

Keller, H. (1908). *The world I live in.* New York: Century. (389)

Kennedy, G. (1963). *The art of persuasion in Greece.* Princeton, NJ: Princeton University Press. (58, 60)

Klein, G. S. (1959). Consciousness in psychoanalytic theory: Some implications for current research in perception. *Journal of the American Psychoanalytic Association, 7*, 5–34. (104, 228)

Klein, G. S. (1962). On inhibition, disinhibition, and "primary process" in thinking. In G. Nielson (Ed.), *Proceedings of the XIV International Congress of Applied Psychology: Vol. 4. Clinical psychology* (pp. 179–198). Copenhagen: Munksgaard. (386)

Klein, G. S. (1967). Peremptory ideation: Structure and force in motivated ideas. In R. R. Holt (Ed.). Motives and thought: Psychoanalytic essays in honor of David Rapaport. *Psychological Issues, 5* (Monograph No. 18/19), 80–128. (167, 173, 180, 186–196, 276, 379)

Klein, G. S. (1970). *Perception, motives and personality.* New York: Knopf. (34, 206, 214, 286)

Klein, G. S. (1972). The vital pleasures. *Psychoanalysis and Contemporary Science, 1*, 181–205. (191)

Klein, G. S. (1976). *Psychoanalytic theory: An exploration of essentials.* New York: International Universities Press. (174, 178, 185, 210, 211, 307, 311, 322, 324, 327, 337)

Klein, G. S., & Holt, R. R. (1960). Problems and issues in current studies of subliminal stimulation. In J. G. Peatman & E. L. Hartley (Eds.), *Festschrift for Gardner Murphy* (pp. 75–93). New York: Harper. (104, 105)

Klein, G. S., Spence, D. P., Holt, R. R., & Gourevitch, S. R. (1958). Cognition without awareness: Subliminal influences upon conscious thought. *Journal of Abnormal and Social Psychology, 57*, 255–266. (104)

Kluckhohn, C. (1959). Recurrent themes in myths and mythmaking. *Daedalus, 88*, 268–279. Also in H. A. Murray (Ed.) *Myth and mythmaking* (pp. 46–60). New York: Braziller, 1960. (389)

Knight, R. P. (1946). Determinism, "freedom," and psychotherapy. *Psychiatry, 9*, 251–262. Also in R. P. Knight & S. Friedman (Eds.), *Psychoanalytic psychiatry and psychology* (pp. 365–381). New York: International Universities Press, 1954. (220)

Kohlberg, L. (1969). Stage and sequence: The cognitive-developmental approach to socialization. In D. A. Goslin (Ed.), *Handbook of socialization, theory and research* (pp. 347–380). Chicago: Rand McNally. (191)

Kohler, I. (1964). The formation and transformation of the perceptual world. *Psychological Issues, 3* (Monograph No. 12). (234–236)

Köhler, W. (1917). *The mentality of apes.* New York: Harcourt, Brace, 1924. (290)

Köhler, W. (1929). *Gestalt psychology.* New York: Liveright. (263)

Kohut, H. (1971). *The analysis of the self.* New York: International Universities Press. (338)

Kohut, H. (1977). *The restoration of the self.* New York: International Universities Press. (338)

Kopit, A. L. (1960). *Oh Dad, poor Dad, Momma's hung you in the closet and I'm feelin' so sad.* New York: Hill & Wang. (227)

Koryé, A. (1956). The origins of modern science: A new interpretation. *Diogenes, 16,* 1–22. (161, 374)

Kris, E. (1952). *Psychoanalytic explorations in art.* New York: International Universities Press. (72, 104, 296)

Kubie, L. S. (1947). The fallacious use of quantitative concepts in dynamic psychology. *Psychoanalytic Quarterly, 16,* 507–518. Also in Symbol and neurosis: Selected papers. *Psychological Issues,* 1978, *11* (Monograph No. 44), 41–51. (160, 181)

Kubie, L. S. (1954). The fundamental nature of the distinction between normality and neurosis. *Psychoanalytic Quarterly, 23,* 167–204. Also in Symbol and neurosis: Selected papers. *Psychological Issues,* 1978, *11* (Monograph No. 44), 127–161. (291)

Kuhn, T. S. (1970). *The structure of scientific revolutions* (rev. ed). Chicago: University of Chicago Press. (46, 207, 212)

Kuklick, B. (1980, January 25). *Harry Stack Sullivan and the American intellectual life.* Paper presented at a conference, "Psychoanalysis 1980: Converging Views," New York. (394)

Laforgue, R. (1926). Verdrängung und Skotomisation. *International Zeitschrift für Psychoanalyse, 12,* 54–65. (287)

La Mettrie, J. O. de (1748). *Man a machine* [*L'homme machine*] (G. C. Bussey & M. W. Calkins, Trans.). Chicago: Open Court, 1927. (146)

Langer, S. K. (1942). *Philosophy in a new key.* New York: Penguin, 1948. (280)

Laplanche, J., & Pontalis, J. B. (1973). *The language of psychoanalysis.* New York: Norton. (16)

Lashley, K. S., & Colby, K. M. (1957). An exchange of views on psychic energy and psychoanalysis. *Behavioral Science, 2,* 231–240. (375)

Laszlo, E. (1971). *Introduction to systems philosophy.* New York: Gordon & Branch. (394)

Laszlo, E. (1972). *The systems view of the world.* New York: Braziller. (229, 239, 394)

Leites, N. (1971). *The new ego.* New York: Science House. (324)

Lévy-Bruhl, L. (1922). *How natives think.* London: George Allen & Unwin, 1926. (389)

Lewin, K. (1935). *A dynamic theory of personality.* New York: McGraw-Hill. (161)

Lewis, H. B. (1981). *Freud and modern psychology* (Vol. 1). New York: Plenum. (244)

Lewis, H. B. (1986). *Freud and modern psychology* (Vol. 2). New York: Plenum. (244)

Lilly, J. C. (1956). Mental effects of reduction of ordinary levels of physical stimuli on intact, healthy persons. *Psychiatric Research Reports, 5,* 1–9. (131)

Lindsley, D. B. (1957). Psychophysiology and motivation. In M. R. Jones (Ed.), *Nebraska Symposium on Motivation* (Vol. 5, pp. 44–105). Lincoln: University of Nebraska Press. (131)

Linton, H. B. (1955). Dependence on external influence: Correlates in perception, attitudes, and judgment. *Journal of Abnormal and Social Psychology, 51,* 502–507. (65)

Lipps, T. (1883). *Grundtatsachen des Seelenlebens.* Bonn: M. Cohn & Sohn. (17)

Loevinger, J. (1966). The meaning and measurement of ego development. *American Psychologist, 21,* 195–206. (300)

Loevinger, J. (1976). *Ego development: Conceptions and theories.* San Francisco: Jossey-Bass. (190, 245, 300)

Loevinger, J., Wessler, R., & Redmore, C. (1970). *Measuring ego development* (2 vols.). San Francisco: Jossey-Bass. (190)

Lorenz, K. (1963). *On aggression.* New York: Harcourt, Brace & World. (184)

Low, B. (1920). *Psycho-analysis: A brief account of Freudian theory.* London: George Allen & Unwin. (125)

Luborsky, L. (1967). Momentary forgetting during psychotherapy and psychoanalysis: A theory and research method. In R. R. Holt (Ed.), Motives and thought: Psychoanalytic essays in honor of David Rapaport. *Psychological Issues, 5* (Monograph No. 18/19), 177–217. (409)

Luborsky, L. (1977). Measuring a pervasive psychic structure in psychotherapy: The core conflictual relationship theme. In N. Freedman & S. Grand (Eds.), *Communicative structures and psychic structures* (pp. 367–395). New York: Plenum. (331)

Luborsky, L. (1984). *Principles of psychoanalytic psychotherapy.* New York: Basic Books. (331, 343)

Mahony, P. (1982). *Freud as a writer.* New York: International Universities Press. (34)

Mainx, F. (1955). Foundations of biology. In O. Neurath, R. Carnap, & C. Morris (Eds.), *International encyclopedia of unified science* (Vol. 1, Part 2, No. 9). Chicago: University of Chicago Press. (158, 162)

Mann, N. (1946). Learning in children. In L. Carmichael (Ed.), *Manual of child psychology* (pp. 370–449). New York: Wiley. (388)

Masson, J. M. (1984). *The assault on truth: Freud's suppression of the seduction theory.* New York: Farrar, Straus & Giroux. (330)

Masters, W. H., & Johnson, V. E. (1966). *Human sexual response.* New York: Little, Brown. (183)

Mayr, E. (1978). Evolution. *Scientific American, 239,* 46–55. (363)

McBurney, J. H. (1936). The place of the enthymeme in rhetorical theory. *Speech Monographs, 3,* 49–74. (58)

McCarley, R. W., & Hobson, J. A. (1977). The neurobiological origins of psychoanalytic dream theory. *American Journal of Psychiatry, 134,* 1211–1221. (112, 368)

McClelland, D. C. (1951). *Personality.* New York: Sloane. (379)

McClelland, D. C., Atkinson, W., Clark, R. A., & Lowell, E. L. (1953). *The achievement motive.* New York: Wiley. (379)

Menninger, K. (1930). *The human mind.* New York: Knopf. (4)

Meynert, T. (1884). *Psychiatry* (B. Backs, Trans.). New York: G. P. Putnam's Sons, 1885. (77, 117)

Miller, J. G. (1978). *Living systems.* New York: McGraw-Hill. (165, 320)

Miller, N. E. (1958). Central stimulation and other new approaches to motivation and reward. *American Psychologist, 13,* 100–108. (131, 381)

Miller, S. C. (1962). Ego-autonomy in sensory deprivation, isolation, and stress. *International Journal of Psycho-Analysis, 43,* 1–20. (126, 131, 224–226, 228, 230, 232)

Modell, A. H. (1963). The concept of psychic energy. *Journal of the American Psychoanalytic Association, 11,* 605–618. (372, 377)

Money, J., & Ehrhardt, A. (1972). *Man and woman, boy and girl.* Baltimore: Johns Hopkins University Press. (193)

Moore, K. C. (1896). The mental development of a child. *Psychological Review Monograph Supplement, 1* (Whole No. 3). (202)

Morgan, C. T. (1959). Physiological theory of drive. In S. Koch (Ed.), *Psychology: A study of a science. Vol. 1. Sensory, perceptual and physiological formulations* (pp. 644–671). New York: McGraw-Hill. (130)

Moyer, K. E. (1973, July). The physiology of violence. *Psychology Today,* pp. 28–35. (192)

Müller, J. (1833-1840). *Handbuch der Physiologie des Menschen [Handbook of human physiology].* Koblenz, West Germany. (149)

Mumford, L. (1970). *The myth of the machine: Vol. 2. The pentagon of power.* New York: Harcourt Brace Jovanovich. (350)

Munro, D. H. (1968). Relativism in ethics. In P. P. Wiener (Ed.), *Dictionary of the history of ideas* (Vol. 4, pp. 70–74). New York: Scribner's. (354)

Murphy, G. (1947). *Personality: a biosocial approach to origins and structure.* New York: Harper. (130)

Murray, H. A. (1940). What should psychologists do about psychoanalysis? *Journal of Abnormal and Social Psychology, 35,* 150–175. (6)

Murray, H. A., et al. (1938). *Explorations in personality.* New York: Oxford University Press. (5, 184, 194, 230)

Nagel, E. (1953). Teleological explanation and teleological systems. In S. Ratner (Ed.) *Vision and action* (pp. 192–222). New Brunswick, NJ: Rutgers University Press. Also in H. Feigl & M. Brodbeck (Eds.), *Readings in the philosophy of science* (pp. 38–56). New York: Appleton-Century-Crofts, 1953. (143, 159, 161, 162)

Nagel, E. (1960). Methodological issues in psychoanalytic theory. In S. Hook (ed.), *Psychoanalysis, scientific method and philosophy* (pp. 38–56). New York: Grove Press. (160)

Nagel, E. (1961). *The structure of science: Problems in the logic of scientific explanation.* New York: Harcourt, Brace & World. (162, 317)

Nietzsche, F. W. (1896). *Also sprach Zarathustra* (5th ed.). Leipzig: Naumann. (382)

Nordenskiöld, E. (1928). *The history of biology: A survey.* New York: Knopf. (374)

Nunberg, H. (1931). The synthetic function of the ego. *International Journal of Psycho-Analysis, 12,* 123–140. Also in H. Nunberg, *Practice and theory of psychoanalysis* (pp. 120–136). New York: Nervous & Mental Diseases, 1948. (41, 96, 389)

Nunberg, H., & Federn, E. (Eds.). (1967). *Minutes of the Vienna Psychoanalytic Society: Vol. 2. 1908–1910* (M. Nunberg, Trans.). New York: International Universities Press. (30, 44)

Olds, J. (1958). Self-stimulation of the brain. *Science, 127,* 315–324. (131)

Olds, J., & Milner, P. (1954). Positive reinforcement produced by electrical stimulation of septal area and other regions of rat brain. *Journal of Comparative and Physiological Psychology, 47,* 419–427. (131)

Olweus, D. (1986). *Mobbning: Vad vi vet och vad vi can göra [Bully/victim problems among school children: what we know and what we can do].* Stockholm: Liber. (261)

Onions, C. T. (Ed.). (1966). *The Oxford dictionary of English etymology.* New York: Oxford University Press. (363)

Ostow, M. (1962). *Drugs in psychoanalysis and psychotherapy.* New York: Basic Books. (160)

Parmelee, A. H., Jr. & Wenner, W. H. (1964, March). *Activated sleep in premature infants.* Paper presented at the fourth annual meeting of the Association for the Psychophysiological Study of Sleep, Palo Alto, CA. (275)

Parmelee, A. H., Jr. & Wenner, W. H. (1965, March). *Sleep states in premature and full-term newborn infants.* Paper presented at the fifth annual meeting of the Association for the Psychophysiological Study of Sleep, Washington, DC. (275)

Paul, I. H. (1967). The concept of schema in memory theory. In R. R. Holt (Ed.), *Motives and thought: Psychoanalytic essays in honor of David Rapaport. Psychological Issues, 5* (Monograph No. 18/19), 219–258. (271, 382, 390)

Pepper, S. C. (1942). *World hypotheses: A study in evidence.* Berkeley: University of California Press. (143, 348, 356, 360, 385)

Pepper, S. C. (1967). *Concept and quality: A world hypothesis.* LaSalle, IL: Open Court. (394)

Pepper, S. C. (1972a). On the case for systems philosophy. *Metaphilosophy, 3,* 151–153. (394)

Pepper, S. C. (1972b). Systems philosophy as a world hypothesis. *Philosophy and Phenomenological Research, 32,* 548–553. (394)

Perry, W. G. (1970). *Forms of intellectual and ethical development in the college years.* New York: Holt, Rinehart & Winston. (353, 355)

Pert, C. (1988, Summer). The material basis of emotions. *Whole Earth Review, 59,* pp. 106–111. (379)

Peterfreund, E. (1971). Information, systems, and psychoanalysis: An evolutionary biological approach to psychoanalytic theory. *Psychological Issues, 7* (Monograph No. 25/26). (181, 307, 314, 336)

Peterfreund, E., & Franceschini, E. (1973). On information, motivation, and meaning. *Psychoanalysis and Contemporary Science, 2,* 220–262. (319, 336)

Piaget, J. (1936). *The origins of intelligence in children* (M. Cook, Trans.). New York: International Universities Press, 1954. (137, 195, 269)

Piaget, J. (1937). *The construction of reality in the child* (M. Cook, Trans.). New York: Basic Books, 1954. (267, 268, 285)

Piaget, J. & Inhelder, B. (1969). *The psychology of the child* (H. Weaver, Trans.). New York: Basic Books. (Original work published 1966) (353)

Pine, F. (1960). Incidental stimulation: A study of preconscious transformations. *Journal of Abnormal and Social Psychology, 60,* 68–75. (104)

Pinloche, A. (1922). *Etymologisches Wörterbuch der Deutschen Sprache.* Paris: Larousse. (77)

Polanyi, M. (1962). *Personal knowledge: Towards a post-critical philosophy* (rev. ed.). Chicago: University of Chicago Press. (160, 310, 375)

Popper, K. R. (1957). *The poverty of historicism.* Boston: Beacon Press. (21, 143, 144)

Popper, K. R. (1963). *Conjectures and refutations: The growth of scientific knowledge.* New York: Harper & Row. (328, 337)

Popper, K. R. (1972). *Objective knowledge: An evolutionary approach.* Oxford: Clarendon Press. (241)

Popper, K. R., & Eccles, J. C. (1977). *The self and its brain: An argument for interactionism.* New York: Springer International. (154)

Pötzl, O. (1917). Experimentelle erregte Traumbilder in ihren Beziehungen zum indirekten Sehen. *Zeitschrift für die gesamte Neurologie und Psychiatrie, 37,* 278–349. (392)

Powers, W. T. (1973). *Behavior: The control of perception.* Chicago: Aldine. (379)

Preyer, W. T. (1882). *Die Seele des Kindes.* Leipzig: Fernan. (202)

Pribram, K. (1962). The neuropsychology of Sigmund Freud. In A. J. Bachrach (Ed.), *Experimental foundations of clinical psychology* (pp. 442–468). New York: Basic Books. (77)

Pumpian-Mindlin, E. (1959). An attempt at the systematic restatement of the libido theory: III. Propositions concerning energetic–economic aspects of libido theory: Conceptual models of psychic energy and structure in psychoanalysis. *Annals of the New York Academy of Sciences, 76,* 1038–1052. (134)

Rado, S. (1956). *Psychoanalysis of behavior* (Vol. 1). New York: Grune & Stratton. (393)

Rado, S. (1962). *Psychoanalysis of behavior* (Vol. 2). New York: Grune & Stratton. (393)

Rapaport, D. (Ed.). (1951a). *Organization and pathology of thought.* New York: Columbia University Press. (72, 73, 101, 104, 163, 212, 256, 258, 293, 383, 386)

Rapaport, D. (1951b). The autonomy of the ego. *Bulletin of the Menninger Clinic, 15,* 113–123. Also in M. M. Gill (Ed.), *The collected papers of David Rapaport* (pp. 357–367). New York: Basic Books, 1967. (223, 228)

Rapaport, D. (1951c). The conceptual model of psychoanalysis. *Journal of Personality, 20,* 56–81. Also in M. M. Gill (Ed.), *The collected papers of David Rapaport* (pp. 405–431). New York: Basic Books, 1967. (271)

Rapaport, D. (1957). Cognitive structures. In *Contemporary approaches to cognition* (pp. 157–200). Cambridge, MA: Harvard University Press. Also in M. M. Gill (Ed.), *The collected papers of David Rapaport* (pp. 631–664). New York: Basic Books, 1967. (100, 104, 256, 272, 277)

Rapaport, D. (1958a). The theory of ego autonomy: A generalization. *Bulletin of the Menninger Clinic, 22,* 13–35. Also in M. M. Gill (Ed.), *The collected papers of David Rapaport* (pp. 772–744). New York: Basic Books, 1967. (100, 126, 223, 224, 226, 228, 231, 380, 381)

Rapaport, D. (1958b). A historical survey of ego psychology. *Bulletin of the Philadelphia Association of Psychoanalysis, 8,* 105–120. Also in M. M. Gill (Ed.), *The collected papers of David Rapaport* (pp. 745–757). New York: Basic Books, 1967. (199)

Rapaport, D. (1959). The structure of psychoanalytic theory: A systematizing attempt. In S. Koch (Ed.), *Psychology: A study of a science. Study 1. Conceptual and systematic. Vol. 3. Formulations of the person and the social context* (pp. 55–183). New York: McGraw-Hill. Also in *Psychological Issues,* 1960, *2* (Monograph No. 6). (14, 90, 105, 129, 130, 153, 158, 163–165, 174, 256, 380)

Rapaport, D. (1960a). Psychoanalysis as a developmental psychology. In B. Kaplan & S. Wapner (Eds.), *Perspectives in psychological theory: Essays in honor of Heinz Werner* (pp. 209–255). New York: International Universities Press. Also in M. M. Gill (Ed.), *The collected papers of David Rapaport* (pp. 820-852). New York: Basic Books, 1967. (212, 266, 272, 385)

Rapaport, D. (1960b). On the psychoanalytic theory of motivation. In M. Jones (Ed.), *Nebraska Symposium on Motivation* (Vol. 8, pp. 173-247). Lincoln: University of Nebraska Press. Also in M. M. Gill (Ed.), *The collected papers of David Rapaport* (pp. 853-915). New York: Basic Books, 1967. (180, 379)

Rapaport, D. (1967). Some metapsychological considerations concerning activity and passivity. In M. M. Gill (Ed.), *The collected papers of David Rapaport* (pp. 530-568). New York: Basic Books. (227, 251, 381)

Rapaport, D., & Gill, M. M. (1959). The points of view and assumptions of metapsychology. *International Journal of Psycho-Analysis, 40,* 153-162. Also in M. M. Gill (Ed.), *The collected papers of David Rapaport* (pp. 795-811). New York: Basic Books, 1967. (15, 86, 165, 171, 213, 256, 325, 372)

Rapaport, D., Gill, M. M., & Schafer, R. (1945-1946). *Diagnostic psychological testing* (2 vols.). Chicago: Year Book Publishers. (Rev. ed., R. R. Holt, Ed. New York: International Universities Press, 1968.) (100, 213, 297, 300)

Rapoport, A. (1962). An essay on mind. In J. M. Scher (Ed.), *Theories of the mind.* Glencoe, IL: Free Press. (143, 149)

Reich, W. (1933). *Character analysis: Principles and techniques for psychoanalysis in practice and training* (3rd ed.). New York: Orgone Institute Press, 1945. (213)

Reiser, M. (1984). *Mind, brain, body: Toward a convergence of psychoanalysis and neurobiology.* New York: Basic Books. (336)

Ricoeur, P. (1970). *Freud and philosophy: An essay on interpretation* (D. Savage, Trans.). New Haven: Yale University Press. (308, 314, 315, 337)

Ricoeur, P. (1978). The question of proof in Freud's psychoanalytic writings. *Journal of the American Psychoanalytic Association, 25,* 835-871. (316)

Rieff, P. (1959). *Freud: The mind of the moralist.* New York: Viking. (340)

Riesen, A. H. (1961). Excessive arousal effects of stimulation after early sensory deprivation. In P. Solomon, P. E. Kubzansky, P. H. Leiderman, J. H. Mendelson, R. Trumbull, & D. Wexler (Eds.), *Sensory deprivation* (pp. 34-49). Cambridge, MA: Harvard University Press. (381)

Riesman, D. (1950). *The lonely crowd.* New Haven: Yale University Press. (65)

Roazen, P. (1975). *Freud and his followers.* New York: Knopf. (38, 43, 65)

Roffwarg, H. P., Dement, W. C., & Fisher, C. (1964). Preliminary observations of the sleep-dream pattern in neonates, infants, children and adults. In E. Harms (Ed.), *Problems of sleep and dream in children* (pp. 60-72). New York: Macmillan. (390)

Rogers, C. R. (1961). *On becoming a person.* Boston: Houghton Mifflin. (376)

Rosenblatt, A. D., & Thickstun, J. T. (1977). Modern psychoanalytic concepts in a general psychology. *Psychological Issues, 11* (Monograph No. 42/43). (308, 319, 322, 324, 336)

Rosenthal, R. (1963). On the social psychology of the psychological experiment: The experimenter's hypothesis as unintended determinant of experimental results. *American Scientist, 51,* 268-283. (30)

Rosenzweig, S. (1938). The experimental study of repression. In H. A. Murray et al., *Explorations in personality* (pp. 472-490). New York: Oxford University Press. (328)

Royce, J. E. (1973). Does person or self imply dualism? *American Psychologist, 28,* 883-886. (379)

Rubinstein, B. B. (1965). Psychoanalytic theory and the mind-body problem. In N. S. Greenfield & W. C. Lewis (Eds.), *Psychoanalysis and current biological thought* (pp. 35-56). Madison: University of Wisconsin Press. (122, 141, 154, 157, 167, 324)

Rubinstein, B. B. (1987a). Explanation and mere description: A metascientific examination of certain aspects of the psychoanalytic theory of motivation. In R. R. Holt (Ed.), *Motives and thought: Psychoanalytic essays in honor of David Rapaport. Psychological Issues, 5* (Monograph No. 18/19), 20-77. (141, 157, 160, 167, 180, 181, 195, 210, 211, 217, 256, 276, 319, 324, 326, 384)

Rubinstein, B. B. (1967b). On the problem of ego autonomy. *International Journal of Psychiatry, 3*, 506–512. (382)

Rubinstein, B. B. (1974). On the role of classificatory processes in mental functioning: Aspects of a psychoanalytic theoretical model. *Psychoanalysis and Contemporary Science, 3* 101–185. (319, 336, 379)

Rubinstein, B. B. (1975). On the clinical psychoanalytic theory and its role in the inference and confirmation of particular clinical hypotheses. *Psychoanalysis and Contemporary Science, 4*, 3–57. (175, 190, 308, 322, 331, 333–336, 377, 386)

Rubinstein, B. B. (1976a). On the possibility of a strictly clinical psychoanalytic theory: An essay in the philosophy of psychoanalysis. In M. M. Gill & P. S. Holzman (Eds.), *Psychology versus metapsychology: Psychoanalytic essays in memory of George S. Klein* (pp. 229–364). *Psychological Issues, 9* (Monograph No. 36). (316, 322, 327, 331, 335)

Rubinstein, B. B. (1976b). Hope, fear, wish, expectation, and fantasy: A semantic–phenomenological and extraclinical theoretical study. *Psychoanalysis and Contemporary Science, 5*, 3–60. (202, 228)

Rubinstein, B. B. (1981, January). *Person, organism, and self: Their worlds and their psychoanalytically relevant relationships.* Paper presented to the New York Psychoanalytic Society. (202, 228)

Russell, B. (1929). *Our knowledge of the external world.* New York: Norton. (382)

Sachs, H. (1945). *Freud, master and friend.* Cambridge, MA: Harvard University Press. (47)

Sandler, J., & Joffe, W. G. (1967). On the psychanalytic theory of autonomy and the autonomy of psychoanalytic theory. *International Journal of Psychiatry, 3*, 512–515. (251)

Schachtel, E. G. (1954). The development of focal attention and the emergence of reality. In E. G. Schachtel, *Metamorphosis* (pp. 251–278). New York: Basic Books, 1959. (388)

Schafer, R. (1954). *Psychoanalytic interpretation in Rorschach testing.* New York: Grune & Stratton. (296)

Schafer, R. (1958). Regression in the service of the ego: The relevance of a psychoanalytic concept for personality assessment. In G. Lindzey (Ed.), *Assessment of human motives* (pp. 119–148). New York: Rinehart. (296)

Schafer, R. (1960). The loving and beloved superego in Freud's structural theory. *Psychoanalytic Study of the Child, 15*, 163–188. (199)

Schafer, R. (1967). Ideals, the ego ideal, and the ideal self. In R. R. Holt (Ed.), *Motives and thought: Psychoanalytic essays in honor of David Rapaport. Psychological Issues, 5* (Monograph No. 18/19), 131–174. (188, 189, 199, 251, 389)

Schafer, R. (1973a). Action: Its place in psychoanalytic interpretation and theory. *Annual of Psychoanalysis, 1*, 159–196. (209, 210)

Schafer, R. (1973b). Concepts of self and identity and the experience of separation–individuation in adolescence. *Psychoanalytic Quarterly, 43*, 42–59. (202, 210)

Schafer, R. (1973c). The idea of resistance. *International Journal of Psycho-Analysis, 54*, 259–285. (210, 211)

Schafer, R. (1976). *A new language for psychoanalysis.* New Haven, CT: Yale University Press. (29, 179, 209, 228, 289, 307, 311, 316, 322, 324, 326, 337, 393)

Schafer, R. (1978). *Language and insight.* New Haven, CT: Yale University Press. (316, 322, 337, 393)

Schilder, P. (1935). *The image and appearance of the human body.* New York: International Universities Press, 1950. (200)

Schimek, J. G. (1975). A critical reexamination of Freud's concept of unconscious mental representation. *International Review of Psycho-Analysis, 51*, 279–297. (288, 391, 392)

Schlick, M. (1953). Philosophy of organic life. In H. Feigl & M. Brodbeck (Eds.), *Readings in the philosophy of science* (pp. 523–536). New York: Appleton-Century-Crofts. (141, 143, 147, 151, 161)

Schneirla, T. C. (1949). Levels in the psychological capacities of animals. In R. W. Sellars, V. J. McGill, & M. Farber (Eds.), *Philosophy for the future: The quest of modern materialism* (pp. 243–286). New York: Macmillan. (159, 162)

Schwartz, F., & Rouse, R. O. (1961). The activation and recovery of associations. *Psychological Issues, 3* (Monograph No. 9). (160, 163)

Sears, R. R. (1943). *Survey of objective studies in psychoanalytic concepts* (Social Science Research Council Bulletin No. 52). (340)

Selvini Palazzoli, M. (1988). *The work of Mara Selvini Palazzoli* (M. Selvini, Ed.; A. J. Pomerans, Trans.). Northvale, NJ: Jason Aronson. (239)

Shakow, D. & Rapaport, D. (1964). The influence of Freud on American psychology. *Psychological Issues, 4* (Monograph No. 13). (10)

Shapiro, D. (1956). Color-response and perceptual passivity. *Journal of Projective Techniques, 20*, 52–69. (381)

Shapiro, D. (1960). A perceptual understanding of color response. In M. A. Rickers-Ovsiankina (Ed.), *Rorschach psychology* (pp. 154–201). New York: Wiley. (381)

Shapiro, D. (1965). *Neurotic styles*. New York: Basic Books. (383)

Sheffield, F. D., & Roby, T. B. (1950). Reward value of a non-nutritive sweet taste. *Journal of Comparative and Physiological Psychology, 43*, 471–481. (130)

Sheffield, F. D., Wulff, J. J., & Barker, R. (1951). Reward value of copulation without sex drive reduction. *Journal of Comparative and Physiological Psychology, 44*, 3–8. (131, 183)

Sherwood, M. (1969). *The logic of explanation in psychoanalysis*. New York: Academic Press. (310, 334)

Shneidman, E. S. (1961). Psycho-logic: A personality approach to patterns of thinking. In J. Kagan & G. S. Lesser (Eds.), *Contemporary issues in thematic apperceptive methods* (pp. 153–190). Springfield, IL: Charles C Thomas. (61)

Silberschatz, G. (1978). *Effects of the analyst's neutrality on the patient's feelings and behavior in the psychoanalytic situation.* Unpublished doctoral dissertation, New York University. (343)

Silverman, L. H. (1967). An experimental approach to the study of dynamic propositions in psychoanalysis: The relationship between the aggressive drive and ego regression—initial studies. *Journal of the American Psychoanalytic Association, 15*, 376–403. (160)

Silverman, L. H. (1982). The subliminal psychodynamic activation method: Overview and comprehensive listing of studies. In J. Masling (Ed.), *Empirical studies of psychoanalytic theory* (Vol. 1, pp. 69–100). Hillsdale, NJ: Erlbaum. (340)

Singer, C. (1959). *A short history of scientific ideas to 1900.* New York: Oxford University Press. (141, 144–151)

Sjöbäck, H. (1988). *The Freudian learning hypotheses.* Lund, Sweden: Lund University Press. (20)

Skinner, B. F. (1948). "Superstition" in the pigeon. *Journal of Experimental Psychology, 38*, 168–172. (269)

Skinner, B. F. (1971). *Beyond freedom and dignity.* New York: Knopf. (249, 311)

Smith, M. B. (1982). Psychology and humanism. *Journal of Humanistic Psychology, 22*, 27–36. (16)

Sokolov, E. N. (1960). Neuronal models and the orienting reflex. In M. A. B. Brazier (Ed.), *The central nervous system and behavior: Transactions of the third conference* (pp. 187–276). New York: Josiah Macy, Jr. Foundation. (189)

Solomon, P., Kubzansky, P. E., Leiderman, P. H., Mendelson, J. H., Trumbull, R., & Wexler, D. (Eds.). (1961). *Sensory deprivation.* Cambridge, MA: Harvard University Press. (131)

Spalding, K. (1952). *An historical dictionary of German figurative usage* (Vol. 1). Oxford: Blackwell. (109)

Spalding, K. (1956). *An historical dictionary of German figurative usage* (Vol. 7). Oxford: Blackwell. (109)

Spehlmann, R. (1953). *Sigmund Freuds neurologische Schriften: Eine Untersuchung zur Vorgeschichte der Psychoanalyse.* Berlin: Springer (English summary by H. Kleinschimidt in *Annual survey of psychoanalysis 1953*, 1957, *4*, 693–706). (174, 370)

Spence, D. P. (1982). *Narrative truth and historical truth: Meaning and interpretation in psychoanalysis.* New York: Norton. (336, 337)

Spiro, A. (1979). Philosophical appraisal of Roy Schafer's *A new language for psychoanalysis. Psychoanalysis and Contemporary Thought, 2,* 253–291. (393)

Steele, R. S. (1979). Psychoanalysis and hermeneutics. *International Review of Psycho-Analysis, 6,* 389–411. (337)

Stellar, E. (1954). The physiology of motivation. *Psychological Review, 61,* 5–22. (130)

Stern, D. (1985). *The interpersonal world of the infant.* New York: Basic Books. (387)

Stevens, S. S. (1939). Psychology and the science of science. *Psychological Bulletin, 36,* 221–263. (13)

Strachey, J. (1957a). Papers on metapsychology: Editor's introduction. *Standard Edition, 14,* 105–107. London: Hogarth Press. (16)

Strachey, J. (1957b). Editor's note [on Freud, S., The unconscious]. *Standard Edition, 14,* 161–165. London: Hogarth Press. (129)

Strachey, J. (1959). Editor's introduction [to Freud, S., Inhibitions, symptoms and anxiety]. *Standard Edition, 20,* 77–86. London: Hogarth Press. (136)

Strachey, J. (1961). Editor's introduction [to Freud, S. The ego and the id]. *Standard Edition, 19,* 3–11. London: Hogarth Press. (203)

Sullivan, H. S. (1953a). *The interpersonal theory of psychiatry.* New York: Norton. (393)

Sullivan, H. S. (1953b). *Conceptions of modern psychiatry.* New York: Norton. (393)

Sullivan, H. S. (1956). *Clinical studies in psychiatry.* New York: Norton. (393)

Sulloway, F. J. (1979). *Freud, biologist of the mind: Beyond the psychoanalytic legend.* New York: Basic Books. (20, 23, 24, 114, 324, 367, 370, 375)

Suppes, P. (1969). *Studies in the methodology and foundations of science.* Dordrecht, The Netherlands: Reidel. (319)

Swales, P. J. (1981, April 27). *Freud, Faust, and cocaine: New light on the origins of psychoanalysis.* Unpublished lecture, New York University. (364)

Swanson, D. R. (1977). A critique of psychic energy as an explanatory concept. *Journal of the American Psychoanalytic Association, 25,* 603–633. (319)

Szasz, T. S. (1952). On the psychoanalytic theory of instincts. *Psychoanalytic Quarterly, 21,* 25–48. (134)

Taine, H. (1864). *On intelligence* (T. D. Haye, Trans.). London: Rewe, 1871. (16, 17, 363)

Teilhard de Chardin, P. (1959). *The phenomenon of man.* New York: Harper & Row. (163)

Thoa, N. B., Eichelman, B., Richardson, J. S., & Jacobowitz, D. (1972). 6-Hydroxydopa depletion of brain norepinephrine and the facilitation of aggressive behavior. *Science, 178,* 75–77. (193)

Triandis, H. C. (1985). Collectivism vs. individualism: A reconceptualization of a basic concept in cross-cultural social psychology. In C. Bagley & G. K. Verma (Eds.), *Personality, cognition, and values: Cross-cultural perspectives of childhood and adolescence.* London: Macmillan. (244)

Vaillant, G. (1977). *Adaptation to life.* Boston: Little, Brown. (343)

Vitz, P. (1988). *Sigmund Freud's Christian unconscious.* New York: Guilford Press. (201, 364)

von Domarus, E. (1944). The specific laws of logic in schizophrenia. In J. S. Kasanin (Ed.), *Language and thought in schizophrenia* (pp. 104–114). Berkeley: University of California Press. (273)

von Eckhardt, B. (1982). Why Freud's research methodology was unscientific. *Psychoanalysis and Contemporary Thought, 5,* 549–574. (330)

von Eckhardt, B. (1985). Adolf Grünbaum: Psychoanalytic epistemology. In J. Reppen (Ed.), *Beyond Freud: A study of modern psychoanalytic theorists* (pp. 353–403). Hillsdale, NJ: The Analytic Press. (327)

von Holst, E., & Mittelstaedt, H. (1950). Das Reafferenzprincip (Wechselwirkungen zwischen Zentralnervensystem und Peripherie). *Naturwissenschaft, 37,* 464–476. (188, 189, 235, 236)

Waelder, R. (1936). The principle of multiple function: Observations on over-determination. *Psychoanalytic Quarterly, 5,* 45–62. (372)

Wallerstein, R. S. (1976). Psychoanalysis as a science: Its present status and its future tasks. In M. M. Gill & P. S. Holzman (Eds.), Psychology versus metapsychology: Psychoanalytic essays in memory of George S. Klein. *Psychological Issues, 9*, (Monograph No. 36), 198–228. (311)

Wallerstein, R. S., & Sampson, H. (1971). Issues in research in the psycho-analytic process. *International Journal of Psycho-Analysis, 52*, 11–50. (343)

Walter, G. (1953). *The living brain.* New York: Norton. (251)

Waters, R. H. (1948). Mechanomorphism: A new term for an old mode of thought. *Psychological Review, 55*, 139–142. (263)

Watzlawick, P., Beavin, J. H., & Jackson, D. (1967). *Pragmatics of human communication.* New York: Norton. (239)

Wayner, M. J., & Carey, R. J. (1973). Basic drives. *Annual Review of Psychology, 24*, 53–80. (177)

Wechsler, D. (1939). *The measurement and appraisal of adult intelligence.* Baltimore: Williams & Wilkins. (36)

Weiss, J., Sampson, H., and the Mount Zion Psychotherapy Research Group. (1986). *The psychoanalytic process: Theory, clinical observation, and empirical research.* New York: Guilford Press. (331)

Weiss, P. A. (1969). The living system: Determinism stratified. *Studium Generale, 22*, 361–400. Also in A. Koestler & J. Smithies (Eds.), *Beyond reductionism* (pp. 3–42). New York: Macmillan, 1969. (229, 246, 385, 394)

Werner, H. (1948). *Comparative psychology of mental development* (rev. ed.). New York: International Universities Press, 1957. (387, 389)

Werner, H., & Kaplan, B. (1963). *Symbol formation.* New York: Wiley. (387)

White, R. W. (1963a). Ego and reality in psychoanalytic theory: A proposal regarding independent ego energies. *Psychological Issues, 3* (Monograph No. 11). (130)

White, R. W. (Ed.). (1963b). *The study of lives: Essays on personality in honor of Henry A. Murray.* New York: Atherton Press. (114)

Whitehead, A. N. (1925). *Science in the modern world* (rev. ed.). New York: Mentor, 1952. (13, 94, 240, 309, 350, 393)

Wiener, N. (1948). *Cybernetics.* New York: Wiley. (166)

Wiener, P. P. (1968). Pragmatism. In P. P. Wiener (Ed.), *Dictionary of the history of ideas* (Vol. 3, pp. 551–570). New York: Scribner's. (354, 356)

Wilson, E., Jr. (1973). The structural hypotheses and psychoanalytic metatheory: An essay on psychoanalysis and contemporary philosophy. *Psychoanalysis and Contemporary Science, 2*, 304–328. (324)

Wilson, E. B. (1897). *The cell in development and inheritance.* New York: Macmillan. (151)

Winnicott, D. W. (1958). *Collected papers: Through pediatrics to psychoanalysis.* New York: Basic Books. (328)

Witkin, H. A. (1949). Perception of body position and of the position of the visual field. *Psychological Monographs, 63* (7, Whole No. 302). (65)

Wolff, P. H. (1960). The developmental psychologies of Jean Piaget and psychoanalysis. *Psychological Issues, 2* (Monograph No. 5). (268–271)

Wolff, P. H. (1967). Cognitive considerations for a psychoanalytic theory of language acquisition. In R. R. Holt (Ed.), Motives and thought: Psychoanalytic essays in honor of David Rapaport. *Psychological Issues, 5* (Monograph No. 18/19), 300–343. (268, 269, 271, 275, 277, 278, 383, 387, 390)

Wynne, L. C., & Singer, M. T. (1963). Thought disorder and family relations of schizophrenics. *Archives of General Psychiatry, 9*, 191–206. (273)

Yankelovich, D. (1981). *New rules: Searching for self-fulfillment in a world turned upside down.* New York: Random House. (32, 244)

Yankelovich, D., & Barrett, W. (1970). *Ego and instinct.* New York: Random House. (178, 324)

Zuckerman, M., Persky, H., Link, K. E., & Basu, G. K. (1968). Experimental and subject factors determining responses to sensory deprivation, social isolation, and confinement. *Journal of Abnormal Psychology, 73*, 183–194. (232)

Index

Absolutism, 352–354, 359 (*see also* Realism, naive)
Action language, 179, 307, 327
Activation of the brain, 74, 130, 167, 230, 393
  activated sleep, 277
Activity and passivity, 225, 227, 229, 252, 278
Actual neurosis, 135, 136
Adaptive/adaptation, 175, 381
  adaptiveness, 161
  behavior, 340
  level, 379
  point of view, 212
Adler, Alfred, 47, 50, 55, 63
Affect, 101, 102, 103, 112, 241
  feedback, 167
  in a phenomenological sense, 112
  signals, 248, 251
  taming of, 101, 369
  theory of, 129
Agassiz, Louis, 151
Aggression, theory of, 132, 184, 192, 193, 379, 385 (*see also* Death instinct/ drive)
Allport, Gordon, 5, 6
Alper, Thelma, 5
Amacher, Peter, 114, 116, 121, 140, 370, 371, 374
Analysis (in methodology), 243, 351, 357
  as dissection, 32, 49
Andreas-Salomé, Lou, 47
Animism, 200, 272, 309, 348, 349, 380
  and religion, 142
  and the soul, 201
  as a theory of life, 143
Annin, S. H., 386–388
Anthropomorphism, 144, 156, 158, 163, 186, 187, 201, 209, 325, 376, 382
  in comparative psychology, 290 (*see also* Personification)
Anticathexes, 89, 90, 93, 97, 98, 102, 103, 227, 369

Antonisen, Nils, 6
Anxiety, 103
  fermentation/toxic theory of, 102, 111, 135
  free vs. bound, 98, 103, 111–113, 369
  instinctual, 245
  signal theory of, 80, 98, 138, 212, 213
  similarity to other "instincts," 179, 184
Apparatus, psychic (*see* Autonomy; Perception; Psychic apparatus)
Aquinas, St. Thomas, 144
Archaeology, 19, 242, 315
Aristotle, 58, 59, 143, 146, 147, 309, 380
Arlow, Jacob, 211
Art/artistic creativity, 291, 296
Atomism, 242, 351
  theory of, 32
  as theory of reality, 143
Attention, 120, 153, 273
  attention cathexis, 87, 103, 106
  bound, 83, 367
  focal, 104, 278, 388
  in infants, 278, 387, 388
Augustine, St., 144
Austen Riggs Foundation, 9, 218
Authoritarianism, cultural, 351, 357
Autistic logic, 273, 299 (*see also* Predicative reasoning)
Automata, 145, 251, 263, 350
Autonomy, ego, 121, 127, 198, 207, 218–252, 244, 380–383
  apparatuses of primary, 223, 238, 266
  as developmental achievement, 245
  family, dependence on/independence from, 246
  from both drive and environment, 250
  from the environment (external reality), 126, 224–227, 245, 250, 277, 278
  from the id (drives), 224, 227
  history of the concept, 220–229
  ideal conception of, 245
  primary, 222, 228

419